Computer Vision
in Medical Imaging

Series in Computer Vision

ISSN: 2010-2143

Series Editor: C H Chen *(University of Massachusetts Dartmouth, USA)*

Series in Computer Vision - Vol. 2

Computer Vision
in Medical Imaging

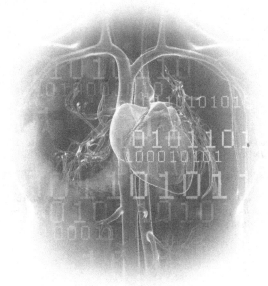

Editor

C H Chen
University of Massachusetts Dartmouth, USA

W World Scientific

NEW JERSEY · LONDON · SINGAPORE · BEIJING · SHANGHAI · HONG KONG · TAIPEI · CHENNAI

Published by

World Scientific Publishing Co. Pte. Ltd.

5 Toh Tuck Link, Singapore 596224

USA office: 27 Warren Street, Suite 401-402, Hackensack, NJ 07601

UK office: 57 Shelton Street, Covent Garden, London WC2H 9HE

British Library Cataloguing-in-Publication Data
A catalogue record for this book is available from the British Library.

Series in Computer Vision — Vol. 2
COMPUTER VISION IN MEDICAL IMAGING

Copyright © 2014 by World Scientific Publishing Co. Pte. Ltd.

ISBN 978-981-4460-93-4

Printed in Singapore

Dedicated in loving memory of

My father (1918-1961)

and

My mother (1917-2012)

PREFACE

The major progress in computer vision allows us to make extensive use of medical imaging data to provide us better diagnosis, treatment and prediction of diseases. In-spite of significant advances in high resolution medical instruments, physicians cannot always obtain the full amount of information directly from the equipment outputs and the large amount of data cannot be easily exploited without computer. Computer vision can make use of texture, shape, contour and prior knowledge along with contextural information from images and image sequences and provide 2-D, 3-D and 4-D information that helps us with better human understanding. Many powerful tools have been available through image segmentation, machine learning, pattern recognition, tracking, and reconstruction to bring us much needed information not easily available by trained human specialists. It is hoped that computer vision does not add cost to the improved health care delivery but would be so much helpful for better medical treatment. Unlike computer vision in other area such as robotics, security, document processing, etc., the main objective of using computer vision in medical imaging is not so much for full automation, but to provide useful results to help physicians for effective diagnosis and treatment.

Although there are a large number of medical imaging journal and conference publications that involve computer vision in medical imaging, this book is probably one of the first to bring together leaders in both computer vision and medical imaging to write chapters of interest to both computer and medical professionals and students. The book should also be useful to system designers who constantly seek for better medical instrumentation.

The areas of medical imaging are very broad and highly interdisciplinary. One prominent issue is perhaps the medical image segmentation. It is not possible for a single volume like this or several volumes to cover them all. The book only provides representative coverage in several areas. However the book does provide insight on what computer vision can achieve in medical imaging and help us project the future capabilities of computer vision in medical imaging.

Chapter 1 provides my general view of computer vision in medical imaging followed by some specific results of our work on segmentation of intravascular ultrasound (IVUS) images. The rest of the book is loosely divided into three parts. The readers re are suggested to go through the entire book to look for some specific information of interest. For example, information on computer vision in MRI (magnetic resonance imaging) is presented in relevant chapters in all three parts. The reason is that the same computer vision technique may be useful in other medical images also.

In part 1, Theory and Methodologies, there are six chapters. Chapter 2 by I. Ben Ayed provides distribution-matching formulations, which enforce some consistency between the feature distribution of the target segment and a given *a prior* learned model. Three different medical imaging segmentation applications are considered: left ventricle segmentation in cardiac images, vertebral-body segmentation in spine images, and brain tumor segmentation. In recent years, computer vision and related computer-aided techniques have had significant impact in medical imaging as clearly shown in Chapter 3 by B. Sabata et al., that introduces the digital pathology and their many benefits. It is good to see that many computer vision, image processing and pattern recognition techniques are now employed in pathology. Chapter 4 by S. Zhang, et al. introduces a robust and efficient shape prior modeling method, Sparse Shape Composition (SSC). A compact and informative shape dictionary is introduced and an on-line learning method is provided to improve the efficiency of SSC in incorporating new training shape instances. Chapter 5 by Y. Song et al. presented a brief review of their recent work on lesion detection and image retrieval for thoracic PET-CT images. For lesion detection, three different methods: region-based feature classification, multi-state discriminative model, and data-adaptive structure estimation are presented. For image retrieval, two different methods: pathological feature description, and spatial encoding are described. Accurate quantitation from phase maps is of critical importance in numerous MRI applications. Chapter 6 by J. Dagher presented a new solution which achieves robust phase estimation, over large dynamic range of phase values, at very high spatial resolutions. Both multi-resolution scheme and active contour model are two important methods for image segmentation in medical imaging. Chapter 7 by Bing Nan Li, et al. constructs Gaussian pyramid for speckle noise reduction and then implemented a phase-based geodesic active contour to refine the boundaries in finer pyramid levels.

In part 2, 2-D, 3-D Reconstructions/imaging Algorithms, Systems & Sensor Fusion, there are seven chapters. Chapter 8 by A. Rosenthal, et al. deals with optoacoustic tomography as a powerful hybrid bioimaging method. They demonstrated the relatively good image quality obtained by regularized model-based inversion as compared to back-projection reconstruction in 2-D and 3-D geometries. Chapter 9 by S.T. Tu, et al. presented a novel, user-friendly system for the fusion of X-ray angiography and IVUS/OCT in 3D for coronary interventions. This important work has the potential of improving outcomes and reducing costs in the treatment of obstructive coronary artery disease. Chapter 10 by B. Hong deals with SPECT, a nuclear emission tomographic imaging technique. An iterative reconstruction of 3D coded aperture SPECT imaging is presented. The clinical application of three or four dimensional ultrasound is gaining importance in medical diagnostics as well as in other areas, such as planning and verification of various therapies. Chapter 11 by S. Koptenko et al. provides an alternative approach for 3-D ultrasound volume reconstruction that makes use of direct frame interpolation (DFI) method which is performed in three major steps. The DFI method based on the linear interpolation between two adjacent image frames satisfies both requirements: high accuracy of the reconstruction and acceptable computational complexity.

In medical image processing, deblurring is an important issue. Chapter 12 by Uvais Qidwai and Umair Qidwai presented blind deconvolution of blurred retinal images using maximum likelihood estimation approach with an initial Gaussian kernel followed by post-processing steps. The enhanced images help the ophthalmologists for diagnosis and treatment of underlying diseases. Medical ultrasound systems require computation of complex algorithms for realtime digital signal processing. Chapter 13 by M. Lewandowski presents methods and systems for implementation of digital signal processing in ultrasonography. The constant development of GPUs, parallel programming tools and methods set the direction for continuous performance improvements. With a similar motivation, Chapter 14 by M. Broxvall and M. Daoutis introduces methods for implementing medical image processing algorithms on GPUs, and methodologies behind designing parallel algorithms for computation in convolution, adaptive filtering and line detections

Part 3, Specific Image Processing and Computer Vision Methods for Different Imaging Modalities Including IVUS, MRI, etc. begins with a tutorial presentation (Chapter 15) of computer vision in interventional cardiology by K.R. Waters. The role of computer vision in IVUS imaging, especially on plaque classification based on IVUS spectral characteristics should be particularly noted though it remains controversial for clinical decision making. Indeed many computer vision techniques in medical imaging have a long way to go from research to the stage that they can be accepted in clinical environments. Chapter 16 by A. Tabesh et al. reviewed several classical and state-of-the-art classifiers, such as the nonlinear support vector classifier, and compared their accuracy in schizophrenia diagnosis based on diffusion MRI. No previous study had determined the impact of the classifier on the accuracy of schizophrenia diagnosis. The authors suggest that further work should investigate whether alternative sparseness constraints and variable selection can further improve classifier performance in schizophrenia diagnosis. Chapter 17 by A. Bilgin, et al. begins with a description of the basic principles of compressed sensing (CS). CS has been used to accelerate dynamic MRI where the goal is to reconstruct a series of temporally varying images. It is clear that CS will enhance the clinical utility of many MR techniques. Several algorithms that can be used to reconstruct MR images from compressive measurements are also presented. Together with CT, MRI is one of the most common ways to visualize the brain, for cerebral structures. The need for an accurate segmentation step which aims to partition the intra-cranial images into different regions of interest is of crucial importance. The characterization of the brain morphology associated with Alzheimer's disease is a good example. Noting the shortcomings of the active contour model, Chapter 18 by J. Cerrolaza, et al. presents a new hierarchical multi-shape segmentation framework to decompose the multi-object structure into levels with different degrees of detail. The automatic segmentation of the set of subcortical brain structures has a clear medical interest. Chapter 19 by D. Turco and C. Corsi traces back to the use of partial differential equations in medical image analysis, as formulation of deformable models with applications to cardiac magnetic resonance imaging data processing, methods in ventricular volume estimation and scar quantification. Chapter 20 by P. Manandhar and C. Chen considers the automated intra-vascular ultrasound image segmentation for diagnosis of coronary heart disease by using active contour model algorithm with special reference to tracking the change in guidewire position such that its effect on IVUS segmentation is minimized.

I am most grateful to the authors for their outstanding contributions to the book. With their valuable inputs I am convinced that much has been achieved with computer vision in medical imaging, while much more have yet to be done in this challenging area. It is useful to keep in mind that the problems considered can be very complex and complicated and we can only make incremental progresses rather than expect for major breakthroughs. The new and more powerful medical devices and instrumentation only bring in additional challenges. We look forward to continued progress on computer vision in medical imaging for many years to come.

C.H. Chen
April 2013

CONTENTS

CHAPTER 1

AN INTRODUCTION TO COMPUTER VISION IN MEDICAL IMAGING

Chi Hau Chen

University of Massachusetts Dartmouth
E-mail: cchen@umassd.edu

There has been much progress in computer vision and pattern recognition in the last two decades, and there has also much progress in recent years in medical imaging technology. Although images in digital form can easily be processed by basic image processing techniques, effective use of computer vision can provide much useful information for diagnosis and treatment. It has been a challenge to use computer vision in medical imaging because of complexity in dealing with medical images. In this chapter a brief introduction of the subject is presented by addressing the issues involved and then focusing on the active contour model for medical imaging.

1. Introduction

There has been enormous progress in medical imaging techniques and modalities in the last decade or so. For example ultrasound has found its use in many areas previously using x-ray or other techniques. Accompanied with the progress is the greatly increased use of computer vision techniques in medical imaging. In computer vision (see e.g. [1][2]) we talk about the low-level processing which involves basic image processing operations like noise filtering, contrast enhancement and image sharpening, the mid-level processing which involves image segmentation and pattern recognition as well as 3D reconstruction and the high-level processing which involves 'making sense' of an ensemble of recognized objects and performing the cognitive functions at the far end of the processing sequence. Medical imaging refers to the techniques and processes used to create images of the human body for clinical purposes, or procedures seeking to reveal, diagnose or examine disease or studying normal anatomy and physiology [3]. Medical imaging evolved from the discovery of x-rays to the newest magnetic resonance image (MRI). The most commonly used techniques these days are x-ray, computer tomography (CT), ultrasound, MRI and positron emission tomography (PET). The emphasis of medical imaging is to help doctors or other trained personal to provide better diagnosis and treatment and thus the low level and mid-level computer vision is particularly important in the medical area. It is evident that medical imaging has significant impact on medicine and computer vision making use of enormous computing power has enormous impact on medical imaging. The following sections will briefly discuss the nature of some of these medical images and the technology behind them. The remaining chapters of the book cover important aspects of computer vision in medical imaging written by leading experts in the field.

2. Some Medical Imaging Methods

2.1. *X-ray*

X-ray is the first and oldest medical technique available to doctors for the visualization of the body without surgery. X-rays were first discovered by Wilhelm Rontgen in 1895. They penetrate most biological tissues with little attenuation and thus provide a comparatively simple means to produce shadow or projection, images of human body. However X-rays have ionizing effects on the body and hence should not be repeatedly used. The X-ray imaging system involves having a film or screen containing a radiation-sensitive material exposed to the x-rays transmitted through the region of the body. The developed film or excited phosphorous screen exhibits a geometric pattern produced by the structures in the beam path [4]. However X-ray imaging is limited as the signal can be reduced due to the scattering of a large percentage of radiation from the body and much detail is lost in the radiographic process with the superposition of 3D structural information onto a 2D surface. Fig. 1 is the X-ray image of the bones. X-ray system has now been greatly improved. Its use for digital mammogram is particularly important (see e.g. Fig. 2, based on our 1996 data base [14]).

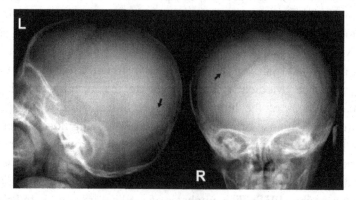

Fig. 1. X-ray image of a skull with a fracture in the right parietal bone.

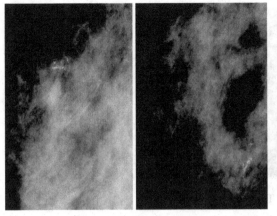

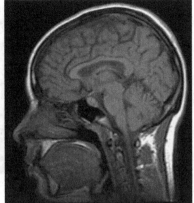

Fig. 2. Mammograms of a patient.   Fig. 3. MRI image of the human head.

2.2. *Magnetic Resonance Image (MRI)*

Magnetic Resonance Image was developed in the early 1970s and has become versatile and clinically useful diagnostic imaging modality [4,5]. MRI is a noninvasive imaging technology that does not use ionizing radiation and provides much more contrast between different soft tissues of the body than computed tomography (CT). It is based on perturbing magnetic fields with radio waves. In MRI, hydrogen nuclei (protons) are imaged due to their strong magnetic moment and prevalence in the soft tissue of the body. The magnetic field is produced by passing an electric current through wire coils in most MRI units. Other coils, located in the machine and in some cases, placed around the part of the body being imaged, send and receive radio waves, producing signals that are detected by the coils. A computer then processes the signals and generates a series of images each of which shows a thin slice of the body. The images can then be studied from different angles by the interpreting physician. Fig. 3 shows the MRI image of the human head. MRI studies brain or body anatomy. More recently, functional MRI has been particularly useful to study brain physiologic function.

2.3. *Intravascular Ultrasound (IVUS)*

Intravascular Ultrasound (or IVUS) allows us to see the coronary artery from the inside-out. This unique picture, Fig. 4, generated in real time, yields information that is not possible with routine imaging methods or even non-invasive Multislice CT scans. A growing number of cardiologists think that new information yielded by IVUS can make a significant difference in how patient is treated and can provide more accurate information which will reduce complications and incidence of heart diseases. Intravascular ultrasound (IVUS) is a catheter-based

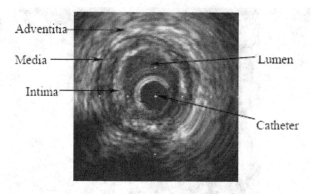

Fig. 4. Typical IVUS image.

technique which provides high-resolution images allowing precise tomographic assessment of lumen area. IVUS uses high-frequency sound waves called ultrasound that can provide a moving picture of your heart. These pictures come from inside the heart rather than through the chest wall. The sound waves are sent with a device called a transducer. The transducer is attached to the end of a catheter, which is threaded through an artery and into your heart. The sound waves bounce off of the walls of the artery and return to the transducer as echoes. The echoes are converted into images on a television monitor to produce a picture of your coronary arteries and other vessels in your body.

In the above IVUS image, the lumen is typically a dark echo-free area adjacent to the imaging catheter and the coronary artery vessel wall mainly appears as three layers: intima, media, and adventitia. As the two inner layers are of principal concern in clinical research, segmentation of IVUS images is a must to isolate the intima-media and lumen boundaries which provides important information about the degree of vessel obstruction as well as the shape and size of plaques. IVUS is only one of many uses of ultrasound in medicine. Actually ultrasonic method is highly versatile, inexpensive and effective in many medical diagnosis uses. Details of the above methods and other medical imaging modalities are well presented in Ref. 5.

3. Roles of Computer Vision, Image Processing and Pattern Recognition

There has been a long history of computers in medicine. The more advanced the medical instrumentation, the more it relies on the computer capability. For medical imaging, computer vision, image processing and pattern recognition techniques are particularly important to provide the required information in diagnosis and treatment. The progress in these techniques is reflected in the sophisticated software tools some of which are commercially available, and others may still be in research and development stage. The software making use of computing power is very useful to deal with the enormous amount of data in medical imaging.

For medical images, the first thing we need to consider is to use image processing techniques (see e.g. [2][6]). They can include image enhancement in spatial and frequency domains, restoration of object from distorted or convoluted images, color image processing, wavelet and mutiresolution image processing, image compression, morphological image processing and image segmentation. Both image enhancement and segmentation can be considered as low level computer vision. For mid-level computer vision, computers can organize the knowledge (information) acquired in the low-level vision to make some useful decisions. For high-level vision, computers must further provide some "thinking" capability like humans do. The above stated division of computer vision tasks may not be precise, but for medical imaging, the low level vision is most important as the results are used for human expert (physicians) to interpret. Thus interactive and 3-D visualization capabilities can be significant. Pattern recognition is closely linked to the image processing and computer vision especially for image segmentation. Some basic tasks in pattern recognition (see e.g. [7][8]) are feature extraction, pattern description (be it statistical, syntactic, structural or else), learning, and decision making process. A major objective in pattern recognition is to make correct decisions or classification with the help of the other three tasks. A good classification is much needed for image segmentation. Though artificial neural networks and support vector machines have made classifier easier, they still cannot be fully relied on in practical recognition problems.

There have been tremendous progress in image processing, pattern recognition and computer vision in the last decades (see e.g. [9-13]) with many applications including the medical area. For images in medical imaging, it is necessary to use the multiple information sources, like intensity, texture, shape, and contextual information within an image and between images. In fact information that captures the dynamics of the medical image patterns can be the key to the success of extracting desired diagnosis information from the images. With greatly improved medical sensors/devices and the use of multiple sensors, it may be necessary to fuse the data from several sources to aid in the diagnosis and treatment.

A note on the performance measure is needed here. The simple percentage correct recognition rate can be highly inadequate. For medical imaging, the ROC (receiver operating characteristics) curve is most popular. It is a plot of recognition rate versus the false alarm rate. Other measures include the sensitivity (true positive rate) versus specificity (true negative rate). The accuracy is probably a major challenge for computer vision/pattern recognition in medical imaging. While there was success in early developments like computer chest X-ray screening for black lungs, the high accuracy desired for medical imaging, such as automated detection and segmentation, and extraction of area or volume information for regions of interest, is still not reached to the author's knowledge. This means that automated method cannot replace the manual operations.

With constant progress in computer vision and pattern recognition, however, the opportunities are really unlimited to reach our goals in medical imaging. Among the large number of signal/image processing techniques have been examined for medical imaging use, the multiresoution image processing stands out to be useful most of the time at it captures the intensity and texture information well and for single image the contextual information also (see e.g. [14]). Effort is much needed to make use of information from a sequence of images to achieve improved segmentation. While other important topics in medical imaging are covered by experts as presented in this book, the rest of this chapter will be focused on the active contours problem for intravascular ultrasound images.

4. Active Contours

The technique of active contours has become quite popular for variety of applications, particularly image segmentation and motion tracking, during the last decade. The active contour model has an advantage of being less sensitive to blurred edges and also avoiding broken contour lines compared to other methods like thresholding and edge-based methods. Active contour models are based on deforming an initial contour C towards the boundary of the object to be detected, through minimizing a functional designed such that its minimum is obtained at the boundary of the object. Energy minimization involves two components, the smoothness of the curve and one for pulling the curve closer to the boundary. The active contour consists of a set of control points connected by straight lines as shown below in Fig. 5. The active contour is defined by the number of control points as well as sequence of each other. However fitting active contours to shapes is an interactive process. The user must suggest an initial contour as shown in Fig. 4 below, which is quite close to the intended shape. Then we have to create an attractor image so that the contour will be attracted to features in the image extracted by internal energy.

There are two main approaches in active contours based on the mathematical implementation: snakes and level sets. The classical snake model was first introduced by Kass et al. [15], while the level sets approach was first proposed by Osher and Sethian [16]. Both are discussed further in the following.

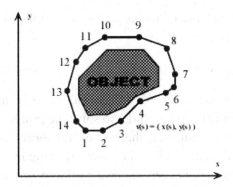

Fig. 5. Basic form of active contour.

4.1. *Snakes*

A snake is an energy minimizing spline guided by external constraint forces and influenced by edges, localizing them accurately. It is also the first model of active contour proposed by Kass et al.

Let us define a contour parameterized by arc s as

$$C(s) \equiv \{ (x(s), y(s)) : 0 \leq s \leq L \} : R \to \Omega$$

where L denotes the length of the contour C, and Ω denotes the entire domain of an image I(x, y). Define an energy function,

$$E(C) = E_{int} + E_{ext} \tag{1}$$

where E_{int} and E_{ext} respectively denote the internal energy and external energy functions. The internal energy function determines the regularity i.e. smooth shape, of the contour. The internal energy is a quadratic functional which is given by:

$$E_{int} \equiv \int_0^L \alpha |C'(s)|^2 + \beta |C''(s)|^2 \, ds \tag{2}$$

where α controls the tension of the contour and β controls the rigidity of the contour.

The external energy on the other hand, determines the criteria of contour evolution depending on the image I (x, y) which is defined as:

$$E_{ext} \equiv \int_0^L E_{img} (C(s)) \, ds \tag{3}$$

where $E_{img}(x, y)$ denotes a scalar function defined on the image plane, so the local minimum of E_{img} attracts the snakes to edges.

A very common example of the edge attraction function is the function of image gradient given by:

$$E_{img}(x, y) = 1/\lambda \, | \nabla^G_\sigma * I(x, y) | \quad : R \rightarrow \Omega \qquad (4)$$

where $^G_\sigma$ denotes a Gaussian smoothing filter with the standard deviation σ and λ is a suitably chose constant. Now in order to solve the problem of snakes we have to find the contour which minimizes the total energy term E with the given set of weights α, β and λ. Also, a set of snake points residing on the image plane are defined in the initial stage and then the next positions of those snake points are determined by local minimum E. The connected form of these particular snake points is called the contour. Fig. 6 shows an example of classic snakes in its initial stage. Fig. 7 shows the final stage.

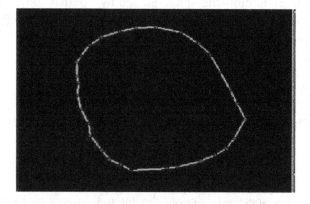

Fig. 6. An example of classic snake in its initial stage.

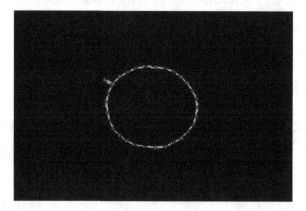

Fig. 7. An example of classic snake in its final stage.

The snake points eventually stop on the boundary of the object. The classic snakes provide an accurate location of the edges only if the initial contour is given sufficiently near the edges as they make use of only the local information along the contour. However, we have a difficult problem estimating a proper position of initial contours without prior knowledge. Also, classic snakes cannot detect more than one boundary simultaneously as the snakes maintain same topology during the evolution stage. The snakes cannot split to multiple boundaries or merge from multiple initial contours. The next model which is the Level set theory has given a solution to this particular problem.

4.2. *Level set methods*

Since the level set method was first proposed by Osher and Sethian, it has become more and more popular theoretical numerical framework within fluid mechanics, graphics, image processing and computer vision. The level set method is basically used for tracking moving fronts by considering the front as the zero level set of an embedding function, called the level set function. It is a widely used tool for image segmentation. Many features can be considered simultaneously such as edges, region statistics, shape and kind of multidimensional data depending upon how propagation speed of the front is defined.

Fig. 8 shows the use of shape prior for segmentation of a partly occluded object. It shows the evolution of the active contour (solid line) with the aid of a prior knowledge of its shape (the dotted line).

The main purpose of the level set methods is to consider the moving interface as a set of zero values of an embedding function Φ. The level set method can be applied to any kind of problem where an interface is moving with a speed F defined on every point.

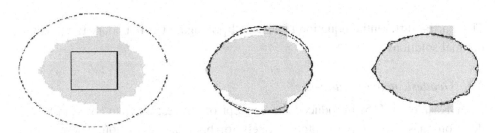

Fig. 8. Examples of the power of the level sets as a segmentation tool.

The level set equation is briefly describes as follows. Let us assume that F is known. Consider an interface г that can be a curve, surface, hyper-surface in R^N, as a boundary between two regions, one inside the boundary and another one outside the boundary. The interface represented as a curve in R^2 is embedded in a level set function Φ and is constituted of all points where the value of the level set function is zero Γ(t) = {x(t) | Φ(x(t), t) = 0}.

In other words, a level set function is constructed around the interface that constitutes the zero value of the embedding function Φ. All other points of the level set function have the value of the distance from the point to the closest point on the boundary. The distance is positive if this point is situated on the outside of the boundary area and negative if it is situated on the inside. The level set function will change with time according to the speed F and the interface is always constituted by the points where the level set function equals zero. The interface, г, embedded by the level set function, Φ, can be expressed as,

$$\Gamma(t) := \{x(t) \mid \Phi(x(t), t) = 0\} \tag{5}$$

where t being the time and x(t) are the points of Φ, Φ < 0 for points lying inside the surface and Φ ≥ 0 for points lying outside the surface.

Computing the time derivative of the level set Φ(x(t), t) by using the chain rule gives:

$$\partial\Phi/\partial t + \nabla \Phi (x(t), t) . dx/dt = 0 \tag{6}$$

where ∇ is the gradient operator.

We introduce F as the speed in the outward normal direction such that F = (dx/dt). n where n = ∇ Φ/ | ∇ Φ |. If the initial level set function is known, Φ (x, t = 0), the level set equation becomes

$$\partial\Phi/\partial t + F \mid \nabla \Phi \mid = 0 \tag{7}$$

This partial differential equation (PDE) will propagate the boundary towards the optimal solution.

4.3. *Geodesic active contours*

After Kass et al. [15] introduced the concept of snakes; extensive research was done on snakes or active contour models for boundary detection. These active contours are examples of general technique of matching deformable model to image data by means of energy minimization. The energy function is basically composed of two components, one controls the smoothness of the curve and another attracts the curve towards the boundary. This particular energy model is not capable of handling changes in the topology of the evolving curve when direct implementations are performed. The Geodesic active contour [18] includes a new component in the curve velocity based on image information that improves the active contour model. The new velocity component accurately tracks boundaries with high variation in their gradient including small gaps. It also allows simultaneous detection of interior and exterior boundaries in several objects without special contour tracking procedures.

4.4. *Region-based active contours*

Chan and Vese [9] have presented a method for segmenting images without edge detection by using a weak formulation of the Mumford-Shah functional. In this method, they separate the image into two regions, one inside the level set function $\Phi < 0$ and the other region on the outside of the boundary $\Phi \geq 0$. Each region is represented by mean intensities over the interior and exterior of the curve. The method extracts the objects by minimizing an energy function using region properties instead of edge properties. Mathematically the energy to be minimized is given by

$$E = \int_{\Omega} (I - u)^2 \, dA + \int_{\Omega'} (I - v)^2 \, dA \tag{8}$$

where Ω and Ω' represent the interior and exterior of the curve, and u and v represent the mean image intensities over Ω and Ω' respectively.

This energy is very robust to noise and curve placement as it looks at integrals of image data rather than image derivatives and although the curve moves locally, it inspects global image statistics rather than just looking along the curve. There are many advantages of region-based approaches than edge-based techniques. However techniques that attempt to model regions using global statistics are not ideal for segmenting heterogeneous objects. As a result region-based active contour may lead to erroneous segmentation.

4.5. *Hybrid evolution method*

The method [19] is to combine both the local based Geodesic active contour and region based active contour method to derive the advantages of both. A hybrid energy is defined and minimized iteratively and a new class of active contour energies should be considered which utilizes local information and also incorporates the benefits of region-based techniques. This hybrid energy is minimized iteratively. Mathematically we begin with the geodesic active contour where the energy of the curve E is given by the following function where C represents the evolving curve and I represent the image data

$$E = \oint_{C(s)} f(I) \, ds \qquad (9)$$

where f is a any positive, decreasing function of the image data and its values from the metric over which the minimum length geodesic will be found as the curve is deformed. The hybrid energy defined below begins with the geodesic energy given in Eq. (9),

$$E = \oint_{C(s)} [\int_{x \in \Omega} (I_\chi(x,s) - u_l(s))^2 + \int_{x \in \Omega'} (I_\chi(x,s) - v_l(s))^2] \, ds \qquad (10)$$

where Ω and Ω' represent the region on the interior and exterior of the curve respectively and the f we chose in Eq. (9) makes use of image data over local regions thus making it similar to the region-based flows. We should select f to be the smallest so that our key assumptions are set. s in the above equation specifies every point along it as the contour integral is evaluated. Also the $u_l(s)$ and $v_l(s)$ are the arithmetic means of points in local neighborhoods around the point C(s). The characteristic function χ defines these neighborhoods and the position of the curve. The χ function evaluates as 1 in a local neighborhood defined by small radius and 0 elsewhere. The contour divides the region selected by function χ into interior local points and exterior local points.

It is noted that there have been much further work on the active contours by increasing the speed, and efficiency and avoiding false contours, etc. The following section deals with IVUS image segmentation using active contour or its variation.

4.6. *IVUS image segmentation*

The raw data of our IVUS images were provided by Brigham Women's Hospital in Boston, MA. By using algorithms developed by Prakash Manandhar, a Ph.D. student in University of Massachusetts at Dartmouth the image data base was used for the segmentation study. The hybrid active contour method was compared to the edge based active contour method using gradient vector flow and region based active contour method. The hybrid model has shown better results compared to the other models. The experiments are conducted on two IVUS images and both of these images are compared to the other active contour models. Both images were segmented correctly using the presented hybrid method compared to other active contour models. The contour extracted is for lumens. One original IVUS image we used is shown in Fig. 9. The lumen was detected correctly after 800 iterations, even though there is presence of guide wire (Fig. 10).

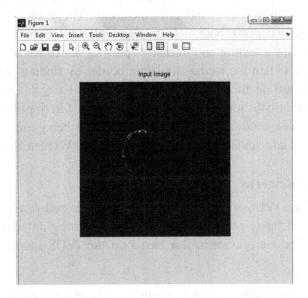

Fig. 9.

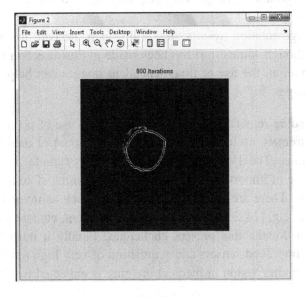

Fig. 10.

The algorithms developed by P. Manandhar, which employ different approach based on active contours are presented in Chapter 20 of this volume. Another approach we have examined and which is a departure from active contours is to use both the texture and intensity information along with radial basis function (RBF) [20] to derive the closed contours for both lumen boundary and outer (Media-Advantita) boundary of the artery. The method uses composite operator [21] which depends both on texture and intensity. Lumen contour can be traced based on finest texture and intensity specifics. Once we have the contour of lumen we can obtain the media-adventitia border by finding the coarse-most texture located outside the lumen border. Once we have this information of the two contour initializations we can use low pass filtering/2D Radial basis functions to obtain smooth 2D contours. The method is being used for automated segmentation of a large database from the Brigham and Women Hospital.

5. Concluding Remarks

The discussion on IVUS image segmentation methods and results show only a very small part of many computer vision in medical imaging activities. Clearly many problem areas are evident, just based on the IVUS image segmentation study.

1. The manual segmentation which presumably is more accurate is very time consuming.
2. Automated algorithms still have a long way to go achieve the desired high accuracy.
3. The 3-D segmentation results are still much needed to be useful for physicians, though some effort has been made in this direction [22]. Even for 2-D segmentation, the use of time-dependent images can help (see [23]) for the IVUS images.

As a concluding remark, computer vision making use of powerful computer resources is extremely useful to deal with a large amount of data for on-line or off-line operations. The IVUS image segmentation example as shown above clearly shows one of important potential and opportunities of computer vision in medical imaging. There are very many other issues such as involving shape, 3D construction (see e.g. [24-26]) and volume measurement, etc. are well within the computer vision domain that present challenges. Finally it must be noted that with constantly improved sensors and acquisition of very high resolution images, the need for computer vision in medical imaging is expected to increase greatly with time.

Acknowledgment

I thank my former graduate students S. Murphy, P. Manandhar, L. Potdar, R. Chittineni, and A. Vaishampayan as well as current graduate student A. R. Gangidi for their constructive participation of the IVUS image segmentation study project.

References

[1] L. Shapiro and G. Stockman, "Computer Vision", Prentice-Hall, 2001.

[2] R.C. Gonzalez and R.C. Woods, "Digital Image Processing", 3rd edition, 2008.

[3] http://en.wikipedia.org/wiki/Medical_imaging

[4] R.A. Robb, Biomedical Imaging, Visualization and Analysis, Wiley, 2000.

[5] A.P. Dhawanm, "Medical Image Analysis", IEEE Press-Wiley, 2003.

[6] U. Qidwai and C.H. Chen, "Digital Image Processing, an algorithmic approach with MATLAB", CRC Press, 2010.

[7] R. Duda, P. Hart, and D.G. Stork, "Pattern Classification", second edition, Wiley, 2001.

[8] S. Theodoridis and K. Koutroumbas, "Pattern Recognition", 4th edition, Academic Press, 2008.

[9] C.H. Chen, L.F. Pau, and P.S.P. Wang, editors, "Handbook of Pattern Recognition", vol. 1, World Scientific Publishing, 1993.

[10] C.H. Chen, L.F. Pau, and P.S.P. Wang, editors, "Handbook of Pattern Recognition", vol. 2, World Scientific Publishing, 1999.

[11] C.H. Chen and P.S.P. Wang, editors, "Handbook of Pattern Recognition", vol. 3, World Scientific Publishing, 2005.

[12] C.H. Chen, editor, "Handbook of Pattern Recognition", vol. 4, World Scientific Publishing, 2010.

[13] C.H. Chen, editor, "Emerging Topics in Computer Vision", World Scientific Publishing, 2012.

[14] C.H. Chen and G.G. Lee, "On digital mammogram segmentation and microcalcification detection using multiresolution wavelet analysis", Graphical Models and Image Processing, vol. 59, no. 5, September 1997, pp. 349–364.

[15] M. Kass, A. Witkin, and D. Terzopoulos, "Snakes: Active contour models", International Journal of Computer Vision, vol. 1, pp. 321–331, 1987.

[16] J.A. Sethian, "Curvature and the evolution of Fronts", Comm. in Math. Phys., 101, pp. 487–499, 1985.

[17] V. Caselles, R. Kimmel, and G. Sapiro, "Geodesic active contours", International Journal of Computer Vision, 22(1), pp. 61–79, 1997.

[18] Tony F. Chan and Luminita A. Vese, "Active contours without edges", IEEE Trans. on Image Processing, vol. 10, no. 2, pp. 266–277, 2001.

[19] C.H. Chen, L. Potdar, and R. Chittineni, "Two novel ACM (active contour model) methods for intravascular ultrasound image segmentation", Review of Quantitative NDE, vol. 29A, American Institute of Physics, 2009.

[20] G. Giannoglou, Y. Chatzizisis, V. Koutkias, I. Kompatsiaris, M. Papadogiorgaki, V. Mezaris, E. Parissi, P. Diamantopoulos, M.G. Strintzis, N. Maglaveras, G. Parcharidis, and G. Louridas, "A novel active contour model for fully automated segmentation of intravascular ultrasound Images: in-vivo validation in human coronary arteries", Computers in Biology and Medicine, September 2007; 37:1292–1302.

[21] A.R. Gangidi, P. Manandhar, and C.H. Chen, "Fast and accurate automated IVUS contour detection and 3D visualization", presented at the 18th Annual Sigma Xi Research Exhibition at UMass Dartmouth, April 30, 2012.

[22] M. Roy Cardinal, "Segmentation of IVUS images", Ph.D. thesis, University of Montreal, 2008.

[23] T. Löfstedt, O. Ahnlund, M. Peolsson, and J. Trygg, "Dynamic ultrasound imaging—A multivariate approach for the analysis and comparison of time-dependent musculoskeletal movements", BMC Medical Imaging, 2012 Sep 27; 12(1):29.

[24] A.C. Kak and M. Slaney, "Principles of Computerized Tomographic Imaging," SIAM (Society of Industrial and Applied Mathematics) Press, 2001.

[25] A.C. Kak, "Computerized tomography with X-ray, emission, and ultrasound sources", Prof. of the IEEE, vol. 67, no. 9, pp. 1245–1273, Sept. 1979.

[26] Y. Sun, I. Liu, and J.K. Grady, "Reconstruction of 3D tree-like structures from three mutually orthogonal projections", IEEE Trans. on Pattern Analysis and Machine Intelligence, vol. 16, pp. 241–248, 1994.

Part 1

Theory and Methodologies

CHAPTER 2

DISTRIBUTION MATCHING APPROACHES TO MEDICAL IMAGE SEGMENTATION

Ismail Ben Ayed

GE Healthcare, London, ON, Canada
University of Western Ontario, London, ON, Canada
E-mails: ismail.benayed@ge.com; ibenayed@uwo.ca

Distribution-matching approaches to semantic image segmentation have recently bestirred an impressive research effort in computer vision and medical imaging. Several recent studies showed that optimizing some measures of affinity between distributions can yield outstanding performances unattainable with standard segmentation algorithms. However, such distribution measures are non-linear (higher-order) functionals, which can be difficult to optimize. The ensuing optimization problems are probably NP-hard and cannot be directly addressed by standard optimizers. The purpose of this chapter is to review some recent developments in this research direction, with focus on both formulation and optimization aspects. The chapter further discusses the usefulness of distribution-matching techniques in various medical image segmentation scenarios, and includes examples from cardiac, spine and brain imaging.

1. Introduction

Segmenting images into meaningful regions, for instance specific organs in medical scans, is a subject of paramount importance in vision and medical imaging for its theoretical and methodological challenges, and various applications. This chapter discusses the problem of segmenting an image into two regions (a target segment and it complement in the image domain), so that some features (e.g., intensity, context or shape) within the target region follows some *a priori* information. Such priors are necessary to obtain semantic segmentations that are unattainable with unsupervised algorithms. We will focus on distribution-matching formulations, which enforce some consistency between the feature distribution of the target segment and a given (*a priori* learned) model. Such formulations have recently sparked a significant research effort in computer vision[1,10,21,26,34,39] and medical imaging[6,3,28,37]. Several recent studies proved that optimizing some measures of affinity between distributions/histograms (e.g, the Kullback-Leibler divergence, Bhattacharyya coefficient or $\mathcal{L}_j$-*distances*) can yield outstanding performances unattainable with standard algorithms, and can be very useful in solving several image partitioning problems, e.g.:

• *Co-segmentation of image pairs*[24,35]: Introduced initially in the well-known work of Rother et al.[41], the problem amounts to finding the same semantic segment in a pair of images. Facilitating segmentation of an image using minimal prior information from another image of the same object of interest, co-segmentation has bestirred several recent investigations[46,24,35] and has shown very useful in object recognition and image retrieval[20,42,16,41], as well as image editing[4] and summarization[17].

• *Interactive image segmentation*[39,3,37]: Interactive segmentation uses minimal user interaction, for instance a few mouse clicks, simple scribbles or bounding boxes, to learn prior information from the current image. Embedding clues on user intention facilitates significantly the segmentation problem, and has led to successful algorithms in vision[39] and medical imaging[3,37].

• *Segmentation with offline learning*[8]: Segmenting a class of images depicting the same object of interest occurs in important applications such as medical image analysis. In this case, offline learning of prior information from segmented training images is very useful[8,15].

• *Tracking*[26,6]: In the context of tracking a target segment (or object) throughout an image sequence, one can segment the current frame using information learned from previously segmented frames.

In general, measures of discrepancy between distributions (or histograms) are non-linear (higher-order) functionals, which can be difficult to optimize[10,21]. The ensuing optimization problems are probably NP-hard and cannot be directly addressed by standard optimizers. As a result, several recent studies focused on designing efficient and reliable optimizers for distribution-matching functionals[10,21,22,26,24,35]. The purpose of this chapter is to review some recent developments in this research direction, with focus on both formulation and optimization aspects. We will further discuss the usefulness of distribution-matching techniques in various medical image segmentation scenarios, and include examples from cardiac, spine and brain imaging.

2. Formulations

Let $\mathbf{F} : \Omega \subset \mathbb{R}^n (n \in \{2, 3\}) \to \mathcal{F} \subset \mathbb{R}^k$ be a function, which maps 3D (or 2D) image domain Ω to a finite set of *feature* values $\mathcal{F}$. $\mathbf{F}$ can be an image-based features, for instance:

• intensity[37]; or
• intensity statistics within several box-shaped image patches of different orientations/scales[3]. Such patch-based features can encode contextual knowledge about the region of interest and its neighboring structures (e.g., size, shape, orientation and relationships to neighboring structures).

Additionally, $\mathbf{F}$ can be a geometry-based feature than encodes:

• the shape of the region of interest[6]; or
• the interactions between different objects[11].

The purpose of distribution-matching formulations is to find an optimal region in Ω, so that (i) the distribution (or histogram) of feature $\mathbf{F}$ within the region most closely matches a given (*a priori* learned) model distribution $\mathcal{M}$; and (ii) the boundary (or surface in the 3D case) of the region is smooth. This amounts to solving an optimization problem of the following general form:

$$\hat{R} = \arg\min_{R \subset \Omega} \underbrace{\mathcal{S}(\mathcal{P}^{\mathbf{F}}(R, .), \mathcal{M})}_{Distribution \;\; matching} + \underbrace{\lambda \mathcal{L}(\partial R)}_{Smoothness} \tag{1}$$

The following is a detailed description of the notations and variables that appear in the optimization problem in Eq. (1):

- For feature $\mathbf{F} : \Omega \subset \mathbb{R}^n (n \in \{2, 3\}) \to \mathcal{F}$, and for any region $R \in \Omega$, $\mathcal{P}^{\mathbf{F}}(R, .)$ is either
  (i) the kernel density estimate of the distribution of $\mathbf{F}$ within region R:

$$\mathcal{P}^{\mathbf{F}}(R, z) = \frac{\int_R \mathcal{K}_z(\mathbf{F}(x)) \, dx}{A(R)} \qquad \forall z \in Z_{\mathcal{F}} \tag{2}$$

with $Z_{\mathcal{F}}$ a set of bins describing feature space $\mathcal{F}$, $A(R)$ the area (or volume) of region R:

$$A(R) = \int_R dx, \tag{3}$$

and $\mathcal{K}_z(\cdot)$ a kernel function, typically Gaussian (σ is the width of the kernel):

$$\mathcal{K}_z(y) = \frac{1}{(2\pi\sigma^2)^{(k/2)}} \exp\left(-\frac{\|z - y\|^2}{2\sigma^2}\right); \tag{4}$$

or
(ii) the histogram of $\mathbf{F}$ within region R:

$$\mathcal{P}^{\mathbf{F}}(R, z) = \int_R \delta(\mathbf{F}(x) - z) \, dx \qquad \forall z \in Z_{\mathcal{F}} \tag{5}$$

where δ is given by:

$$\delta(y) = \begin{cases} 1 & \text{if} \quad y = 0 \\ 0 & \text{if} \quad y \neq 0 \end{cases} \tag{6}$$

Note that, in (4), replacing the kernel function by δ yields the normalized histogram.

- $\mathcal{S}(f, g)$ is a measure of discrepancy between distributions or histograms, e.g., the Kullback-Leibler divergence[21,10,33], the negative Bhattacharyya coefficient[40,39,5], the Earth Mover's Distance[1], or an $\mathcal{L}_j$-*distance*[26,35]. In section 4, we will show and discuss medical imaging applications of model

(1) using the Bhattacharyya coefficient as an example of discrepancy measure:

$$\mathcal{S}(\mathcal{P}^{\mathbf{F}}(R,.),\mathcal{M}) = -\mathcal{B}(\mathcal{P}^{\mathbf{F}}(R,.),\mathcal{M})$$

$$= -\sum_{z \in Z_{\mathcal{F}}} \sqrt{\mathcal{P}^{\mathbf{F}}(R,z)\mathcal{M}(z)} \qquad (7)$$

The Bhattacharyya coefficient $\mathcal{B}$ is always in $[0, 1]$, with 1 indicating a perfect match between the distributions and 0 a total mismatch. Therefore, $\mathcal{B}$ has a fixed (normalized) range that affords a conveniently practical appraisal of the similarity.

- $\mathcal{M}$ is a model distribution of features. $\mathcal{M}$ can be learned from the current testing image (i.e., the image to be segmented) using minimal user inputs, e.g., a few mouse clicks, simple scribbles or bounding boxes[3,37,39]. Alternatively, $\mathcal{M}$ can be learned from training images different from the testing image. For instance, in the context of tracking an object in an image sequence[26,6], one can segment the current frame using a model distribution learned from previously segmented frames. Similarly, in the context of co-segmentation algorithms[35,41], the model used to segment one image is learned from other images depicting the same object.

- $\mathcal{L}(\partial R)$ denotes the length of the boundary (or surface in the 3D case) of region R. Minimization of such standard length-based term enforces smoothness of the solutions. It penalizes irregular boundaries as well as small and isolated regions in the solution.

- λ is a positive constant that balances the relative contribution of each of the terms in the functional.

3. Optimization Aspects

In general, measures of discrepancy between distributions (or histograms) are non-linear (higher-order) functionals, which can be difficult to optimize[21,10]. The ensuing optimization problems are probably NP-hard and cannot be directly addressed by powerful global optimizers such as graph cuts[13] or convex-relaxation techniques[47]. In the following, we will discuss different options for optimizing distribution-matching terms.

3.1. *Specialized optimizers*

Several recent studies investigated specialized optimizers for particular forms of distribution-matching functionals[41,35,26]. For instance, Rother et al.[41] investigated optimization of the $\mathcal{L}_1$-*distance* between histograms via graph cuts[13]. Following concepts from trust-region techniques in continuous optimization[12], they computed a sequence of parametric linear approximations of the functional, and performed optimization over the approximation parameter. They further proposed a submodular-supermodular procedure[36] for initialization of the sequence, which assumes the functional is supermodular, and proved that this holds for the $\mathcal{L}_1$-*distance*. It is worth noting that the algorithm in[41] is not applicable to other distribution-matching functionals. Another related study in[35] proposed to replace the $\mathcal{L}_1$ by the $\mathcal{L}_2$-*distance* because the latter affords some interesting combinatorial properties, which is amenable to powerful graph cut optimization. After linearizing the $\mathcal{L}_2$-*distance*, the authors of[35] rewrote the problem as the optimization of a quadratic pseudo-boolean function (QPBF). Although non-submodular, such QPBF form allows roof-duality relaxation that can be solved by graph cuts[29]. It is worth noting that such relaxation yields only partial solutions with some pixels left unlabeled. Furthermore, the solution in[35] uses specific properties of the $\mathcal{L}_2$-*distance* and, therefore, cannot be applied to other distribution-matching functionals.

The authors of[5] built a bound optimizer for the Bhattacharyya measure. They divided the problem into a sequence of sub-problems, each corresponding to a bound of the functional. Within each sub-problem, a global optimum can be obtained with a graph cut[13]. The solution obtained from each graph cut guarantees that the functional decreases. The bound optimizer in[5] yielded very rapid convergences (it requires a few graph cuts, typically less than 5) and competitive accuracies/optima. Also, it was successfully applied to interactive color image segmentation[39]. It is worth noting, however, that the bound derivation in[5] is based on particular properties of the Bhattacharyya coefficient, which precludes its application to other distribution-matching functionals.

3.2. *Derivative-based optimizers*

This section discusses derivative-based approaches to optimizing distribution-matching functionals. Such approaches use the first-order Gateâux derivative of the functional. This is the case of standard active-curve/level-set techniques[33,2,19,1], which use functional derivatives to compute gradient flows, or the recently proposed line search and trust region methods[22,21], which use first-order approximations of the functionals within a graph cut framework.

3.2.1. *Active curves and level sets*

Active-curve/level-set techniques can address arbitrary differentiable functionals[33]. Therefore, they were commonly used in the literature to deal with distribution-matching terms[33,2,19,1]. In the active-curve/level-set framework, minimization of any differentiable functional is carried out by computing a partial differential equation (PDE), which governs the evolution of the boundary of region R. The curve evolution equation is obtained by a local gradient descent and the first-order derivative of the functional. Therefore, the ensuing solutions may correspond to weak local minima[5]. Furthermore, in the case of distribution-matching functionals, active curves may result in computationally intensive algorithms[5,33], more so when the image dimension is high (3D or higher). This may limit significantly their application in medical imaging. For example, the curve flow optimizing the Bhattacharyya measure is incremental[5,33], and requires a large number of iterative updates of computationally costly distributions. Moreover, the robustness of active curve methods inherently relies on a user initialization of the contour close to the target region and the choice an approximating numerical solution that is controlled by several crucial parameters (e.g., step size).

3.2.2. *Line search and trust region methods*

In the recent studies in[22,21], Gorelick et al. proposed iterative line-search and trust-region methods, which can deal with arbitrary differentiable functionals. Within each iteration, they optimized a first-order approximation of the functional via graph cuts. These methods can make larger moves in the gradient-descent direction than active curves, thereby resulting in much more efficient algorithms. However, similarly to active curves, they are not applicable to non-differentiable functionals, e.g., the $\mathcal{L}_1$-*distance* between histograms[41].

3.3. *Bound optimizers*

Let $\mathcal{E}(R)$ be a segmentation functional to be optimized over some region R. Bound-optimization algorithms build and optimize *auxiliary functionals* of $\mathcal{E}$, whose optimization is easier than the original functional:

Definition 1: Given an auxiliary variable R^i, $\mathcal{A}(R|R^i)$ is an auxiliary functional of $\mathcal{E}$ if it verifies the following conditions:

$$\mathcal{E}(R) \leq \mathcal{A}(R|R^i) \tag{8a}$$

$$\mathcal{E}(R) = \mathcal{A}(R|R) \tag{8b}$$

Instead of minimizing $\mathcal{E}$, one can minimize iteratively a sequence of auxiliary functionals:

$$R^{i+1} = \arg\min_R \mathcal{A}(R|R^i), \quad i = 1, 2, \ldots \tag{9}$$

Using the conditions in (8a) and (8b), and by definition of minimum in (9), one can prove that the solutions in (9) correspond to decreasing functional $\mathcal{E}$ during iterations: $\mathcal{E}(R^i) = \mathcal{A}(R^i|R^i) \geq \mathcal{A}(R^{i+1}|R^i) \geq \mathcal{E}(R^{i+1})$.

Bound optimization algorithms are derivative- and parameter-free; they do not require the functional to be differentiable, neither do they use optimizer parameters such as step sizes. Furthermore, they never worsen the functional. They can be very efficient because they turn difficult and, in some instances, very complex optimization problems into easier ones[48]. Bound optimization yielded efficient solver for difficult problems in Nonnegative Matrix Factorization[31] and computational statistics[30], and is gaining interest in machine learning[48]. For instance, the study[48] demonstrated the power of bound optimization in solving AdaBoost and logistic regression models.

The main difficulty in bound optimization is in building an appropriate auxiliary functional. On the one hand, the bound should be close enough to the original functional. On the other hand, a good auxiliary functional should be amenable to fast and global solvers. The study in[5] proposed an efficient bound optimizer specific for the Bhattacharyya measure. In the next section, we will see the application of this optimizer in various medical image segmentation scenarios. More recently, Ben Ayed et al.[10] proposed a generalization of the Bhattacharyya auxiliary functional in[5] to more general forms of higher-order functionals, including the Kullback-Leibler divergence and the $\mathcal{L}_j$-*distances*. The auxiliary functionals in[5,10] have the following general forms:

$$\mathcal{A}(R|R^i) = \int_R f(x, R^i) + \int_{\Omega \setminus R} g(x, R^i) + \lambda \mathcal{L}(\partial R) \tag{10}$$

where $f(., R^i) : \Omega \to \mathbb{R}$ and $g(., R^i) : \Omega \to \mathbb{R}$ are scalar functions defined over the image domain. R^i is a constant segmentation region, which does not depend on variable region R (R^i is obtained from the previous iteration). The general form in (10) is amenable to powerful and global solvers such as graph cuts[13] or convex-relaxation techniques[47].

3.3.1. *Graph cuts*

In combinatorial optimization, functionals of the form (10) can be solved globally and efficiently in low-order polynomial time with a graph cut by solving an equivalent max-flow problem[13]. In the next section, we will show some experimental examples based on graph cut bound optimization via the well-known max-flow algorithm of Boykov and Kolmogorov[13]. Here we omit the details of the max-flow algorithm. Such details are well-known in the literature, and can be found in[13].

3.3.2. *Convex-relaxation techniques*

An alternative to graph cuts would be to use recent convex-relaxation techniques[47,40]. Unlike graph-cut approaches, convex-relaxation techniques can be easily parallelized to reduce substantially the computational time for 3D domains (or higher) and extends easily to high dimensions, which makes them appealing for medical image segmentation. In the next section, we will show some experimental examples based on convex relaxation and bound optimization.

4. Medical Imaging Applications

This section discusses the usefulness of distribution-matching techniques in three different medical image segmentation scenarios.

4.1. *Left ventricle segmentation in cardiac images*

Accurate detection of the left ventricle (LV) boundaries (the endo- and epicardium) in cardiac Magnetic Resonance (MR) time sequences is an essential step in diagnosing various cardiovascular abnormalities. Such boundaries results in LV dynamics which translate into extensive clinical information[14], e.g., the ejection fraction, ventricular enlargement, aneurysms, regional wall motion, and myocardium scars. The problem consists of segmenting each frame into three regions: the LV cavity, myocardium, and background (Refer to the examples in Fig. 1). However, manual segmentations of all the images in cardiac sequences is time-consuming[a]. Therefore, automatic or semi-automatic solutions are highly desired and are still being intensively investigated, despite the impressive research effort that has been devoted to LV segmentation in the last decade (A comprehensive review on LV segmentation methods can be found in[38]). In general, LV segmentation algorithms use strong geometric priors, e.g., statistical shape models or atlases[38]. Strong priors remove the need for user interventions at the price of a time-consuming training step, which builds a large, manually-segmented set of sequences to train the algorithms. Although very effective in some cases, these training-based algorithms may have difficulty in capturing the substantial variations encountered in a clinical context[9,6,27,7], with the results often being dependent on the choice of a specific training set. For instance, a pathological case outside the set of learned shapes may not be recovered, and intensity models have to be updated for new acquisition protocols and sequences. Furthermore, manual segmentations of a large set of subjects during a training phase can be time-consuming and requires trained experts, which may be difficult to implement in routine clinical use.

One way to remove the need for intensive external training would be to use a manually segmented frame in each cardiac sequence to create training models and compute segmentations for the rest of the sequence[6,49,7,23]. Based only on the current data, these methods allow more flexibility in clinical use, although at the price of a user initialization. In this connection, distribution-matching formulations were shown to be very useful[6]. In the remainder of this section, we will discuss the distribution-matching method in[6]. Within each frame, the algorithm in[6] seeks the LV cavity and myocardium regions consistent with subject-specific model distributions learned from the first frame in the sequence. As we will illustrate with an experimental example later, the distribution-matching formulation in[6] has the following advantages over standard LV segmentation algorithms:

- It removes the need of external learning from a large training set;
- It handles intrinsically geometric variations of the LV without biasing the solution towards a set of template shapes; and
- It removes the need of costly pose optimization (or registration) procedures.

---

[a]A cardiac MRI data set of a single subject typically contains 200 images.

Consider a MR cardiac sequence containing J image functions $I^j : \Omega \subset \mathbb{R}^2 \rightarrow \mathbb{R}, j \in [1..J]$. The algorithm in[6] finds the cavity and myocardium regions within the domain of each frame j. The problem is posed as the minimization two functionals, one for the cavity and the other for the myocardium. Each functional contains two distribution-matching terms, one intensity-based and the other distance-based. For each target region (cavity or myocardium), let us assume that a manual segmentation of first frame I^1 is provided by the user. Using prior information from frame I^1 and the user input, intensity and distance models of the target region (cavity or myocardium) are learned and embedded in the following functional:

$$\hat{R} = \arg \min_{R \subset \Omega} \underbrace{-\mathcal{B}(\mathcal{P}^{I^j}(R, .), \mathcal{M}^I)}_{Intensity\ matching} \underbrace{-\mathcal{B}(\mathcal{P}^D(R, .), \mathcal{M}^D)}_{Distance\ matching} + \underbrace{\lambda \mathcal{L}(\partial R)}_{Smoothness} \qquad (11)$$

where

- $D = \frac{\|x - O\|}{N_D} : \Omega \rightarrow [0, 1]$ a function measuring the normalized distance between each point x and a fixed point O, which corresponds to the centroid of cavity region in the learning frame. N_D a normalization constant which is computed systematically in order to restrict the values of distance function D within interval $[0; 1]$. $\mathcal{M}^D$ be the model distribution of distances learned from the cavity region in the learning frame. The purpose of the distance matching term in (11) is to constrain the segmentation with prior geometric information (shape, scale, and position of the cavity) obtained from the learning frame. Note that this distance prior is invariant to rotation, and embeds implicitly uncertainties with respect to scale via parameter σ that controls the kernel width in the kernel density estimate in (4). The higher σ, the more scale variations allowed.
- $\mathcal{M}^I$ is a model distribution of intensity learned from the manual segmentation of the first frame.

The solution of (11) is obtained efficiently with bound optimization and graph cuts[6].

4.1.1. *Example*

In Fig. 1, we give tracking examples from a cardiac sequence of one subject, including mid-cavity and apical slices. The green and red curves (colors better perceived on the screen) depict the automatic endo- and epicardium boundaries, respectively. The yellow discontinuous curves depict the ground-truth boundaries. The proposed method prevented the papillary muscles from being included erroneously in the myocardium. This task is challenging[18] because the papillary muscles and the myocardium are connected and have almost the same intensity. The second row of the Figure depict apical frames, where it is difficult to segment the cavity because of the small size of the structures and moving artifacts. The example further shows how the formulation handles implicitly significant variations in the scale of the cavity,

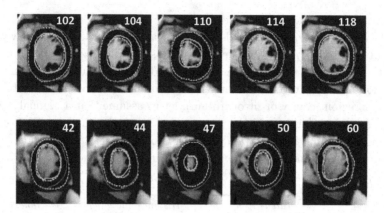

Fig. 1.   Example of tracking the left ventricle boundaries in a cardiac MRI sequence using the distribution matching model in (11). The frame number is indicated on each of the images.

although neither an additional optimization over geometric transformations nor a large training set are required.

4.2. Vertebral-body segmentation in spine images

In this section, we show the potential of distribution-matching formulations in segmenting the vertebral bodies (VBs) in spine MRI. Accurate segmentations of the VBs in MRI is an essential step towards diagnosing spine deformities[25,32]. However, the problem is quite challenging because of the weak edges between the VBs and their neighboring structures, the strong noise which results in intensity inhomogeneity within the VBs, and numerous acquisition protocols with different resolutions and noise types. Most of the existing VB segmentation algorithms require an intensive external training from a large, manually-segmented training set and/or costly pose-estimation procedures[25,44]. Although effective in some cases, training-based algorithms may have difficulty in capturing the substantial variations in a clinical context. The ensuing results are often bounded to the choice of a training set and a specific type of MRI data.

One way to remove the need for intensive external training would be to use simple user inputs to learn a VB model and pose VB segmentation as a distribution-matching problem[3]. In the remainder of this section, we will discuss the distribution-matching method in[3].

For each point $x \in \Omega$, the method in[3] computes a vector of features $\mathbf{F}(x)$ containing image statistics within several box-shaped image patches of different orientations/scales. Such patch-based features can encode contextual knowledge about the region of interest and its neighboring structures (e.g., size, shape, orientation and relationships to neighboring structures). First, the method estimates a model $\mathcal{M}$ from features $\mathbf{F}$ within a rectangular approximation of one VB in a single 2D mid-sagittal slice of Ω (refer to the example in Fig. 2). Such approximation is obtained from a very simple user input, which amounts to a few points (clicks). Given $\mathcal{M}$, VB segmentation in the whole 3D domain is posed as a distribution-matching problem of the from (1). Then, the optimization of (1) is performed efficiently using a bound optimizer combined with a convex-relaxation technique[47].

The distribution-matching formulation in[3] has the following advantages over the existing spine segmentation algorithms:

- It does not require a complex external learning from a large manually-segmented training set. Therefore, the ensuing results are independent of the choice of a training set and a specific type of MRI data; and
- It removes the need of costly pose optimization (or registration) procedures.

4.2.1. *Example*

Fig. 2 depicts an example using a lumbar spine MR volume of the type T2-weighted. The left-hand side of the figure depicts the user input in a single 2D mid-sagittal slice. The right-hand side of the figure depicts the obtained results, including the 3D surfaces of the lumbar (L1 to L5) and T12 VBs as well as one of the corresponding 2D-slice results. For this example, the feature vector at each point x of the image domain is of dimension 3: $\mathbf{F}(x) = (\mathbf{F}_1, \mathbf{F}_2, \mathbf{F}_3)$, with $\mathbf{F}_1$ the mean of intensity within a $21 \times 7 \times 1$ rectangular-shaped, vertically-oriented patch, $\mathbf{F}_2$ the mean of intensity within a $7 \times 21 \times 1$ rectangular-shaped, horizontally-oriented patch, and $\mathbf{F}_3$ the mean intensity within a $7 \times 7 \times 1$ square-shaped patch, all centered at point x. The feature distributions were estimated using 32 bins.

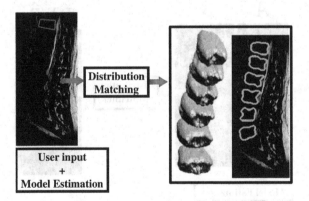

Fig. 2.   An example of vertebral-body segmentation using a distribution matching approach.

4.3. *Brain tumor segmentation*

In this section, we discuss the potential of distribution-matching formulations for brain tumor segmentations. Segmenting accurately brain tumors in MRI is an essential step towards assessing the disease. Manual segmentation is prohibitively time-consuming, and is not reproducible. Therefore, automatic or semi-automatic algorithms are highly desirable. Although several studies addressed automating this task (see[37] and the references therein), the problem is still acknowledged to be difficult. Most of the existing algorithms are still not fast and flexible enough for realistic clinical scenarios. This is due to the difficulties inherent to brain tumor segmentation. In general, brain tumors have shape and intensity characteristics that may vary dramatically from one subject to another, which impedes building reliable models from training data. For instance, the shape of a brain tumor may be arbitrary, and do not necessarily fall within a category (or class) of shapes that can be learned from a finite set of training subjects, as is the case in many other medical image segmentation problems. Furthermore, in some cases, tumors might have intensity profiles that are very similar to the other normal regions within the image. In this section, we discuss a distribution-matching, data-driven formulation of brain tumor segmentation[37], which promises to solve the problem. The distribution-matching method in[37] does not require an external learning from a large, manually-segmented training set. It uses only the image information and a simple user input. Fig. 3 illustrates the algorithm in[37]. The user input is three points, two to divide the brain into two symmetric parts (A and B in the figures) and one to identify the normal part, i.e., the part that does not contain the tumor (part A in the figure). The method computes a model $\mathcal{M}$ from the intensity data within the normal part (refer to sub-domain A in the figure).

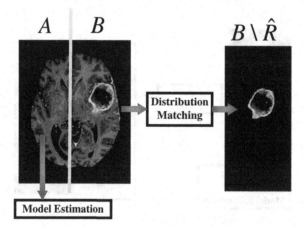

Fig. 3.   An example of brain tumor segmentation using a distribution matching approach.

Thus, $\mathcal{M}$ contains prior information on the intensity within the normal regions in the considered brain image. The purpose of the algorithm is to find within the abnormal part (sub-domain B in the figure) an optimal region $\hat{R}$ whose intensity distribution most closely matches model $\mathcal{M}$. This can be stated as a distribution matching problem following the general formulation in (1), with feature $\mathbf{F}$ corresponding to intensity and Ω corresponding to sub-domain B. The solution $\hat{R}$ yields the complement of the tumor in the abnormal part. This gives us the target tumor region: $B \setminus \hat{R}$.

5. Conclusion and Outlook

In this chapter, we reviewed some recent distribution-matching approaches to semantic image segmentation. We discussed both formulation and optimization aspects pertaining to distribution-matching algorithms, and demonstrated their potential in various medical image segmentation scenarios, including examples from cardiac, spine and brain imaging. It is worth noting that these works still have some limitations, and can bear several interesting extensions. For instance, in the general formulation in (1), we assume prior model distribution $\mathcal{M}$ is an accurate description of the target segment, which may not be the case in several applications. Possible extensions includes embedding some uncertainties in model $\mathcal{M}$ or using multiple prior models.

Other interesting extensions include embedding distribution-matching constraints on the boundary (or surface) of the segment of interest, e.g., shape-distribution constraints[43,45]. Such constraints contain pose-invariant information about the shape of the region of interest, and can be very useful in both segmentation and recognition scenarios.

References

1. Adam, A., Kimmel, R., Rivlin, E.: On scene segmentation and histograms-based curve evolution. IEEE Transactions on Pattern Analysis and Machine Intelligence 31(9), 1708–1714 (2009)
2. Ayed, I.B., Lu, Y., Li, S., Ross, I.G.: Left ventricle tracking using overlap priors. In: MICCAI (1). pp. 1025–1033 (2008)
3. Ayed, I.B., Punithakumar, K., Minhas, R., Joshi, R., Garvin, G.J.: Vertebral body segmentation in mri via convex relaxation and distribution matching. In: MICCAI (1). pp. 520–527 (2012)
4. Batra, D., Kowdle, A., Parikh, D., Luo, J., Chen, T.: icoseg: Interactive co-segmentation with intelligent scribble guidance. In: CVPR (2010)
5. Ben Ayed, I., Chen, H.M., Punithakumar, K., Ross, I., Li, S.: Graph cut segmentation with a global constraint: Recovering region distribution via a bound of the bhattacharyya measure. In: CVPR. pp. 3288–3295 (2010)
6. Ben Ayed, I., Chen, H.M., Punithakumar, K., Ross, I., Li, S.: Max-flow segmentation of the left ventricle by recovering subject-specific distributions via a bound of the bhattacharyya measure. Medical Image Analysis 16, 87–100 (2012)
7. Ben Ayed, I., Li, S., Ross, I.: Embedding overlap priors in variational left ventricle tracking. IEEE Transactions on Medical Imaging 28(12), 1902–1913 (2009)
8. Ben Ayed, I., Li, S., Ross, I.: A statistical overlap prior for variational image segmentation. International Journal of Computer Vision 85(1), 115–132 (2009)
9. Ben Ayed, I., Punithakumar, K., Li, S., Islam, A., Chong, J.: Left ventricle segmentation via graph cut distribution matching. In: Medical Image Computing and

Computer-Assisted Intervention (MICCAI 2009). vol. 1, pp. 901–909. London, UK (2009)

10. Ben Ayed, I., Gorelick, L., Boykov, Y.: Auxiliary cuts for general classes of higher order functionals. In: CVPR (2013)

11. Ben Ayed, I., Punithakumar, K., Garvin, G.J., Romano, W., Li, S.: Graph cuts with invariant object-interaction priors: Application to intervertebral disc segmentation. In: IPMI. pp. 221–232 (2011)

12. Bertsekas, D.P.: Nonlinear Programming. Athena Scientific, 2nd edition edn. (1999)

13. Boykov, Y., Kolmogorov, V.: An experimental comparison of min-cut/max- flow algorithms for energy minimization in vision. IEEE Transactions on Pattern Analysis and Machine Intelligence 26(9), 1124–1137 (2004)

14. Cerqueira, M.D., Weissman, N.J., D, V., Jacobs, A.K., Kaul, S., Laskey, W.K., Pennell, D.J., Rumberger, J.A., Ryan, T., Verani, M.S.: Standardized myocardial segmentation and nomenclature for tomographic imaging of the heart: A statement for healthcare professionals from cardiac imaging committee of the council on clinical cardiology of the american heart association. Circulation 105, 539–542 (2002)

15. Chen, S., Radke, R.J.: Level set segmentation with both shape and intensity priors. In: ICCV (2009)

16. Cho, M., Shin, Y.M., Lee, K.M.: Co-recognition of image pairs by data-driven monte carlo image exploration. In: ECCV(4). pp. 144–157 (2008)

17. Cui, J., Yang, Q., Wen, F., Wu, Q., Zhang, C., Gool, L.V., Tang, X.: Transductive object cutout. In: CVPR (2008)

18. El-Berbari, R., Bloch, I., Redheuil, A., Angelini, E.D., Mousseaux, É., Frouin, F., Herment, A.: Automated segmentation of the left ventricle including papillary muscles in cardiac magnetic resonance images. In: Functional Imaging and Modeling of the Heart (FIMH 2007). pp. 453–462. Salt Lake City, UT, USA (2007)

19. Freedman, D., Zhang, T.: Active contours for tracking distributions. IEEE Transactions on Image Processing 13, 518–526 (2004)

20. Gallagher, A.C., Chen, T.: Clothing cosegmentation for recognizing people. In: CVPR (2008)

21. Gorelick, L., Schmidt, F.R., Boykov, Y.: Fast trust region for segmentation. In: CVPR (2013)

22. Gorelick, L., Schmidt, F.R., Boykov, Y., Delong, A., Ward, A.: Segmentation with non-linear regional constraints via line-search cuts. In: ECCV. pp. 583–597 (2012)

23. Hautvast, G., Lobregt, S., Breeuwer, M., Gerritsen, F.: Automatic contour propagation in cine cardiac magnetic resonance images. IEEE Transactions on Medical Imaging 25(11), 1472–1482 (Nov 2006)

24. Hochbaum, D.S., Singh, V.: An efficient algorithm for co-segmentation. In: ICCV (2009)

25. Huang, S., Chu, Y., Lai, S., Novak, C.: Learning-based vertebra detection and iterative normalized-cut segmentation for spinal mri. IEEE Trans. on Medical Imaging 28(10), 1595–1605 (2009)

26. Jiang, H.: Linear solution to scale invariant global figure ground separation. In: CVPR. pp. 678–685 (2012)

27. Jolly, M.P.: Automatic recovery of the left ventricular blood pool in cardiac cine mr images. In: Medical Image Computing and Computer-Assisted Intervention (MICCAI 2008). vol. 1, pp. 110–118. New York, NY, USA (2008)

28. Kang, S.M., Wan, J.W.L.: A multiscale graph cut approach to bright-field multiple cell image segmentation using a bhattacharyya measure. In: SPIE Medical Imaging (2013)

29. Kolmogorov, V., Rother, C.: Minimizing nonsubmodular functions with graph cuts-a review. IEEE Transactions on Pattern Analysis and Machine Intelligence 29(7), 1274–1279 (2007)

30. Lange, K., Hunter, D.R., Yang, I.: Optimization transfer using surrogate objective functions. Journal of Computational and Graphical Statistics 9(1), 1–20 (2000)

31. Lee, D.D., Seung, H.S.: Algorithms for non-negative matrix factorization. In: NIPS. pp. 556–562 (2000)

32. Michopoulou, S., Costaridou, L., Panagiotopoulos, E., Speller, R., Panayiotakis, G., Todd-Pokropek, A.: Atlas-based segmentation of degenerated lumbar intervertebral discs from mr images of the spine. IEEE Trans. on Biomedical Engineering 56(9), 2225–2231 (2009)

33. Mitiche, A., Ben Ayed, I.: Variational and Level Set Methods in Image Segmentation. Springer, first edition edn. (2010)

34. Mukherjee, L., Singh, V.: Scale invariant cosegmentation for image groups. In: CVPR (2011)

35. Mukherjee, L., Singh, V., Dyer, C.R.: Half-integrality based algorithms for cosegmentation of images. In: CVPR. pp. 2028–2035 (2009)

36. Narasimhan, M., Bilmes, J.A.: Submodular-supermodular procedure with applications to discriminative structure learning. In: UAI. pp. 404–412 (2005)

37. Njeh, I., Ayed, I.B., Hamida, A.B.: A distribution-matching approach to mri brain tumor segmentation. In: ISBI. pp. 1707–1710 (2012)

38. Petitjean, C., Dacher, J.N.: A review of segmentation methods in short axis cardiac mr images. Medical Image Analysis 15, 169–184 (2011)

39. Pham, V.Q., Takahashi, K., Naemura, T.: Foreground-background segmentation using iterated distribution matching. In: CVPR. pp. 2113–2120 (2011)

40. Punithakumar, K., Yuan, J., Ayed, I.B., Li, S., Boykov, Y.: A convex max-flow approach to distribution-based figure-ground separation. SIAM J. Imaging Sciences 5(4), 1333–1354 (2012)

41. Rother, C., Minka, T.P., Blake, A., Kolmogorov, V.: Cosegmentation of image pairs by histogram matching - incorporating a global constraint into mrfs. In: CVPR. pp. 993–1000 (2006)

42. Russell, B., Freeman, W., Efros, A., Sivic, J., Zisserman, A.: Using multiple segmentations to discover objects and their extent in image collections. In: CVPR. pp. 1605–1614 (2006)

43. Salah, M.B., Ayed, I.B., Mitiche, A.: Active curve recovery of region boundary patterns. IEEE Trans. Pattern Anal. Mach. Intell. 34(5), 834–849 (2012)

44. Seifert, S., Wachter, I., Schmelzle, G., Dillmann, R.: A knowledge-based approach to soft tissue reconstruction of the cervical spine. IEEE Transactions on Medical Imaging 28(4), 494–507 (April 2009)

45. Toshev, A., Taskar, B., Daniilidis, K.: Object detection via boundary structure segmentation. In: CVPR. pp. 950–957 (2010)

46. Vicente, S., Kolmogorov, V., Rother, C.: Cosegmentation revisited: Models and optimization. In: ECCV(2). pp. 465–479 (2010)

47. Yuan, J., Bae, E., Tai, X.C.: A study on continuous max-flow and min-cut approaches. In: CVPR (2010)

48. Zhang, Z., Kwok, J.T., Yeung, D.Y.: Surrogate maximization/minimization algorithms and extensions. Machine Learning 69, 1–33 (2007)

49. Zhu, Y., Papademetris, X., Sinusas, A.J., Duncan, J.S.: Segmentation of the left ventricle from cardiac mr images using a subject-specific dynamical model. IEEE Transactions on Medical Imaging 29(4), 669–687 (2010)

CHAPTER 3

DIGITAL PATHOLOGY IN MEDICAL IMAGING

Bikash Sabata, Chukka Srinivas, Pascal Bamford, and Gerardo Fernandez
Digital Pathology and Workflow
Roche Tissue Diagnostics (Ventana Medical Systems)
Mountain View, CA, USA
{bikash.sabata, chukka.srinivas, pascal.bamford, jerry.fernandez}@ventana.roche.com

Pathologists have practiced medicine in a relatively unchanged manner over the last century to render the diagnosis of disease. However, over the last decade, the practice of pathology has started to undergo a foundational change. In addition to major advances in diagnostic biomarkers, we are seeing a ground-swell in new imaging technologies. This new image-based technology offers significant opportunities to the practice. However it comes at a cost that only recently has been offset by advances in the underlying technology and new compelling applications that imaging makes possible. Pathology lags behind other medicine practice such as radiology in the adoption of digital workflow. Recently, significant advances have been made in the capture and management of the whole slide images used in pathology practice and this is leading to an explosion in the data volume that completely eclipses the vast quantities of data being produced in radiology. Another area of technology challenges is related to the analysis of imaged data for detection, identification, recognition and quantification of the pathology in the slide. Hardware and software solutions being developed will enable a paradigm shift in the practice and clinical importance of Pathology.

1. Introduction

Twenty five years ago, staining automation and instruments became routinely adopted by anatomic pathology (AP) laboratories to help standardize processes and increase efficiency under the rising demand of clinical patient testing. Today's laboratory is inconceivable without these instruments. However, a key step in the AP laboratory process has undergone little change in centuries: pathologists reviewing glass slides under a microscope. This is now changing, after several decades in the making, as the introduction of digital pathology (DP) revolutionizes clinical practice. To illustrate this emerging field, we take the example of breast cancer care and compare it in today's manual workflow to the new digital workflow. Figure 1 commences with a symptomatic patient, or a patient with an abnormal screening result, that is referred to a diagnostic imaging center. The various modalities of MRI, X-Ray, CT and ultrasound are known collectively as radiological imaging. X-Ray devices in particular, like consumer cameras, underwent a revolution two decades ago when they converted from analogue film to digital imagery. The ability to efficiently store, rapidly access and process digital radiology images has improved patient care by enabling rapid case history review, remote consultation and computer aided diagnosis (CAD) applications. In addition, also spawned several novel clinical applications, such as multi-modality fusion and tomo synthesis, made possible only due to digitization.

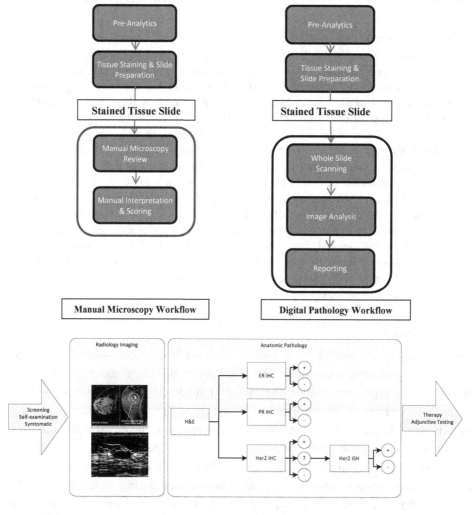

Figure 1. Breast cancer triage and workflow (adapted from NCCN guidelines [16]).

The introduction of Digital Pathology is often compared to this difficult, but ultimately highly successful transition in radiology. A key difference, however, between these fields is that the 'film' in pathology is the glass slide and cannot be removed, yet, from the process. While digitization in radiology started by scanning film, it migrated to eliminating the film altogether and using high end monitors, with fine pixel-spacing, for diagnostic interpretation. In pathology, as shown below, the stained tissue on the glass slide *is* the signal to be digitized. Therefore while the benefits of adopting DP are numerous, and likely far more potent than in radiology as we will discuss here, the field has until relatively recently fallen short at the very first obstacle in adoption: being competitive to the microscope for routine applications.

In this chapter, we use the breast cancer example to describe the digital pathology workflow. A suspicion of breast cancer via radiology is confirmed and further stratified at the Anatomic Pathology (AP) laboratory. A biopsy section of breast tissue is removed from the patient, in the area identified in the radiological imagery, and is then sent to the AP laboratory for processing. Very thin sections (typically 4-6um) of tissue are prepared onto glass slides, stained using a combination of hematoxylin and eosin (H&E) – see figure 2 for examples. In today's manual workflow, the glass slide is usually compiled with several others in a cardboard folder, along with printed patient data, that is then delivered to the pathologist. The pathologist is then able to immediately review the slide in a matter of seconds to render a diagnosis of disease. Herein lies one of the greatest challenges in the digitization of the AP laboratory. DP inserts additional processes, hardware, networking and storage requirements into today's manual workflow. As the scanning of slides to digital images is an additional introduced step, much of the focus by commercial and academic efforts has been to explore novel methods to minimize this impact. Hence today's scanners accept large numbers of slides for bulk processing so this can occur overnight or in an unsupervised manner and are engineered to match the workflow demands of even the busiest laboratories. Sub-minute scan times are now routinely achieved and made possible only recently with modern fast camera data transfer rates and computing powerful enough to stitch, compress and store these images as fast as they are produced. The inconvenience associated with the introduction of this step is however offset by the immediacy with which the image is then available, anywhere in the world, for review within an informatics environment that is able to present all the necessary patient data to complete a diagnosis. The next challenge to widespread DP adoption is efficient digital slide review. As previously mentioned, a pathologist today is able to do this extremely quickly and efficiently, generally within the time it would take to decompress the huge DP images generated by scanning a specimen at high resolution (often several

GBs uncompressed and several hundred MB compressed.) Therefore the most common architecture for enabling this is the client/server model whereby only the imagery requested by the pathologist, as he navigates the specimen, are sent, decompressed and presented on-screen. However the inherent latencies in this process continue to be a major barrier to adoption for routine daily use and is a major focus for the field. For other lower volume and more specialized applications such as remote tele-consultation, remote frozen sections and tumor boards, DP has seen far greater acceptance and market penetration. Ever increasing networking and computation power will reduce these latencies; however algorithms that automatically highlight abnormal areas, or even eliminate the need to review normal slides, will alter the cost/benefit ratio of DP entirely. Such applications have already achieved significant clinical success in cytopathology and have enabled more accurate and more efficient diagnosis, made possible only by first scanning and digitizing glass slides.

Figure 3 illustrates the major components of a DP solution. While the scanning hardware is an essential first component to the digital workflow, image and workflow management enables applications not previously possible. The integration of a single patient-centric view is enabled, allowing the medical practitioner to review all information from patient history, to radiology images and results, pathology whole slide images and image analysis results to better inform and direct medical decision making. This layer is generally implemented on top of established enterprise application framework technologies, but with additional modules and services designed to serve and process huge DP images. For example, this layer may include an image management service and an image processing service running on separate servers in different locations.

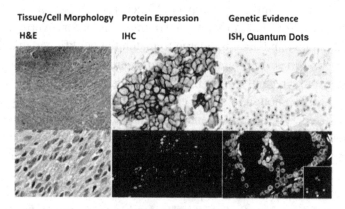

Figure 2. Examples of tissue staining. H&Es provide basic information regarding tissue and cell morphology, IHCs are used to query the protein expression and genetic evidence is obtained by ISH and Quantum Dot labelled probes.

A. Subtyping and the role of digital pathology

In the context of a breast biopsy specimen, the H&E slide confirms the presence of cancer in the breast. Subsequent to this primary diagnosis, additional tests are ordered that allow the pathologist to further confirm the diagnosis of cancer, and to quantify disease specific characterstic that enable the oncologist to recommend treatment by cancer subtype. A common set of tests applied at this stage use what are known as immunohistochemical (IHC) stains that have a colorimetric tag and target specific proteins in the cell. As shown in Figure 1, a set of these tests are often ordered together as a 'breast panel' consisting of Her2, estrogen receptor (ER) and progesterone receptor (PR). Histopathology has developed numerous "grading algorithms" to guide the pathologist to provide quantified information for these assays. Examples of such scoring are TMN scores in breast cancer, Gleason scores in prostate cancer, prognostic "quantification algorithms" that include - ASCO/CAP scoring for Her2 breast tumor, and percent positivity score for nuclear markers (such as ER and PR).

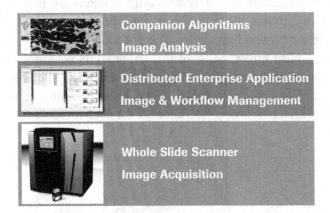

Figure 3. Complete Digital Pathology solution requires the technology stack consisting of image acquisition, image and workflow management, and image analysis.

ASCO/CAP Her2 Scoring Guidelines

Score 3+: Uniform intense membrane staining of more than 30% of invasive tumor cells

Score 2+: Complete membrane staining that is non-uniform or weak but with obvious circumferential distribution in at least 10% of cells, or intense complete membrane staining in 30% or less of tumor cells

Score 1+: Weak, incomplete membrane staining in any proportion of invasive tumor cells, or weak, complete membrane staining in less than 10% of cells.

Score 0: No staining is observed in invasive tumor cells

The grading and scoring algorithms have been laboriously developed by researchers and pathologists using experimental data and understanding of the cancer mechanisms. In the manual workflow, the pathologist uses his training to assign a category to the visual representation of the glass slide. However, although primary diagnosis based on H&E staining focuses on cancer detection, grading of the cancer tumor requires the pathologist to quantify using many subjective criteria. Such quantifications can vary from pathologist to pathologist and also with the same pathologist at different times. DP has the distinct advantage of being highly reproducible and thus promises to make the task of quantification, and subsequent decision making, more consistent.

B. *Quantification of IHC markers*

With the emergence of IHC stains, the need for precise quantification of protein expression levels is critical. IHC stains are used by pathologists to evaluate the expression of specific proteins as a result of normal or mutated genes. The stains are typically accompanied with a hematoxylin counterstain that highlights the tissue structure to provide the pathologist with the tissue context. Humans are extremely good at detection but precise quantification is laborious and prone to a high degree of human errors. Most of the DP analysis solutions in the market with FDA approvals fall within this category of Intended Use. Figure 4 below shows an example system developed by Roche Tissue Diagnostics (Ventana) that assists the pathologist to score an IHC slide with a nuclear marker.

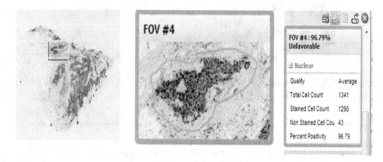

Figure 4. Pathologist selects the Field of View for quantification and the algorithm scores it by counting the tumor cells with positive and negative stains and calculating the ratio.

In the digital workflow the pathologist is able to select regions, or even the entire slide, to quantify. For markers such as ER and PR, the scoring criteria are based on the percentage of positively stained cells divided by the total number of (positively and non-stained) cells. This is often done by experience in the manual workflow and works very well for assays for which there are 'simple' thresholds. For example, the ER assay result is considered positive if there are greater than 1% of cells within an area stained. At this low threshold, any staining generally indicates positivity and is simple to determine by eye. Around these thresholds however, and for assays for which a clinically proven threshold may be more difficult to determine (e.g. 10%), the DP imaging tool is critical in its ability to accurately count cells and divide with complete precision – without room for interpretation. The clinical validation of assays like the breast panel were done prior to the widespread clinical use of imaging tools. Hence to date these tools have necessarily been developed and considered accurate only once compared to a ground truth that is human determined. As this field matures, we will see imaging used not only for its inherent reproducibility but also for its accuracy in the determination of thresholds and ultimately what constitutes a positive or negative result [17].

C. Tissue and stain variability

DP is the last process in the AP lab system. As a pathologist must in today's manual workflow, DP must be able to accept the tolerance stack associated with different tissue preparation techniques from the moment the tissue is handled once it is out of the body. The quality of images under the microscope is strongly dependent on these pre-analytic steps, the thickness of tissue cut and any staining variation or preferences a laboratory may have. The introduction of automated processes at each of the processing steps is giving the laboratory better control on the quality of the final slide that the pathologist will use for diagnosis. Furthermore vendors that offer a complete line of co-optimized tools have the benefit of minimizing such variability. Once the glass slide is prepared; the calibration of the scanning imaging device must also be controlled or could be a further source of image appearance variations. At the current time, however, it is accepted practice that color variability due to these upstream processes is unavoidable and imaging solutions must be robust to this potential source of error. This is the area where the human eye/brain combination is able to compensate for dramatic variability, but where automated image analysis finds its greatest challenges.

The image analysis challenges in histopathology images at the foundational level are no different from the pattern recognition challenges faced in other imagery related domains. The language of computer vision only has to adapt to the domain specific semantics and many of the standard techniques transfer over. However, there are some unique characteristics that require the development of additional new techniques.

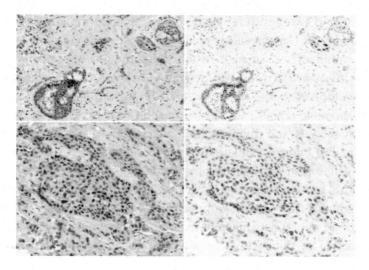

Figure 5. Examples of ER tissue stain variation.

The analysis of images in DP answers the questions about detection – "there is a positive signal associated with the image"; recognition – "the region of interest has pattern similar to cancer"; and identification – "the evidence quantifies the cancer to be Her2 3+."

Broadly, to automate the slide interpretation and scoring process, the following computer vision tasks have to be solved.

a) Robust detection of the tissue objects such as nuclei, membrane and glands
b) Segmentation of the image into epithelial and stromal regions
c) Accurate classification of the tissue objects and quantification.

The main challenge in developing automated solutions is to compensate for the inherent variability in the scanned slide. Apart from the stain color variability, the nuclei vary in size, shape and orientation and the glandular regions have irregular outlines and consist of overlapping nuclei and with significant variability in the tissue morphology and background context.

D. Rules-based segmentation and identification

Since the tissue preparation for interpretation is geared towards the assessment of staining patterns in the tissue, the first generation of image analysis algorithms relied on color processing and threshold based techniques to render the diagnosis. Additional post processing steps were added to account for morphological information. However, all these techniques had challenges related to robustness (Figure 6).

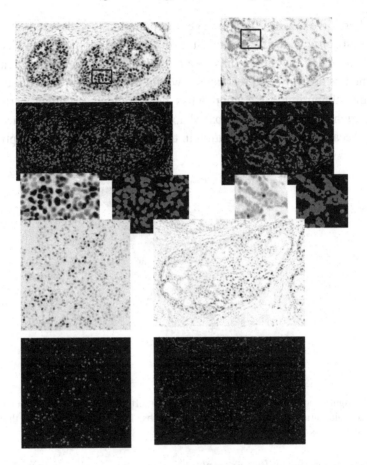

Figure 6. The color thresholds tuned to generate acceptable output for these training images, although yields acceptable color segmentation results for the images above, output nuclei objects with distorted shape outlines resulting in nuclei misclassification.

These "bottoms-up" color-based image segmentation methods suffer from several limitations. Although it is straight forward enough to custom define a rule set or parameter set, with a trial and error iterative experimentation, to yield acceptable results on a small set of training slides there is no guarantee that the resultant solution generalizes, as shown below. Given the image variability, there is no easy way to specify a robust set of rules and/or parameter sets to work on a wide range of images. Additionally, the low-level segmentation methods are not guaranteed to preserve the tissue object shape outlines and the segmentation errors are image-specific, rules-specific and unpredictable. This makes it challenging to translate expert interpretation process of a pathologist to a set of workable rule sets and algorithm parameters.

The alternative to rules-based image interpretation is to develop methods that model the specific pattern of interest using a-priori domain knowledge. The model-based vision paradigm has been used in many other domains where *a-priori* models are built and recognized within the image. In structured domains such as manufacturing, such approaches have yielded excellent performance. However, such purely knowledge-based approach has not been very successful in pathology because of the vast variation in the tumor and disease description.

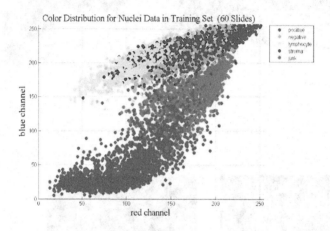

Figure 7. The figure shows the distribution of color for different objects of interest in the tissue images due to stain variability across instruments and labs. There is no single color threshold that can separate the objects.

E.   Learning from image data examples

Statistical models are another way to build a-priori models for interpretation. Here instead of using domain knowledge to represent and build models of anatomical objects, a pattern is learned from data to identify cancer or disease specific image regions.

Similarly, image patch learning algorithm for gland detection and classification in PIN-4 stained prostate needle biopsies have been developed earlier. An Ada-Boost classifier is trained on a large set of image patches for glandular regions and non-gland regions, based on the features computed from a sliding image patch followed with a graph-based gland identification and classification method.

The classifier models are as good as the training data and the features used to represent the image data. The success of the statistical models within pathology is very dependent on the feature engineering exercise to define the representation. In some sense, the feature engineering encodes the domain knowledge of the histopathology images.

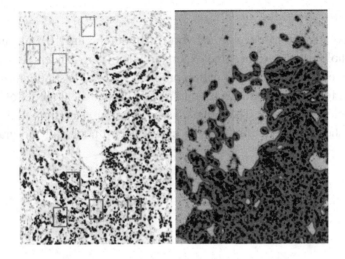

Figure 8. The system is shown positive and negative image patch examples (left) and the statistical models are built to interpret (right).

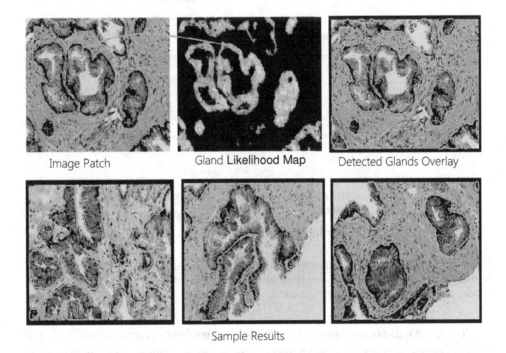

Figure 9. An Ada-Boost classifier trained on a large dataset. For each image patch on the target image a gland likelihood map is generated that is used for the gland segmentation.

F.   *Object-based learning models*

A third alternative is to develop a hybrid method (Figure 10) that mimics the training pathologists use to become experts in identifying cancer. As an example, nuclear segmentation and classification problem for ER/PR slide interpretation is presented. A top down method is used to develop a statistical model of primitives such as nuclei and cells. The object based learning paradigm then uses the features of the identified primitives to classify the tumor and the grade of the cancer.

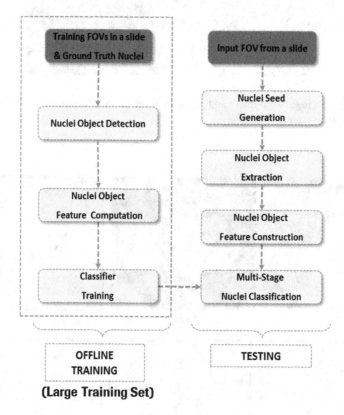

Figure 10. Top-down object-based supervised learning methodology trains a classifer based on features extracted from identified low-level anatomical primitives such as nuclei and cells. The learned model is then used for interpretation.

To detect cell nuclei a perceptual model of a nucleus is constructed. This will include visual features such as shape and stain colors. Training data will include touching and overlapping cells, stain variations, background contexts, and variations within the nuclei. A shape prior based seed detection algorithm then identifies shape preserving blobs for nuclei seeds.

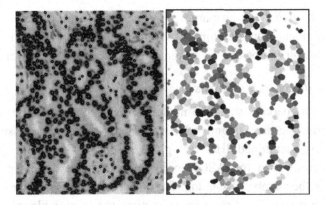

Figure 11. Shape prior based seed detection algorithm that identifies shape preserving blobs for nuclei seeds.

The features of the detected nuclei are then used in a multistage classifier to identify the type of each candidate nucleus (Figure 12). Such methods have proven to be very robust to a large amount of variations in pathology images.

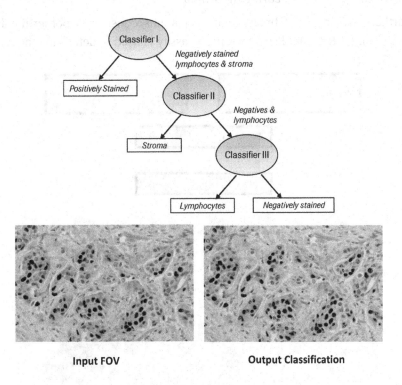

Figure 12. Features of the detected nuclei are used in a multistage classifier to identify each nucleus as belonging to a specific type. The class labels are then used for quantifications such as percent positivity score.

This object-based learning paradigm is very powerful and generalizable to other recognition and identification tasks in histopathology. The primitive objects in addition to nuclei can be cell membranes, glands, and blood vessels.

G. Membrane detection algorithms

Whereas ER, PR markers stain the nuclei, HER2 tumor marker stains the cell membrane, reflecting the amount of HER2 receptor protein on the surface of the cancer cells. As mentioned IHC test gives a score of 0 to 3+, as shown in Figure 13, according to the ASCO guideline based on the intensity and the completeness of the membrane staining. The nuclei are stained with the Hemotoxlyin counter stain. For automated slide interpretation, the scoring algorithm translates to an image analysis task of nuclei and membrane detection, cross validation of detection results at cellular level and scoring. For nuclei detection, the algorithm mentioned above is used. The membrane detection algorithms range from positive stain color image segmentation to tangential tensor-voting methods [15].

H. HER2 Dual ISH slide scoring algorithm

For further assessment of breast cancers patients considered borderline HER2 positive (2+), HER2 Dual ISH DNA probe assay is used to determine the number

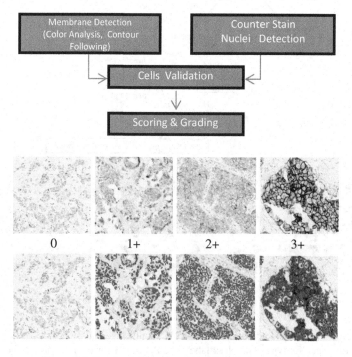

Figure 13. Scoring of membrane markers in breast tissue.

of copies of HER2 gene in tumor tissue by enumeration of the gene status ratio of the HER2 gene to Chromosome 17, where the HER2 (silver) and Chromosome 17 (red) probes are stained using two different colors. A ratio of greater than 2.2, is considered HER2-positive. A set of tumor cells with high amplification in a given slide are considered to compute the ratio. In a DP workflow, as shown below, the whole slide is scanned and regions annotated for analysis. Automation of the scoring process translates to two major image analysis tasks a) cell segmentation and selection and b) probe dot detection and classification. For cell segmentation and selection, dynamic programming methods can be used.

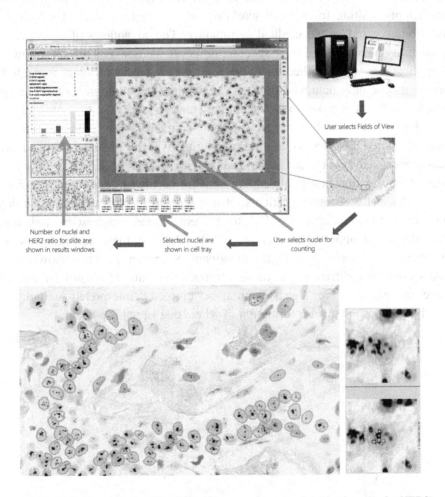

Figure 14. Dynmaic programming based algorithm to segment and select the cells for HER2 gene ratio computation. Results from a DoG-based algorithm to detect and count red and black dots.

To detect the probe dots, several popular dot detection algorithms, like DoG operator etc., from the computer vision literature are used. Different supervised learning classifiers are used to classify dots into HER2 and Chromosome 17 probe categories. For cell-segmentation, different region segmentation algorithms such as region growing, active contours and dynamic programming are useful.

2. DP Enabled Applications

Digital pathology has to date been highly successful in providing robust automated quantification tools to the pathologist for existing assays such as the breast panel. It could be argued that these are relatively simple applications that were simply waiting for the DP workflow to mature to a level at which they would be accepted by the medical community. The advantages of accuracy and repeatability have ensured their success; however we now embark on a new era of applications where either the workflow can be made efficient enough for clinical use or only achieved through DP imaging technologies. One example application that will prove to be a stepping stone to this era is the application of tissue heterogeneity to breast cancer risk assessment. Today's breast panel has achieved incredible success in improving the lives of patients afflicted with breast cancer. However there is increasing evidence that by extracting a second order of information that is already present in the breast panel, new predictive assays can better subtype patients. There are two fundamental technology approaches to this; applying DP to current tissue prognostics and using molecular-based approaches such as qPCR. Both of these technologies will find synergistic application in the treatment of cancer patients. However, to underscore a key difference in these approaches Figure 15 shows an example where an ER positive signal cannot be correctly interpreted without the underlying morphological information of where that signal is present.

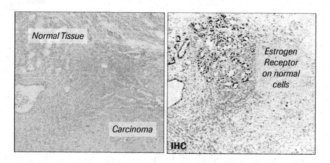

Figure 15. Preserving tissue morphology prevents a false ER positive as the signal is present in normal cells, not the area of abnormality.

Such cases strongly suggest that preserving the tissue context and using DP for quantification will continue to be a major component in patient care. Furthermore, it is becoming increasingly apparent that there are many different subtypes of cancer that must be accurately identified to ensure optimal treatment. The clinician is therefore interested in the simultaneous analysis of morphology, gene and protein status within the tissue context of the tumor. In addition the expression of multiple markers within the same tumor is important for the recognition of heterogeneity of the cancer. These have direct impact on the treatment plan for the patient and therefore the outcome.

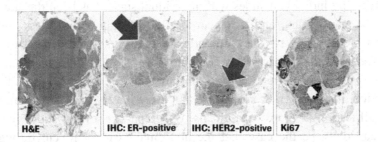

Figure 16. The H&E shows the tumor context while the ER and Her2 clearly show that the tumor is hetrogeneous and the Ki67 indicates a high degree of proliferation. This analysis guides the therapy that includes both ER and Her2 targets rather than only one of the two.

Figure 16 demonstrates the case of a breast cancer patient who has a significant probability of incomplete prognosis and therefore a treatment plan that would be ineffective. The pathologist recognizes the heterogeneity of the tumor only when reviewing the case in the registered panel of tumor images. DP is a key enabling technology in the presentation of such views to assist the pathologist in reviewing multiple testing on several sections of the tissue block.

Inter-marker image registration further enables contextual data to be viewed but is also critical for automated correlation and fusion of evidence. Rigid (template) and deformable models ensure that higher order data across tissue sections, and various staining modalities, is being analyzed from the same area. Algorithms for such registration are unique to pathology tissue images because of the image size and the type of distortions observed in real data. Unlike image matching problems in radiological imaging, where template matching and mutual information based methods are typically used, as shown in Figure 17 to register pathology digital slides the matching has to rely on structural matching of the underlying tissue ignoring the stain color intensity information.

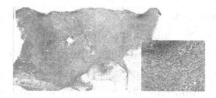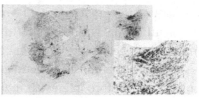

Figure 17. Regions for analysis selected by a pathogist on a H&E slide are automatically identified and mapped to similar regions in the ER whole slide from an adjacent serial section. The zoomed region shown an example of mapping a tumorous region.

3. Multiplexed Quantification

While preparing individual slides with individual stains has been the standard of practice for many years, and the incorporation of data across these sources is greatly enabled by DP, two key limitations are driving a movement to clinical multiplexed assays. These assays combine several tests onto the same tissue specimen and use multiple colors (chromagens or fluorophores) for their visualization. Firstly, it is often the case that there is very little cancer material to perform all testing in biopsy specimens. By preparing several slides for unique tests, it can often be the case that the abnormal material it 'cut through' and simply no longer present, preventing an entire panel to be executed. A second motivation is by having all the signals present on one slide, spatial and morphological information is trivially present without the need for registration and potentially irreconcilable slides (which are prepared by hand). A unique application of DP is the interpretation of these multiplexed assays. Traditional methods of analysis are limited to a few quantifications such as stage, grade, size, and expression of a few clinical markers. E.g. in breast cancer the TNM grade, the percentage positivity of ER, PR, Ki67, p53 nuclear markers and the score in HER2 expression. This information is used to propose a treatment plan for the patient. However, as the understanding of cancers is improving it is becoming clear that the tumor micro environment has a significantly larger amount of information about the nature of the tumor. This elicitation of the information requires the use of multiplexing to query the status of multiple biomarkers at the same time. Novel multiplexing techniques are being developed and the corresponding imaging algorithms are sought. Multiplexing is one area where imaging based solutions are the only option as the detection and interpretation of 6-10 signal multiplexing is almost impossible for manual inference.

The most common form of multiplexing today is applied in the field of in-situ hybridization, where generally more than one probe is applied to the genetic target and visualized using different colors. In breast cancer care, a situation can arise where the Her2 protein status is equivocal and not possible to determine as a positive or negative result (Figure 1). In these cases, the patient sample is further tested for genetic status via a pair of probes that target the Her2 gene and the chromosome 17 control. Generally this test is able to adjudicate equivocal Her2 status which is essential in the decision of whether to recommend the drug Tamoxifen. DP can assist the interpretation of such assays by automating tedious counting of gene signals that such an assay demands.

An alternate technology for multiplexing is the use of organic dyes or Quantum Dot probes that are attached to genetic events using in-situ hybridization techniques [10]. The challenges of very high degree of multiplexing are exciting and difficult. The imaging technologies typically used are multi-spectral imaging with fluorescence tagging. Information corresponding to different genetic or protein events is present in different spectral channels.

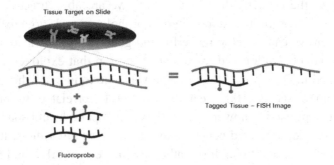

Figure 18. The basic process of tagging inserts a fluorescent probe into the cellular nuclei which then attaches to a targeted section of the gene or protein.

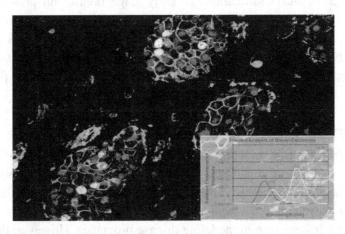

Figure 19. Quantum Dot based multiplexed assay in Breast tissue. ER is marked with QD585, Ki67 with QD605, PR with QD625, p53 with QD655 and Her2 with QD705. The spectral signatures of each Quantum Dot is in the right corner inset.

The imaging challenge is to untangle the signal in the multiple channels acquired with noise. The noise is as a result of the sensor and background phenomenon within the tissue that is excited and emit in the same wavelength as the signals. In addition, the spectral signatures of the probes also vary from lot to lot and in the specific environment the tissue is imaged. All these variations need to be accounted for when doing a quantification of markers for diagnostic and prognostic inference.

4. Quantification Algorithms

In addition to the above routine use of image analysis for scoring, a new paradigm shift is happening in the discovery of novel algorithms by using sophisticated image and data analysis. A foundational principle of histopathology is that the tissue morphology and the tumor environment are directly correlated to the biology of the cancer cells. Therefore, if we are able directly correlate the cancer patterns within the tumor cell morphology and organization to the outcomes then we can develop powerful and generic prognostication algorithms for cancer characterization and treatment. A system that exploited this principle was developed in [11]. The C-Path system was able to identify the most relevant features from a set of 6000 features that best correlated to breast cancer outcomes. The predictive power of C-Path was comparable and sometimes better than other very sophisticated genetic expression based algorithms. It is expected that the inclusion of additional histopathology images with IHC and ISH markers will only improve the robustness of such algorithms. The importance of the discovery of such algorithms is realized when we see statistics that indicate the percentage of misclassifications of early stage breast and prostate cancer. Many commercial algorithms such as OncotypeDX, Mammostrat, Femtelle, and Mammaprint, have been introduced that typically combine the scores associated with each IHC marker and other molecular test scores. There is continued interest in the medical community to find simple pathology tests that can predict the prognosis of disease and also of disease recurrence.

5. Summary

As cancer treatment is moving into the era of personalized medicine new methods of analysis of diagnostic information is needed that provide robust characterization of the disease. Digital pathology has entered into the field by providing a key enabling technology for the inclusion of image based histopathology information in modeling disease prognosis. However, the field of pathology image analysis is still at a very early stage and there is increasing demand to develop solutions that are robust and generalizable.

Infrastructure challenges are no less important than the discovery of new algorithms for accurate prognostication. The performance of these distributed systems will be critical to the widespread adoption of digital pathology solutions. The adoption will set the stage for transformative changes to the practice of medicine. As the decade progresses, we anticipate breakthroughs in medical informatics and "Big-Data" analysis will enable the large volumes of multi-scale, multi-dimensional data to be used in insightful information to drive the discovery of personalized companion algorithms for treatment planning.

Digital pathology is making advances in areas of image acquisition and image analysis that complements the incessant search for novel biomarkers that identify and characterize the specific cancer. The collaboration between instrumentation, image analysis and assay development is a unique cross disciplinary development that promises to lead to breakthroughs that would not otherwise be possible. Use of novel ISH probes for both fluorescence and brightfield imaging allows the pathologist to query molecular events within the tissue context. Hyper-spectral technologies and unmixing allow sensing of multiplexed information within the cellular compartment.

On the image analysis front, the focus has been on developing robust algorithms that work within a large operating range of stain variability. A combination of techniques that learn from data and model the patterns that are known about the domain shows the most promise in providing a framework for algorithm development in digital pathology. In the early stages of adoption the focus will be on aiding the pathologist to improve the repeatability and consistency of scoring and consequently making the workflow more efficient. But as the field matures, we anticipate the development of additional *computational pathology* capabilities that go beyond improving efficiency to adding insights that are not available by mere inspection of histopathology images. The development of C-Path type of systems is exciting and a new frontier. Such systems need to move through multiple levels of clinical trials for validation. Once these algorithms reach that level of validation, the pathology community will have low barriers to adoption and the pathologist will be able to weld a powerful weapon that combines the centuries old morphometric interpretation with cutting edge advances in genomics and bioinformatics in the war on cancer.

Acknowledgment

We would like to thank the Imaging and Analysis group at Ventana Digital Pathology. Many novel and sophisticated algorithms are being developed in the

B. Sabata et al.

team and this review has benefited from numerous discussions and interactions with Anindya Sarkar, Olcay Sertel, Jeorg Brendo, Lou Dietz, and Jim Martin.

The opinions expressed in this article are the views of the individuals only and not of the employer.

References

[1] D. Evanco, A. Heinrichs, and C.K. Rosenthal, "Milestones in Light Microscopy," May 14, 2011; published by Nature on the web at:
     http://www.nature.com/milestones/milelight/index.html

[2] A.H. Coons, "The beginnings of immunofluorescence," *J. Immunol*, 87:499-503, 1961.

[3] J.W. Lichtman and J.A. Conchello, "Fluorescence Microscopy," *Nature Methods*, 2(12):910-919, Dec 2005.

[4] J.H. Price, A. Goodacre, *et. al.*, "Advances in Molecular Labeling, High Throughput Imaging and Machine Intelligence Portend Powerful Functional Cellular Biochemistry Tools," *J. Cellular Biochemistry Supplement*, 39:194-210, 2002.

[5] C. Demir and B. Yener, "Automated Cancer Diagnosis Based on Histopathological Images: A Systematic Survey", *Technical Report*, Rensselaer Ploytechnic Institute, Dept of Computer Science, TR-05-09.

[6] N. Orlov, J. Johnston, *et. al.*, "Computer Vision for Microscopy Applications," In *Vision Systems: Segmentation and Pattern Recognition*, Ed. G. Obinata and A. Dutta, pp546. June 2007.

[7] L.A.D. Cooper, A.B. Carter, *et. al.*, "Digital Pathology: Data Intensive Frontier in Medical Imaging," Technical Report, Center for Comprehensive Informatics, Emory University, CCI-TR-2011-5, Aug 2011.

[8] G. Alexe, J. Monaco, *et. al.*, "Towards Improved Cancer Diagnosis and Prognosis Using Analysis of Gene Expression Data and Computer Aided Imaging," *Experimental Biology and Medicine*, 234(8):860-879, Aug 2009.

[9] A.C. Ruifrok and D.A. Johnston, "Quantification of histochemical staining by color deconvolution," *Anal Quant Cytol Histol*, 23:291-299.

[10] R.Y. Tsien, "The green fluorescent protein," *Annu Rev Biochem*, 67:509-544, 1998.

[11] A.H. Beck, A.R. Sangoi, *et. al.*, "Systematic analysis of breast cancer morphology uncovers stromal features associated with survival," *Sci Transl Med* 3:108ra113, 2011.

[12] Yang, Q., Parvin, B.: Perceptual organization of radial symmetries. Proc. of IEEE Int. Conf. on Computer Vision and Pattern Recognition (CVPR) 1, 320-325 (2004).

[13] Gurcan, M.N., Boucheron, L., Can, A., Madabhushi, A., Rajpoot, N., Yener, B.: Histopathological image analysis: A review. IEEE Reviews in Biomedical Engineering 3, 147-171 (2009).

[14] Jemal, A., Siegel, R., Xu, J., Ward, E.: Cancer statistics, 2010. CA: A Cancer Journal for Clinicians 60, 277-300 (2010).

[15] Leandro Loss, Bebis G, Parvin B, Iterative Tensor Voting for Perceptual Grouping of Ill-Defined Curvilinear Structure, IEEE Transactions on Medical Imaging, 30(8), 1503-1613, 2011.

[16] NCCN Guidelines, National Comprehensive Cancer Network,
     http://www.nccn.org/clinical.asp

[17] Mitch Dowsett, Torsten O. Nielsen, Roger A'Hern, John Bartlett, R. Charles Coombes, Jack Cuzick, Matthew Ellis, N. Lynn Henry, Judith C. Hugh, Tracy Lively, Lisa McShane, Soon Paik, Frederique Penault-Llorca, Ljudmila Prudkin, Meredith Regan, Janine Salter, Christos Sotiriou, Ian E. Smith, Giuseppe Viale, Jo Anne Zujewski, Daniel F. Hayes, "Assessment of Ki67 in Breast Cancer: Recommendations from the International Ki67 in Breast Cancer Working Group," J Natl Cancer Inst 2011;103:1656-1664.

CHAPTER 4

ADAPTIVE SHAPE PRIOR MODELING VIA ONLINE DICTIONARY LEARNING

Shaoting Zhang[1,*], Yiqiang Zhan[2], Yan Zhou[3], and Dimitris Metaxas[1]

[1]*Computer Science Department, University of North Carolina at Charlotte*
Charlotte, NC, USA
[2]*CAD R&D, Siemens Healthcare, Malvern, PA, USA*
[3]*Elekta Inc., Maryland Heights, MO, USA*
*E-mail: szhang16@uncc.edu

"Shape" and "appearance", the two pillars of a deformable model, complement each other in object segmentation. In many medical imaging applications, while the low-level appearance information is weak or mis-leading, shape priors play a more important role to guide a correct segmentation. The recently proposed Sparse Shape Composition (SSC) [49,51] opens a new avenue for shape prior modeling. Instead of assuming any parametric model of shape statistics, SSC incorporates shape priors on-the-fly by approximating a shape instance (usually derived from appearance cues) by a sparse combination of shapes in a training repository. Theoretically, one can increase the modeling capability of SSC by including as many training shapes in the repository. However, this strategy confronts two limitations in practice. *First*, since SSC involves an iterative sparse optimization at run-time, the more shape instances contained in the repository, the less run-time efficiency SSC has. Therefore, a compact and informative shape dictionary is preferred to a large shape repository. *Second*, in medical imaging applications, training shapes seldom come in one batch. It is very time consuming and sometimes infeasible to re-construct the shape dictionary every time new training shapes appear. In this chapter, we introduce an online learning method to address these two limitations. Our method starts from constructing an initial shape dictionary using the K-SVD algorithm. When new training shapes come, instead of re-constructing the dictionary from the ground up, we update the existing one using a block-coordinates descent approach. Using the dynamically updated dictionary, sparse shape composition can be gracefully scaled up to model shape priors from a large number of training shapes without sacrificing run-time efficiency. Our method is validated on lung localization in X-Ray and cardiac segmentation in MRI time series. Compared to the original SSC, it shows comparable performance while being significantly more efficient.

1. Introduction

Sparse Shape Composition (SSC) [50,49,51] is a recently proposed method for shape prior modeling. Different from previous methods, which often assume a parametric model for shape statistics, SSC is a non-parametric method that approximates an input shape usually derived from low level appearance features, by a sparse combination of other shapes in a repository. Specifically, SSC models shape priors based on two sparsity observations: 1) Given a large shape repository of an organ, a shape instance of the same organ can be approximated by the composition of a sparse set of instances in the shape repository; and 2) a shape instance derived by local appearance cues might have gross errors but these errors are sparse in spatial space. Shape prior modeling is then formulated as a sparse optimization problem. More specifically, an input shape instance, which is usually derived from local appearance cues, is approximated by a sparse combination of other shapes in a repository. In this way, shape priors are incorporated on-the-fly. Thanks to the incorporation of two sparsity priors, SSC is able to correct gross errors of input shape and can preserve shape details even they are not statistically significant in the training repository.

Theoretically, the more shape instances contained in the shape repository, the more shape modeling capacity SSC has. However, a repository including a large number of shapes adversely affects the efficiency of SSC, which iteratively performs sparse optimization at run-time. A large shape repository not only increases the computational cost of each round of sparse optimization, but also decreases the convergency speed. Hence, it induces the low run-time efficiency of SSC, which is not acceptable in many applications. In fact, owing to the similar shape characteristics across the population, this large number of shape instances usually contain lots of redundant information. Therefore, a natural solution is to learn a compact and informative dictionary from the large number of training shapes in the repository. Unfortunately, dictionary learning sometimes confronts another limitation. In real world applications, a large number of training shape instances seldom come in one batch. If the dictionary needs to be completely re-learned every time new training shapes come, the learning process will become very time consuming and sometimes infeasible.

In this chapter, we introduce an on-line learning method to address these two limitations [48]. Our method starts from learning an initial dictionary off-line using available training shapes. K-SVD method is employed to learn the initial dictionary due to its flexibility and accelerated convergency. When new training shapes come, instead of re-constructing the dictionary from the ground up, we use an on-line dictionary learning method [25] to update the shape dictionary on-the-fly. More specifically, based on stochastic approximation, this online learning algorithm exploits the specific structure of the problem and updates the dictionary efficiently using block-coordinates descent. In this way, our shape dictionary can be gracefully scaled-up to contain a very large number of training shapes. Although the shape dictionary has much less number of atoms compared to the size of training samples, these atoms can still well approximates a shape instance through sparse combination. Hence, rather than using the complete shape repository, our sparse shape composition can be performed on this shape dictionary efficiently without sacrificing the shape modeling capability. This proposed method has been validated on two applications: 1) 2D lung segmentation in X-Ray images, 2) 2D cardiac segmentation in MRI time series. Compared with traditional SSC, this online dictionary learning based method has similar shape modeling performance with much higher run-time efficiency.

2. Relevant Work

We aim to improve the robustness of deformable model-based segmentation methods using shape priors. In various applications of medical image segmentation, deformable models have achieved tremendous success [19,39,6,5,28,32,17], thanks to the combined use of shape and appearance characteristics. While appearance features provide low level clues of organ boundaries, shapes impose high level knowledge to infer and refine deformable models. Therefore, shape prior modeling is crucial to the performance of segmentation methods.

Related studies can be traced to two categories, shape modeling and sparse dictionary learning. In the former category, most previous studies [6,15,18,20,35,41,42,60] aim to model shape priors using a parametric model, e.g., multi-variant Gaussian [6] and hierarchical diffusion wavelet [20]. Following the seminal work on active shape models, many of these methods have been proposed to alleviate problems in three categories 1) complex shape variations [4,29,35,41,61,60,12,53], 2) gross errors of input [9,21,40,31], and 3) loss of shape details [36,7].

SSC is the first shape modeling method to handle the above-mentioned three challenges in a unified framework. It is based on the sparse representation theory. Sparsity methods have been widely investigated recently. It has been shown that a sparse signal can be recovered from a small number of its linear measurements with high probability [2,8]. These sparsity priors are employed in many computer vision applications, such as, but not limited to, robust face recognition [38], image restoration [26], image bias estimation [56], MR reconstruction [24,16], atlas construction [34], resolution enhancement [54], image bias estimation [57,56] and automatic image annotation [47,13]. Sparsity methods have been proved to be very effective at handling gross errors or outliers.

To improve the computational efficiency, sparse dictionary learning methods have also been extensively studied in signal processing domain. Popular ones include optimal direction (MOD) [11] and K-SVD [1]. While these methods require the access of all training samples, a recently proposed online dictionary learning [25] allows an efficient dictionary update only based on new samples. Although dictionary learning has been successfully applied on low level image processing tasks, to the best of our knowledge, the proposed method is the first one to employ them for high-level shape prior modeling.

3. Methodology

In this section, we will first briefly introduce standard Sparse Shape Composition. Dictionary learning technologies that aims to tackle the two limitations of SSC will be presented afterwards.

3.1. *Sparse Shape Composition*

SSC is designed based on two observations: 1) After being aligned to a common canonical space, any shape can be approximated by a sparse linear combination of other shape instances in the same shape category. Approximation residuals might come from inter-subject variations. 2) If the shape to be approximated is derived by appearance cues, residual errors might include gross errors from detection/segmentaion errors. However, such errors are sparse as well. Accordingly, shape priors can be incorporated *on-the-fly* through shape composition, which is formulated as a sparse optimization problem as follows. Fig. 1 shows an example of the SSC-based shape prior modeling.

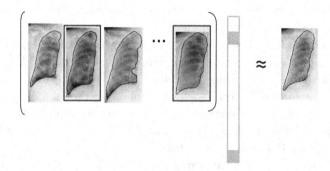

Fig. 1.   An illustration of the SSC-based shape prior modeling. Two instances from the training samples are selected to approximate the input shape.

In SSC, a shape is represented by a contour (2D) or a triangle mesh (3D) which consists of a set of vertices. Denote the input shape as $\mathbf{v}$, where $\mathbf{v} \in \mathbf{R}^{\mathfrak{D}N}$ is a vector concatenated by coordinates of its N vertices, where $\mathfrak{D} = \{2, 3\}$ denotes the dimensionality of the shape modeling problem. (In the remainder of this chapter, any shape instance is defined as a vector in the same way.) Assume $D = [\mathbf{d}_1, \mathbf{d}_2, ..., \mathbf{d}_K] \in \mathbf{R}^{\mathfrak{D}N \times K}$ is a large shape repository that includes K accurately annotated and pre-aligned shape instances $\mathbf{d}_i$. The approximation of $\mathbf{v}$ by D is then formulated as an optimization problem:

$$\arg\min_{\mathbf{x}, \mathbf{e}, \beta} \|T(\mathbf{v}, \beta) - D\mathbf{x} - \mathbf{e}\|_2^2 + \lambda_1 \|\mathbf{x}\|_1 + \lambda_2 \|\mathbf{e}\|_1, \tag{1}$$

where $T(\mathbf{v}, \beta)$ is a global transformation operator with parameter β, which aligns the input shape $\mathbf{v}$ to the common canonical space of D. The key idea of SSC lies in the second and third terms of the objective function. In the second term, the $L1$-norm of $\mathbf{x}$ ensures that the nonzero elements in $\mathbf{x}$, i.e., the linear combination coefficients, is sparse [2]. Hence, only a sparse set of shape instances can be used to approximate the input shape, which prevents the overfitting to errors from missing/misleading appearance cues. In the third term, the same sparse constraint applies on $\mathbf{e} \in \mathbf{R}^{\mathfrak{D}N}$, the large residual errors, which incorporates the observation that gross errors might exist but are occasional.

Eq. 1 is optimized using an Expectation-Maximization (EM) style algorithm, which alternatively optimizes β ("E" step) and $\mathbf{x}$, $\mathbf{e}$ ("M" step). "M" step is a typical sparse optimization, which employs a typical convex solver, e.g., interior-point convex solver [27] in this study.

By optimizing Eq. 1, shape priors are in fact incorporated *on-the-fly* through shape composition. Compared to traditional statistical shape models, e.g., active shape model, this method is able to remove gross errors from local appearance cues and preserve shape details even if they are not statistically significant. However, on the other hand, the optimization of Eq. 1 increases the computational cost, hence, limits the run-time efficiency of the SSC.

3.2. Shape Dictionary Learning

Theoretically, the more shape instances in D, the larger shape modeling capacity SSC has. However, the run-time efficiency of SSC is also determined by the size of the shape repository matrix $D \in \mathbf{R}^{\mathcal{D}N \times K}$. More specifically, the computational complexity of the interior-point convex optimization solver is $\mathcal{O}(N^2K)$ per iteration [27], which means the computational cost will increase quickly with the increase of K, the number of the shape instances in the shape repository. Note that $\mathcal{O}(N^2K)$ is the computational complexity for *one* iteration. Empirically, with larger K, it usually takes more iterations to convergency, which further decreases the algorithm speed.

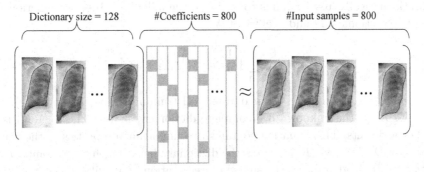

Fig. 2. An illustration of dictionary learning for 2D lung shapes. The input data contains 800 training samples, and a size 128 compact dictionary is generated. Each input shape can be approximately represented as a sparse linear combination of dictionary elements. Note that dictionary elements are "virtual shapes", which are not the same as any input shape but can generalize them well.

In fact, owing to the similar shape characteristics across the population, these K shape instances usually contain lots of redundant information. Instead of including all of them, D should only contain "representative" shapes. This is exactly a dictionary learning problem, which has been extensively investigated in signal

---

Algorithm 1 The framework of the OMP algorithm.

Input: Dictionary $D \in \mathbf{R}^{n \times k}$, input data $y_i \in \mathbf{R}^n$.
Output: coefficients $x_i \in \mathbf{R}^k$.
$\Gamma = \emptyset$.
repeat

   Select the atom which most reduces the objective

$$\arg \min_j \left\{ \min_{x'} |y_i - D_{\Gamma \cup \{j\}} x'|_2^2 \right\} \qquad (2)$$

   Update the active set: $\Gamma \leftarrow \Gamma \cup \{j\}$.
   Update the residual using orthogonal projection

$$r \leftarrow \left(I - D_\Gamma (D_\Gamma^T D_\Gamma)^{-1} D_\Gamma^T \right) y_i \qquad (3)$$

   where r is the residual and I is the identity matrix.
   Update the coefficients

$$x_\Gamma = (D_\Gamma^T D_\Gamma)^{-1} D_\Gamma^T y_i \qquad (4)$$

until Stop criteria

---

processing community. More specifically, a well learned dictionary should have a compact set of "atoms" that are able to sparsely approximate other signals. In our study, shape dictionary is learned using K-SVD [1,52], a popular dictionary learning method because of its accelerated converging speed.

Mathematically, K-SVD aims to optimize the following objective function with respect to dictionary D and coefficient X:

$$\arg \min_{D,X} \frac{1}{K} \sum_{i=1}^{K} \left(\frac{1}{2} \|y_i - Dx_i\|_2^2 + \|x_i\|_1 \right) \qquad (7)$$

where $y_i, i \in [1, K]$ represents all dataset (all training shapes in our case), $D \in \mathbf{R}^{n \times k} (k \ll K)$ is the unknown overcomplete dictionary, matrix $x_i, i \in [1, K]$ is the sparse coefficients. This equation contains two important properties of the learned dictionary D. *First*, $k \ll K$ indicates the dictionary has a much more compact size. *Second*, $\forall i, \|x_i\|_1$ guarantees the sparse representation capability of the dictionary.

In K-SVD algorithm, Eq. 7 is optimized by two alternative steps, sparse coding and codebook update. Sparse coding is a greedy method which can approximate an input data by finding a sparse set of elements from the codebook. Codebook update is used to generate a better dictionary given sparse coding results. These two steps are alternately performed until convergence.

Sparse coding stage: K-SVD algorithm starts from a random D and X and the sparse coding stage uses pursuit algorithms to find the sparse coefficient x_i for each signal y_i. OMP [3] is employed in this stage. OMP is an iterative greedy algorithm that selects at each step the dictionary element that best correlates with

---

Algorithm 2 The framework of the K-SVD algorithm.

Input: dictionary $D \in \mathbf{R}^{n \times k}$, input data $y_i \in \mathbf{R}^n$ and coefficients $x_i \in \mathbf{R}^k$.

Output: D and X.

repeat

    Sparse coding:

    use OMP to compute coefficient x_i for each signal y_i, to minimize

$$\min_{x_i}\{\|y_i - Dx_i\|_2^2\} \; subject \; to \; \|x_i\|_0 \leq L \tag{5}$$

    Codebook update:

    for $i = 1, 2, ..., k$, update each column d_i in D and also x_T^i (*i*th row)

        Find the group using d_i ($x_T^i \neq 0$), denoted as ω_i

        Compute error matrix E_i

        Restrict E_i by choosing columns corresponding to ω_i. The resized error is denoted as E_i^R

        Apply SVD and obtain

$$E_i^R = U\Sigma V^T \tag{6}$$

    Update d_i as the first column of U. Update nonzero elements in x_T^i as the first column of V multiplied by $\Sigma(1,1)$

until Stop criterions

---

the residual part of the signal. Then it produces a new approximation by projecting the signal onto those elements already selected [37]. The pseudo-codes of OMP is listed in Algorithm 1.

Codebook update stage: In the codebook update stage K-SVD aims to update D and X iteratively. In each iteration D and X are fixed except only one column d_i and the coefficients corresponding to d_i (*i*th row in X), denoted as x_T^i. Eq. 7 can be rewritten as

$$\left\| Y - \sum_{j=1}^{k} d_j x_T^j \right\|_F^2 = \left\| \left(Y - \sum_{j \neq i} d_j x_T^j \right) - d_i x_T^i \right\|_F^2 \tag{8}$$

$$= \left\| E_i - d_i x_T^i \right\|_F^2 \tag{9}$$

We need to minimize the difference between E_i and $d_i x_T^i$ with fixed E_i, by finding alternative d_i and x_T^i. Since SVD finds the closest rank-1 matrix that approximates E_i, it can be used to minimize Eq. 8. Assume $E_i = U\Sigma V^T$, d_i is updated as the first column of U, which is the eigenvector corresponding to the largest eigenvalue. x_T^i is updated as the first column of V multiplied by $\Sigma(1,1)$. The updated x_T^i may not always guarantee sparsity. A simple but effective solution is to discard the zero entries corresponding to the old x_T^i. The detail algorithms of K-SVD are listed in the Algorithm 2.

Algorithm 3 Online learn and update dictionary, using mini-batch mode.

Input: Initialized dictionary $D_0 \in \mathbf{R}^{n \times k}$, input data $Y = [y_1, y_2, ..., y_K], y_i \in \mathbf{R}^n$, number of iterations T, regularization parameter $\lambda \in R$.

Output: Learned dictionary D_T.

$A_0 = 0, B_0 = 0$.

for $t = 1 \to T$ **do**

    Randomly draw a set of $y_{t,1}, y_{t,2}, ..., y_{t,\eta}$.

    for $i = 1 \to \eta$ **do**

        Sparse coding: $x_{t,i} = \arg\min_{x \in \mathbf{R}^k} \frac{1}{2} \|y_{t,i} - D_{t-1}x\|_2^2 + \lambda \|x\|_1$.

    end for

    $A_t = \beta A_{t-1} + \sum_{i=1}^{\eta} x_{t,i} x_{t,i}^T$, $B_t = \beta B_{t-1} + \sum_{i=1}^{\eta} y_{t,i} x_{t,i}^T$,

    where $\beta = \frac{\theta + 1 - \eta}{\theta + 1}$, and $\theta = t\eta$ if $t < \eta$, $\theta = \eta^2 + t - \eta$ otherwise.

    Dictionary update: Compute D_t, so that:

    $\arg\min_{D} \frac{1}{t} \sum_{i=1}^{t} \frac{1}{2} \|y_i - Dx_i\|_2^2 + \lambda \|x_i\|_1 =$

    $\arg\min_{D} \frac{1}{t} \left(\frac{1}{2} Tr\left(D^T D A_t\right) - Tr(D^T B_t) \right)$.

end for

The learned dictionary D will be used in Eq. 1 at run-time. It is worth noting that an element in D might not be the same as any shape instances in the training set. In other words, the learned shape dictionary consists of virtual shape instances which might not exist in the real world. However, these virtual shapes do have sparse composition capabilities with a significantly more compact size, which can highly improve the run-time efficiency of our sparse shape composition. Fig. 2 shows an illustration of dictionary learning for 2D lung shapes. Ap compact dictionary is generated from input samples, such that each input sample can be approximately represented as a sparse linear combination of dictionary elements. This compact dictionary is used as data matrix D for our model.

3.3. *Online Shape Dictionary Update*

Using the compact dictionary derived by K-SVD, the run-time efficiency of SSC is dramatically improved, as the number of atoms in D is much less than the number of training shapes. However, K-SVD requires all training shapes available in the "dictionary update" step, which can not be satisfied in a lot of medical applications. For example, owing to the expensive cost, manual annotations of anatomical structures often come gradually from different radiologists/technicions. Re-construction of the dictionary D with every batch of new training shapes is very time consuming and not always feasible. To tackle this problem, we employ a recently proposed online dictionary method [25] to update the shape dictionary.

Algorithm 3 shows the framework of online dictionary learning for sparse coding. Starting from an initial dictionary learned by K-SVD, it iteratively employs two stages until converge, sparse coding and dictionary update. Sparse coding aims to find the sparse coefficient x_i for each signal y_i:

$$x_i = \arg\min_{x \in \mathbf{R}^k} \frac{1}{2}\|y_i - Dx\|_2^2 + \lambda\|x\|_1 \tag{10}$$

where D is the initialized dictionary or dictionary computed from the previous iteration. LARS-Lasso algorithm [10] is employed to solve this step. The dictionary update stage aims to update D based on all discovered $x_i, i \in [1, K]$:

$$\arg\min_{D} \frac{1}{K} \sum_{i=1}^{K} \frac{1}{2}\|y_i - Dx_i\|_2^2 + \lambda\|x_i\|_1 \tag{11}$$

Based on stochastic approximation, the dictionary is updated efficiently using block-coordinates descent. It is a parameter-free method and does not require any learning rate tuning. It is important to note that the "dictionary update" step in Algorithm 3 is significantly different from that of K-SVD. Instead of requiring all training shapes, it only exploits a small batch of newly coming data (i.e., $x_i, i \in [1, \eta]$). The dictionary update thereby becomes much faster than K-SVD, as $\eta \ll K$. In this way, we can efficiently update the shape dictionary online by using new data as selected x_i.

Using this online updated dictionary, SSC obtains two additional advantages. 1) The run-time efficiency of shape composition is not sacrificed with much more training shapes. 2) SSC can be gracefully scaled-up to contain shape priors from, theoretically, infinite number of training shapes.

4. Experiments

We validate our algorithm in two applications, lung localization in Chest X-ray, and left ventricle tracking in MRI.

4.1. *Lung Localization*

Chest radiography (X-ray) is a widely used medical imaging modality because of the fast imaging speed and low cost. Localization of lungs in chest radiography not only provides lung shapes, which are critical clues for pathology detection, but also paves the way for other medical image analysis tasks, e.g., cardiac measurements. On one hand, owing to the relatively cheap cost of manual/semi-automatic annotations of lungs in X-ray images, it is possible to get a large number of lung shapes for training. On the other hand, however, training lung shapes seldom come in one batch in clinical practices. Instead, clinicians often verify and correct auto-localization results and prefer a system that has self-improvement ability using these corrected shapes as new training shapes. Therefore, lung localization in chest X-ray becomes an ideal use case to test the effectiveness of our online dictionary method.

Our lung localization system starts from a set of auto-detected landmarks around the lung (e.g., the bottom-left lung tip) using learning-based methods [55,23,44,45,43,51],

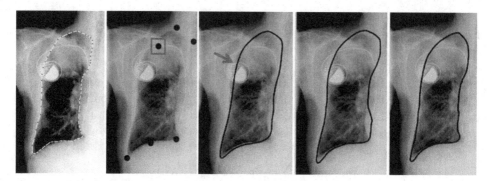

Fig. 3.   Comparisons of the localization results. From left to right: manual label, detection results, PCA, SSC, and the online learning based shape refinement results. Due to the erroneous detection (marked by the box), PCA result moves to the right and is not on the boundary (see the arrow). Zoom in for better view.

Table 1.   Quantitative comparisons of the lung localization using shape priors. P, Q, DSC stand for the sensitivity, specificity, and dice similarity coefficient (%), respectively.

	P	Q	DSC
PCA	87.5 ± 5.2	96.0 ± 3.1	90.1 ± 4.0
SSC	86.7 ± 4.8	**96.6 ± 2.4**	89.4 ± 3.9
Ours	**94.3 ± 4.6**	96.2 ± 2.3	**94.5 ± 3.6**

based on which lung shapes are inferred using shape priors. Note that various factors, e.g., imaging artifacts, lung diseases, etc., might induce missing/wrong landmark detection, which should be corrected by shape prior models. Although the overall system performance depends on multiple components, including initial landmark detection, shape prior modeling and the following deformable segmentation, our comparison focuses on the shape prior modeling part, i.e., other components remain the same in comparsions. Our experimental dataset includes 367 X-ray images from different patients. 32 of them are used as training data to construct the initial data matrix/dictionary D in Eq. 1. Note that simply stacking more training shapes into D can also improve the capability of shape representation. However, it dramatically reduces the computational efficiency, which highly depends on the scale of D when solving Eq. 1 [27].

Three shape prior methods are compared, 1) the PCA based prior as used in Active Shape Model [6], 2) SSC [49], and 3) our method. Fig. 3 shows an example of using these methods to infer shapes from auto-detected landmarks. This case is challenging due to the misplaced medical instrument, which causes erroneous detections (marked by a box in Fig. 3). Although all three methods achieve reasonable accuracy, the whole shape of PCA result shifts slightly to the right (where the arrow points in Fig. 3), because PCA is sensitive to outliers. Benefited by the sparse

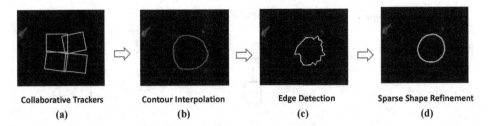

Collaborative Trackers	Contour Interpolation	Edge Detection	Sparse Shape Refinement
(a)	(b)	(c)	(d)

Fig. 4.   Tracking pipeline of our method. It includes collaborative tracking, contour interpolation, edge detection and sparse shape refinement.

representation and $L1$-norm constraint, SSC and our method can both handle erroneous detections. However, since the initial shape dictionary may not be generative and representative enough, the inferred shape from SSC is not as accurate as the proposed method, which updates the dictionary on-the-fly and improves its capability of shape representations. Table 1 shows the quantitative accuracy (compared to experts' annotations) of the three methods, in terms of the sensitivity, specificity, and dice similarity coefficient (DSC). In general, our method achieves significantly better sensitivity, while slightly worse specificity than SSC. The reason is that SSC under-segments some images, which results in low sensitivity but high specificity. Our method achieves much better performance in terms of DSC, which is a more comprehensive measurements (includes both sensitivity and specificity) for localization accuracy. The experiments are performed on a PC with 2.4GHz Intel Quad CPU, 8GB memory, with Python 2.5 and C++ implementations. The whole framework is fully automatic and efficient. The shape inference step takes 0.2-0.3s, with around 0.06s as an overhead to update the dictionary online, which is negligible. In contrast, re-training the dictionary using K-SVD needs around 15-40s each time.

4.2. *Real-time Left Ventricle Tracking*

Extraction of the boundary contour of a beating heart from cardiac MRI image sequences plays an important role in cardiac disease diagnosis and treatments. MRI-guided robotic intervention is potentially important in cardiac procedures such as aortic valve repair. One of the major difficulties is the path planning of the robotic needle, which requires accurate contour segmentation of the left ventricle on a *real-time* MRI sequence. Thus, the algorithm should be robust, accurate and fast. We use a shape prior based tracking framework to solve this problem. Note that the left ventricle segmentation has been widely investigated [30]. Our intent is not to provide a thorough accuracy comparison with state-the-art techniques on standard datasets. Instead, we aim to demonstrate that the proposed method can efficiently deal with this real-time task by incorporating it into a tracking framework. In our method, a collaborative trackers network is employed to provide a deformed mesh and then generate a rough contour as the initialization at each time step [58]. Next, this initialized shape model deforms based on low level image appearance. Appearance-based

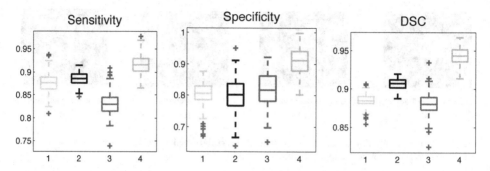

Fig. 5.   Box plots for quantitative comparisons. From left to right of each figure: results from the deformation, PCA, SSC, and the proposed method, respectively.

deformation may not be accurate since the image information can be ambiguous and noisy. Thus, the shape prior model is employed to refine the deformed contour [59]. Fig. 4 shows the cardiac tracking pipeline of our method. Based on this framework, we compare the performance of (a) deformable model based on image appearance, (b) PCA based, (c) SSC based and (d) the online dictionary based shape refinement methods. For computational efficiency consideration, the dictionary size of (b) and (c) is fixed as a small number 8. The SSC method constantly uses this initial dictionary, while the proposed method (c) updates the dictionary on-the-fly by using acquired tracking results as the mini-batch input of Algorithm 3.

Fig. 5 shows the quantitative evaluations, in terms of the sensitivity, specificity, and the dice similarity coefficient. Appearance-based deformation results produces inconsistent results when the image information is ambiguous. SSC based shape refinement may not improve the accuracy of the deformed result due to the small size of dictionary. PCA based method achieves good performance. However, it is not able to handle certain new shapes which cannot be generalized from the current PCA results. In general, the proposed method achieves the most accurate result, since it updates the dictionary on-the-fly using newly acquired information. Thus it is more generic and adaptive to new data. Online updating the dictionary takes around 0.03s, which causes very small overhead for the whole system. To track total of 189 frames, our system takes 23.7s. Re-training the dictionary using K-SVD takes around 12s each time, which is not feasible for realtime applications.

5. Conclusions

In this chapter, we introduce a robust and efficient shape prior modeling method, Sparse Shape Composition (SSC). Contrary to traditional shape models, SSC incorporates shape priors on-the-fly through sparse shape composition. It is able to handle gross errors, to model complex shape variations and to preserve shape details in a unified framework. Owing to the high computational cost of standard SSC, a straightforward integration might has low runtime efficiency, which impedes the segmentation system being clinically accepted. Therefore, we designed two strategies to improve the computational efficiency of the sparse shape composition. First, given a large number of training shape instances, K-SVD is used to learn a much more compact but still informative shape dictionary. Second, when new shapes come, online dictionary learning method is used to update the dictionary on-the-fly. With the dynamic updated dictionary, SSC is adaptive and gracefully scaled-up to contain shape priors from a large number of training shapes without losing the run-time efficiency. The proposed method was validated on two medical applications. Compared to standard SSC, it achieved better shape modeling performance with a much faster speed. It is worth noting our shape prior method can also be coupled with other segmentation algorithms, such as registration-based and patch-based methods [14,62,33,46,22,29]. In the future, we would like to apply this shape prior method to more applications such as registration.

References

1. Aharon, M., Elad, M., Bruckstein, A.: K-SVD: An algorithm for designing overcomplete dictionaries for sparse representation. In: IEEE Transaction on Signal Processing. pp. 4311–4322 (2006)
2. Candes, E., Romberg, J., Tao, T.: Robust uncertainty principles: Exact signal reconstruction from highly incomplete frequency information. IEEE Transactions on Information Theory 52(2), 489–509 (2006)
3. Chen, S., Billings, S.A., Luo, W.: Orthogonal least squares methods and their application to non-linear system identification. In: International Journal of Control. pp. 1873–1896 (1989)
4. Cootes, T.F., Taylor, C.J.: A mixture model for representing shape variation. In: Image and Vision Computing. pp. 110–119 (1997)
5. Cootes, T., Edwards, G., Taylor, C.: Active appearance models. In: ECCV. pp. 484–498 (1998)
6. Cootes, T., Taylor, C., Cooper, D., Graham, J.: Active shape model - their training and application. Computer Vision and Image Understanding 61, 38–59 (1995)
7. Davatzikos, C., Tao, X., Shen, D.: Hierarchical active shape models, using the wavelet transform. IEEE Transactions on Medical Imaging 22(3), 414–423 (2003)
8. Donoho, D.L.: Compressed sensing. IEEE Transactions on Information Theory 52(4), 1289–1306 (2006)
9. Duta, N., Sonka, M.: Segmentation and interpretation of MR brain images. an improved active shape model. IEEE Transactions on Medical Imaging 17(6), 1049–1062 (1998)
10. Efron, B., Hastie, T., Johnstone, I., Tibshirani, R.: Least angle regression. The Annals of statistics 32(2), 407–499 (2004)
11. Engan, K., Aase, S., Hakon Husoy, J.: Method of optimal directions for frame design. In: ICASSP. vol. 5, pp. 2443–2446 (1999)
12. Etyngier, P., Segonne, F., Keriven, R.: Shape priors using manifold learning techniques. In: International Conference on Computer Vision. pp. 1–8 (2007)
13. Gao, S., Chia, L., Tsang, I.: Multi-layer group sparse codingfor concurrent image classification and annotation. In: IEEE Conference on Computer Vision and Pattern Recognition. pp. 2809–2816. IEEE (2011)

14. Han, X., Fischl, B.: Atlas renormalization for improved brain mr image segmentation across scanner platforms. IEEE Transactions on Medical Imaging 26(4), 479–486 (2007)
15. Heimann, T., Meinzer, H.P.: Statistical shape models for 3D medical image segmentation: A review. Medical Image Analysis 13(4), 543–563 (2009)
16. Huang, J., Zhang, S., Metaxas, D.: Efficient MR image reconstruction for compressed MR imaging. Medical Image Analysis 15(5), 670–679 (2011)
17. Huang, X., Metaxas, D.: Metamorphs: Deformable shape and appearance models. IEEE Transactions on Pattern Analysis and Machine Intelligence 30(8), 1444–1459 (2008)
18. Hufnagel, H., Pennec, X., Ehrhardt, J., Handels, H., Ayache, N.: Shape analysis using a point-based statistical shape model built on correspondence probabilities. In: Ayache, N., Ourselin, S., Maeder, A. (eds.) MICCAI 2007, Part I, LNCS, vol. 4791, pp. 959–967. Springer, Heidelberg (2007)
19. Kass, M., Witkin, A., Terzopoulos, D.: Snakes: Active contour models. International Journal of Computer Vision 1, 321–331 (1987)
20. Langs, G., Paragios, N., Essafi, S.: Hierarchical 3D diffusion wavelet shape priors. In: ICCV. pp. 1717–1724 (2010)
21. Lekadir, K., Merrifield, R., zhong Yang, G.: G.-z.: Outlier detection and handling for robust 3D active shape models search. IEEE Transaction on Medical Imaging 26, 212–222 (2007)
22. Li, H., Shen, T., Smith, M., Fujiwara, I., Vavylonis, D., Huang, X.: Automated actin filament segmentation, tracking and tip elongation measurements based on open active contour models. In: IEEE International Symposium on Biomedical Imaging: From Nano to Macro. pp. 1302–1305. IEEE (2009)
23. Ling, H., Zhou, S., Zheng, Y., Georgescu, B., Suehling, M., Comaniciu, D.: Hierarchical, learning-based automatic liver segmentation. In: IEEE Conference on Computer Vision and Pattern Recognition. pp. 1–8. IEEE (2008)
24. Lustig, M., Donoho, D., Pauly, J.: Sparse MRI: The application of compressed sensing for rapid MR imaging. Magnetic Resonance in Medicine 58(6), 1182–1195 (2007)
25. Mairal, J., Bach, F., Ponce, J., Sapiro, G.: Online dictionary learning for sparse coding. In: ICML. pp. 689–696 (2009)
26. Mairal, J., Bach, F., Ponce, J., Sapiro, G., Zisserman, A.: Non-local sparse models for image restoration. In: ICCV. pp. 2272–2279 (2009)
27. Nesterov, Y., Nemirovsky, A.: Interior point polynomial methods in convex programming. Studies in applied mathematics 13, 1993 (1994)
28. Paragios, N., Deriche, R.: Geodesic active contours and level sets for the detection and tracking of moving objects. IEEE Transactions on Pattern Analysis and Machine Intelligence 22(3), 266–280 (2000)
29. Pohl, K., Warfield, S., Kikinis, R., Grimson, W., Wells, W.: Coupling statistical segmentation and pca shape modeling. Medical Image Computing and Computer-Assisted Intervention pp. 151–159 (2004)
30. Radau, P., Lu, Y., Connelly, K., Paul, G., Dick, A., Wright, G.: Evaluation framework for algorithms segmenting short axis cardiac MRI. The MIDAS Journal, Cardiac MR Left Ventricle Segmentation Challenge (2009)
31. Rogers, M., Graham, J.: Robust active shape model search. In: European Conference on Computer Vision, pp. 289–312 (2006)
32. Shen, D., Davatzikos, C.: An adaptive-focus deformable model using statistical and geometric information. IEEE Transactions on Pattern Analysis and Machine Intelligence 22(8), 906–913 (2000)

33. Shen, T., Li, H., Huang, X.: Active volume models for medical image segmentation. IEEE Transactions on Medical Imaging 30(3), 774–791 (march 2011)
34. Shi, F., Wang, L., Wu, G., Zhang, Y., Liu, M., Gilmore, J., Lin, W., Shen, D.: Atlas construction via dictionary learning and group sparsity. Medical Image Computing and Computer-Assisted Intervention pp. 247–255 (2012)
35. Shi, Y., Qi, F., Xue, Z., Chen, L., Ito, K., Matsuo, H., Shen, D.: Segmenting lung fields in serial chest radiographs using both population-based and patient-specific shape statistics. IEEE Transactions on Medical Imaging 27(4), 481–494 (2008)
36. Sjostrand, K., Rostrup, E., Ryberg, C., Larsen, R., Studholme, C., Baezner, H., Ferro, J., Fazekas, F., Pantoni, L., Inzitari, D., Waldemar, G.: Sparse decomposition and modeling of anatomical shape variation. TMI 26(12), 1625–1635 (2007)
37. Tropp, J.A.: Greed is good: Algorithmic results for sparse approximation. In: IEEE Transaction Information Theory. pp. 2231–2242 (2004)
38. Wright, J., Yang, A., Ganesh, A., Sastry, S., Ma, Y.: Robust face recognition via sparse representation. TPAMI 31(2), 210–227 (2009)
39. Xu, C., Prince, J.: Snakes, shapes and gradient vector flow. IEEE Transaction on Image Processing 7, 359–369 (1998)
40. Yan, P., Xu, S., Turkbey, B., Kruecker, J.: Discrete deformable model guided by partial active shape model for trus image segmentation. IEEE Transactions on Biomedical Engineering 57(5), 1158–1166 (2010)
41. Yan, P., Kruecker, J.: Incremental shape statistics learning for prostate tracking in trus. In: Jiang, T., Navab, N., Pluim, J.P.W., Viergever, M.A. (eds.) MICCAI 2010, Part II. LNCS, vol. 6362, pp. 42–49. Springer, Heidelberg (2010)
42. Yeo, B.T., Yu, P., Grant, P.E., Fischl, B., Golland, P.: Shape analysis with overcomplete spherical wavelets. In: MICCAI. pp. 468–476 (2008)
43. Zhan, Y., Dewan, M., Zhou, X.S.: Cross modality deformable segmentation using hierarchical clustering and learning. In: the 12th International Conference on Medical Image Computing and Computer Assisted Intervention. pp. 1033–1041 (2009)
44. Zhan, Y., Shen, D.: Deformable segmentation of 3D ultrasound prostate images using statistical texture matching method. IEEE Transaction on Medical Imaging 25(3), 256–272 (2006)
45. Zhan, Y., Zhou, X.S., Peng, Z., Krishnan, A.: Active scheduling of organ detection and segmentation in whole-body medical images. In: the 11th International Conference on Medical Image Computing and Computer Assisted Intervention. pp. 313–321 (2008)
46. Zhang, D., Wu, G., Jia, H., Shen, D.: Confidence-guided sequential label fusion for multi-atlas based segmentation. Medical Image Computing and Computer-Assisted Intervention pp. 643–650 (2011)
47. Zhang, S., Huang, J., Huang, Y., Yu, Y., Li, H., Metaxas, D.: Automatic image annotation using group sparsity. In: IEEE Conference on Computer Vision and Pattern Recognition. pp. 3312–3319. IEEE (2010)
48. Zhang, S., Zhan, Y., Zhou, Y., Uzunbas, M., Metaxas, D.: Shape prior modeling using sparse representation and online dictionary learning. Medical Image Computing and Computer-Assisted Intervention pp. 435–442 (2012)
49. Zhang, S., Zhan, Y., Dewan, M., Huang, J., Metaxas, D., Zhou, X.: Deformable segmentation via sparse shape representation. In: Fichtinger, G., Martel, A., Peters, T. (eds.) MICCAI 2011, Part II. LNCS, vol. 6892, pp. 451–458. Springer, Heidelberg (2011)
50. Zhang, S., Zhan, Y., Dewan, M., Huang, J., Metaxas, D., Zhou, X.: Sparse shape composition: A new framework for shape prior modeling. In: IEEE Conference on Computer Vision and Pattern Recognition. pp. 1025–1032 (2011)

51. Zhang, S., Zhan, Y., Dewan, M., Huang, J., Metaxas, D., Zhou, X.: Towards robust and effective shape modeling: Sparse shape composition. Medical Image Analysis 16(1), 265–277 (2012)
52. Zhang, S., Zhan, Y., Metaxas, D.N.: Deformable segmentation via sparse representation and dictionary learning. Medical Image Analysis 16(7), 1385–1396 (2012)
53. Zhang, W., Yan, P., Li, X.: Estimating patient-specific shape prior for medical image segmentation. In: International Symposium on Biomedical Imaging. pp. 1451–1454. IEEE (2011)
54. Zhang, Y., Wu, G., Yap, P.T., Feng, Q., Lian, J., Chen, W., Shen, D.: Hierarchical patch-based sparse representation - a new approach for resolution enhancement of 4d-ct lung data. IEEE Transactions on Medical Imaging 31(11), 1993–2005 (nov 2012)
55. Zheng, Y., Barbu, A., Georgescu, B., Scheuering, M., Comaniciu, D.: Four-chamber heart modeling and automatic segmentation for 3D cardiac CT volumes using marginal space learning and steerable features. IEEE Transaction on Medical Imaging 27, 1668–1681 (2008)
56. Zheng, Y., Gee, J.: Estimation of image bias field with sparsity constraints. In: IEEE Conference on Computer Vision and Pattern Recognition. pp. 255–262. IEEE (2010)
57. Zheng, Y., Grossman, M., Awate, S., Gee, J.: Automatic correction of intensity nonuniformity from sparseness of gradient distribution in medical images. Medical Image Computing and Computer-Assisted Intervention pp. 852–859 (2009)
58. Zhou, Y., Yeniaras, E., Tsiamyrtzis, P., Tsekos, N., Pavlidis, I.: Collaborative tracking for MRI-guided robotic intervention on the beating heart. In: Jiang, T., Navab, N., Pluim, J., Viergever, M. (eds.) MICCAI 2010, Part III. LNCS, vol. 6363, pp. 351–358. Springer, Heidelberg (2010)
59. Zhou, Y., Zhang, S., Tsekos, N., Pavlidis, I., Metaxas, D.: Left endocardium tracking via collaborative trackers and shape prior. In: IEEE International Symposium on Biomedical Imaging. pp. 784–787. IEEE (2012)
60. Zhu, Y., Papademetris, X., Sinusas, A., Duncan, J.: Segmentation of the left ventricle from cardiac MR images using a subject-specific dynamical model. TMI 29(3), 669–687 (2010)
61. Zhu, Y., Papademetris, X., Sinusas, A., Duncan, J.: A dynamical shape prior for LV segmentation from RT3D echocardiography. In: International Conference on Medical Image Computing and Computer Assisted Intervention. pp. 206–213 (2009)
62. Zhuang, X., Rhode, K., Razavi, R., Hawkes, D., Ourselin, S.: A registration-based propagation framework for automatic whole heart segmentation of cardiac MRI. IEEE Transactions on Medical Imaging 29(9), 1612–1625 (2010)

CHAPTER 5

FEATURE-CENTRIC LESION DETECTION AND RETRIEVAL IN THORACIC IMAGES

Yang Song[1], Weidong Cai[1], Stefan Eberl[2], Michael J Fulham[2,3],
and David Dagan Feng[1]

[1]*Biomedical and Multimedia Information Technology (BMIT) Research Group,
School of Information Technologies, University of Sydney, Australia*
[2]*Department of PET and Nuclear Medicine, Royal Prince Alfred Hospital,
Sydney, Australia*
[3]*Sydney Medical School, University of Sydney, Australia*
E-mail: yson1723@uni.sydney.edu.au

Advances in medical digital imaging have greatly benefited patient care. Computer-aided diagnosis is increasingly being used to facilitate semi- or fully-automatic medical image analysis and image retrieval. While different tasks involve different methodologies in this domain, these tasks normally require image feature extraction as an essential component in the algorithmic framework. In this Chapter, we focus on image feature modeling in lesion detection and image retrieval for thoracic images. For both tasks, we first review the state-of-the-art and then present some of our own work in more detail.

1. Lesion Detection

Lung cancer is the most common cause of cancer-related death. Non-small cell lung cancer (NSCLC) is the most prevalent type of lung cancer, and it accounts for about 80% of all cases.[1] Staging, which assesses the degree of spread of the cancer from its original source, is critical in determining prognosis and choosing the most appropriate treatment. In the 'tumor, node, metastasis' (TNM) staging system, the size and spatial extent of the primary lung tumor and the degree of involvement of regional lymph nodes are critical factors.

Positron emission tomography – computed tomography (PET-CT) with [18]*F-fluoro-deoxy-glucose* (FDG) tracer is now accepted as the best imaging technique for non-invasive staging of NSCLC.[2] In PET-CT, the CT scan provides anatomical information; it has relatively low soft tissue contrast which causes difficulties in separating lesions from the surrounding tissues. On the other hand, the PET scan has high contrast and reveals increased metabolism in structures with rapidly growing cancer cells, but the localization of these foci of increase metabolism is limited by the low spatial resolution in PET. The integrated PET and CT scan thus provides complementary functional and anatomical information. In current routine clinical workflow, the detection of abnormalities is performed manually. There may be many such abnormalities in a patient with NSCLC. To assist this time-consuming process and potentially provide a second opinion to the reading physicians, an automated system that can provide fast and robust lesion detection is desirable.

The objective is thus to design a fully automated methodology to detect primary lung tumors and disease in regional lymph nodes from PET-CT images of the thorax. Examples of lesion detection are shown in Fig. 1. There are two main challenges. First, tumor metabolism detected in PET relates to uptake of the tracer FDG; this uptake can be expressed semi-quantitatively as the standard uptake value (or SUV). The SUV normally exhibits high intra- and inter-patient variances, and can highlight non-pathological areas (e.g. in myocardium). Second, separation of the primary lung tumors from abnormal lymph nodes can be difficult, especially in complex cases where tumors invade the mediastinum or lymph nodes in the pulmonary hilar regions. In this section, we review the state-of-the-art in lesion detection, and describe our approaches[3–5] to tackle this problem.

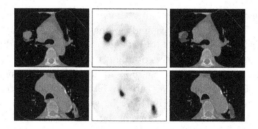

Fig. 1. Examples of primary lung tumors and involved lymph nodes.[4] Each row shows one example, using a transaxial slice view for easier visualization. The left column shows the CT slices, the middle column the PET slices, and the right column shows the lung tumors (dark gray) and involved lymph nodes (light gray).

1.1. *Review of State-of-the-art*

Currently there are no published data on the simultaneous detection of lung tumors and disease in regional lymph nodes, apart from our own studies. Existing work is mainly on lung tumor detection, without considering the involvement of lymph nodes. By first segmenting the lung fields, a threshold and fuzzy-logic based approach is then used to detect the lung tumors,[6] but the detection performance is quite sensitive to the delineation accuracy of the lung fields. Another approach attempts to handle tumors lying close to the edge of lung fields by incorporating the location, intensity, and shape information,[7] but the method could potentially result in a large number of false positives with the predefined SUV thresholds. False positives are usually detected in the mediastinum with elevated SUV. To reduce such false positives, learning-based techniques with tumor-specific features have been proposed,[8,9] but the methods are based on empirical studies of SUV distributions and tumor sizes, and do not seem to consider abnormal lymph nodes in the thorax.

Another category of lesion detection is to detect all instances from PET images, regardless of their types. Such approaches include a texture-based classification method,[10] and a water-shed based algorithm integrated with morphological measures.[11] A common drawback with these techniques is that they operate on user-selected volume-of-interest (VOI) or potential lesions. Fully automated lesion detection has also been studied,[12] and we have previously reported several methods[13–15] based on subject-level contrast features. However, differentiation of lung tumors from abnormal lymph nodes is not investigated in these studies.

1.2. *Region-based Feature Classification*

In our work, we first proposed a region-based feature classification method[3] to detect the primary lung tumors and the abnormal lymph nodes, in a three-step approach.

1.2.1. *Region Type Identification*

A modified fuzzy c-means (FCM) approach is first used to cluster each PET-CT slice into regions of various sizes and shapes.[16] Based on anisotropic diffusion filtering (ADF),[17] Gabor and shape features, each region is then represented by a 12-dimensional feature vector F: mean and variance of ADF/Gabor filtered CT values; mean and variance of ADF/Gabor filtered PET SUVs; the size; the eccentricity; and the centroid x and y coordinates.

Next, the regions are classified into 5 types: lung field, mediastinum, involved regional lymph node (N), tumor in the lung, and border area surrounding the tumor. The last two represent the T type. The classification is based on feature F with a multi-class linear-kernel support vector machine (SVM).[18] The feature weights for each region type are also derived from the support vectors, resulting in a 5×12 matrix of feature weights w.

1.2.2. *Region Type Refinement*

The region types identified are often misclassified, particularly in terms of correct T and N classifications. Since both could be characterized by high CT values and high SUVs, the feature vector F is not sufficient to differentiate the two types. A major difference between T and N, however, could be modeled by the spatial relationships between regions. For example, T is within lung fields while N is in the mediastinum or the hilar nodal area.

We thus refine the region classifications based on spatial information. The region delineation step normally formulates several near-concentric regions at the T/N area, and several large regions corresponding to the lung fields and mediastinum surrounding the T/N area. Therefore, for each region, R_i, initially classified as T or

N, its spatial information could be defined by the regions inside and outside of R_i: $\langle R_j, R_k \rangle$. A 36-dimensional feature vector FS is hence computed by concatenating the feature vectors of R_i, R_j and R_k.

A second multi-class SVM is then trained to classify the regions based on the feature vector. The final region type is determined by combining the margins computed from both multi-class SVMs. The output with the maximum combined margin is chosen as the region type.

1.2.3. *3D Object Localization*

Given the T or N regions identified from each PET-CT slice pair, we then attempt to localize the 3D T or N objects within a case. Because not all T or N areas are correctly identified from the slices due to errors from the classification and the region delineation step, we design a voting-based method for the localization. Specifically, two scores S_I^T and S_I^N are assigned to each slice I in a case:

$$S_I^{T/N} = \exp\left[-min(d(I, J), d(I, K))\right] \tag{1}$$

J and K are the slices spatially nearest to I (above and below) with detected T/N regions; and d is the normalized weighted (w) Euclidean distance between the feature vectors of the T/N regions. For each case, the mean score value and median locations of the T/N regions are computed from its set of images. T/N regions with scores higher than the mean score value are marked as valid locations.

1.3. *Multi-stage Discriminative Model*

A drawback of the region-based classification method[3] is that it requires a separate class of tumor border, to work around the issue that the surrounding areas of tumors in the lung are often misclassified as mediastinum. Such a tumor-border class complicates the training process, which is unnatural for a clinical workflow. Our later work[19] avoids this issue as we use a multi-level discriminative model and more comprehensive spatial features. However, this method requires the surrounding regions of tumors and abnormal lymph nodes to be accurately classified, involving a heuristic-based grouping operation to separate the surrounding regions from the mediastinum. In addition, the regions belonging to a tumor or an abnormal lymph node are classified individually, which could result in inconsistent labeling within a 3D volume. Therefore, we then proposed a multi-stage discriminative model,[4] as detailed in the following.

1.3.1. *Abnormality Detection*

In the first stage, after preprocessing for background removal,[20] each transaxial PET-CT slice of a 3D image set is clustered into regions using quick-shift clustering.[21] Represent each 3D image set by N_r regions from all slices $V = \{r_i : i =$

$1, ..., N_r$}. Each region r_i is then classified into lung fields (L), mediastinum (M) or abnormality (ROI) categories based on low-level and high-level features.

Two types of low level features are computed: intensity and neighborhood. To describe the intensity features, a two-dimensional intensity vector is computed: (i) average CT density and (ii) average normalized SUV of r_i. While the average CT density is based on the raw values, for PET, we perform an extra SUV normalization $\|u_i\|$ with a sigmoid function:

$$\|u_i\| = \frac{C_1}{1 + \exp(-(u_i - \theta_V)/\theta_V)} \tag{2}$$

where u_i is the average SUV of r_i, θ_V is the adaptive reference value computed for each 3D image set V in a similar approach to our previous work,[13] and C_1 is a scaling constant controlling the range of the normalized SUV. The normalization is to rescale the SUVs across patients within a similar range, and in the process, boost the separations between the ROIs and the mediastinum. To describe the neighborhood features, the average CT density and normalized SUV of the neighboring area of region r_i in the adjacent slices (one above and one below) are also computed, to incorporate 3D information.

In some cases, the SUVs of ROIs and the mediastinum are relatively close, and some false positive ROIs could be detected in the mediastinum with the low-level features. We thus exploit the high-level features, by computing the contrast between the detected ROIs and the lung fields and mediastinum. To do this, we first classify the regions into lung fields, mediastinum and ROI – {R_L, R_M, R_O}, based on the low-level features. Let u_L, u_M and u_O be the average normalized SUVs of R_L, R_M and R_O, a four-dimensional high-level feature is then computed for each ROI region r_i: {$u_r/u_L, u_r/u_M, u_r/u_O, u_r$}, where u_r is the average normalized SUV of r_i.

Any misclassification at this stage would be propagated to later stages. Thus we use soft labeling to create a vector of probabilities, rather than labeling every region with a single category (L, M or ROI), to reduce the impact of possible misclassifications. The soft labeling vector, denoted as $p_i = \{p_i^L, p_i^M, p_i^O\}$ for region r_i, is obtained by combining the probability estimates of the SVM classification based on both low- and high-level features.

1.3.2. *Tumor and Lymph Node Differentiation*

In the second stage, the detected abnormalities are differentiated as tumors or abnormal lymph nodes, as illustrated in Fig. 2. A conditional random field (CRF)[22] model integrated with SVM and a comprehensive set of features are designed to achieve an accurate discrimination between the two types of abnormalities (SVM), and minimize any misclassification by exploiting 3D correlations (CRF). The use of CRF allows us to incorporate the structural information in addition to the region-based features, so that a 3D ROI volume could be classified collectively.

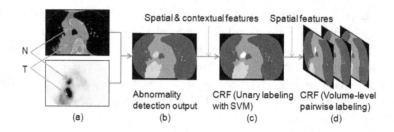

Fig. 2.   Illustration of tumor and lymph node differentiation.[4] (a) A transaxial PET-CT slice. (b) The abnormality detection output with two ROIs detected. (c) Region-level labeling with the unary term based on spatial and contextual features, showing the two ROIs labeled as T (gray) and N (white). (d) Volume-level labeling with the pairwise term based on 3D spatial features.

Based on the outputs of the first stage, the abnormalities detected from a 3D image set V are represented as N_O regions $\{r_i : i = 1, ..., N_O\}$. Rather than individual regions created at the clustering step, r_i here represents a large ROI region created by merging regions that are labeled as ROI and spatially connected in the same slice. A set of 3D connected $\{r_i\}$ (i.e. across slices) then form a 3D ROI volume, and V could contain multiple ROI volumes, e.g. a primary lung tumor and several abnormal lymph nodes.

The objective is then to assign each r_i a binary label $a_i \in \{T, N\}$; and the probability of a labeling set $A = \{a_i : i = 1, ..., N_O\}$ is modeled as a conditional distribution in the CRF framework:

$$P(A|V) = Z^{-1} \exp(-E(A|V)) \tag{3}$$

where Z is the partition function. We define the energy $E(A|V)$ as a linear combination of a set of unary features $F_k(a_i, V)$ and a pairwise feature $G(a_i, a_{i'}, V)$:

$$E(A|V) = \sum_i \sum_k \lambda_k F_k(a_i, V) + \sum_{i,i'} \mu G(a_i, a_{i'}, V) \tag{4}$$

where λ_k is the weight of the kth feature, i and i' index the 3D connected regions (in different slices), and μ is the weight of the pairwise feature. The unary features are computed for each r_i and are the most decisive factor for labeling $a_i \in \{T, N\}$, while the pairwise features are to exploit the 3D structural information for a consistent labeling throughout an ROI volume.

The idea is then to search for a labeling combination for V, so that the total energy cost is minimum, leading to a labeling set that would be optimized for the whole 3D volume. Graph cut[23] is used to derive the most probable labeling A^* that minimizes the energy function: $A^* = \operatorname{argmin}_A E(A|V)$.

Unary Term:

The unary term $\sum_k \lambda_k F_k(a_i, V)$ (denoted as $\psi(a_i)$) indicates the labeling preference of individual region r_i. Specifically, given label a_i for region r_i, a higher $\psi(a_i)$ means a higher cost (i.e. lower probability) of r_i belonging to a_i. The unary term could thus be considered as a binary classifier for r_i. We design a highly discriminative feature set describing the spatial and contextual features, and derive the unary cost $\psi(a_i)$ from the classifier output (SVM).

The main distinctive feature between T and N is the location information. In particular, it is generally true that T is in the lung fields while N is in hilar region or in mediastinum. However, quite often T might invade into the mediastinum and appear to be outside of the lung fields. For T that is near to the mediastinum, mislabeling of its surrounding areas would cause T to appear outside of the lung fields. In addition, N could be adjacent to the lung fields, appearing similar to T.

Based on these considerations, we design three types of features to extract from each region r_i that is detected as ROI: (i) Quad-radial global histogram: four radial lines are drawn at $\pm 45°$ and $\pm 135°$, from the geometric center of r_i, and a 12-dimensional histogram H_g is then created to compute the distribution of L, M and ROI in the four radials. (ii) Surrounding contour histogram: a closed contour is drawn outside of r_i, with a displacement of d from the boundary of r_i, and a three-dimensional histogram H_s is then created to count the percentages of L, M and ROI in the surrounding contour. (iii) Pleural distances: a four-dimensional vector D containing the distances between r_i and the lateral, medial, anterior, and posterior sides of the nearest lung field are computed.

To compute the unary cost, a binary SVM is used to classify r_i to T or N categories based on its feature vector $\{H_g, H_s, D\}$, with a probability estimate p_{a_i} for each category. The unary cost is then computed as $\psi(a_i) = 1 - p_{a_i}$, to produce two cost values for each r_i. Furthermore, we observe that the regions nearer to the boundary of the ROI volume are more prone to mislabeling. Therefore, the unary cost is refined with a Gaussian weight ω_i based on the distance between r_i and the volume center:

$$\psi(a_i) = \omega_i(1 - p_{a_i}); \quad \omega_i = \exp(-\frac{(z_i - z_c)^2}{2\sigma^2}) \tag{5}$$

where z_i and z_c are the z coordinates of r_i and the center of the volume, and σ is calculated as $1/2$ of the size of the volume.

Pairwise Term:

The pairwise term $\mu G(a_i, a_{i'}, V)$ (denoted as $\phi(a_i, a_{i'})$) is useful in promoting spatial consistency between spatially connected regions r_i and $r_{i'}$. Specifically, a cost is assigned as $\phi(a_i, a_{i'})$ if r_i and $r_{i'}$ are labeled differently. The regions r_i and $r_{i'}$ are considered spatially connected if they are part of the same 3D ROI volume. The pairwise term thus explores the inter-slice and volume-level information for refined labeling.

We define the pairwise cost as:

$$\phi(a_i, a_{i'}) = \delta(a_i - a_{i'}) \cdot x'; \quad x' = \frac{1}{1 + \exp(-C(x - 0.5))} \tag{6}$$

where $\delta(a_i - a_{i'})$ is 0 or 1 indicating the same or different labelings of r_i and $r_{i'}$, and x' is the cost value, which is a sigmoid normalization of the actual cost: $x = \alpha(r_i, r_{i'}) \cdot \beta(r_i, r_{i'})$.

The factor $\alpha(r_i, r_{i'})$ measures the spatial distances between the two regions. The value of $\alpha(r_i, r_{i'})$ is in $[0, 1]$ range, and is larger if the distance between r_i and $r_{i'}$ is smaller. Such a computation is similar to the usual CRF formulation, but is based on the spatial distances, rather than intensity differences; and the pairwise cost is computed between all pairs of regions of a 3D ROI volume, rather than only for those neighboring regions. The factor $\beta(r_i, r_{i'})$ is computed as the degree of overlap in the xy plane between the two regions in different slices. This factor is introduced because in some cases, adjacent T and N volumes could actually form into one 3D volume. With the $\alpha(r_i, r_{i'})$ factor alone, the regions in T and N would be all correlated, and the lowest energy solution would tend to produce a single label for the joint volume.

1.3.3. *Tumor Region Refinement*

In the third stage, we identify high uptake in the myocardium as a false positive tumor volume and update its labeling to M. This is based on the usual assumption that images showing a high SUV in the myocardium should be considered normal, and a tumor detected in such an area should be ignored.[12]

Given a detected tumor volume T_q, if it is at the left half of the thorax, a CRF model is employed to classify T_q to either M or T category, depending on the likelihood of T_q representing a high-uptake in the myocardium or a lung tumor. Defining T_q as a series of regions $\{r_i : i = 1, ..., N_O\}$, with each r_i representing a set of connected T regions in a slice, the CRF model is designed based on the same construct as in the second stage, but with a different set of features for the unary term: (i) Pleural Distances: the signed distances between r_i and the four sides of the left lung field is computed. (ii) Shape of Lung Field: a HOG descriptor[24] is used to describe the shape of the left lung field that r_i is adjacent to. A binary SVM is then used to classify r_i to either M or T, and the unary cost is computed from the probability estimates of the classifier.

1.3.4. *Experimental Results*

The dataset used in this study comprised image scans from 85 patients diagnosed with NSCLC, acquired using a Siemens TrueV 64 PET-CT scanner at the Royal Prince Alfred Hospital, Sydney. A total of 93 lung tumors and 65 abnormal lymph nodes were annotated. During the preprocessing, the PET images were linearly interpolated to the same voxel size as the CT images, and FDG uptake normalized into SUV based on the injected dose and patient's weight.

We compared our results to the previous method,[19] which was the only work that addressed the detection of tumor and involved lymph nodes. Since the original

Table 1. Performance comparison with other methods. * indicates rerun results on current dataset. R means recall and P means precision.

Method	Test size	# T	# N	T-R	T-P	N-R	N-P
Proposed method	85 cases	93	65	97.9	88.4	86.2	88.9
Song et.al.[19]	50 cases	53	36	84.4	83.8	77.8	76.9
Song et.al.[19]*	85 cases	93	65	89.3	79.1	72.3	82.5

work[19] was evaluated on a different dataset, we repeated the test on the current dataset. As shown in Table 1, our method exhibited clear improvements, which were mainly attributed to three factors: (i) fewer abnormal lymph nodes mislabeled as tumors, especially for those nodes lying close to the lung fields, with the spatial and contextual features (unary term); (ii) fewer tumors mislabeled as abnormal lymph nodes, especially those previously caused by inconsistent labeling of regions in one tumor volume, with the spatially-smoothed 3D volume labeling (pairwise term); and (iii) fewer high-uptake areas in the myocardium mislabeled as abnormalities.

1.4. *Data Adaptive Structure Estimation*

While the multi-stage discriminative model is fairly effective for lesion detection, it relies mainly on complicated and domain-specific feature design. These features are designed based on domain knowledge and empirical studies, and so their effectiveness may be restricted to the limited scenarios available in the datasets, and might be difficult to generalize to a larger variation of cases.

Therefore, we proposed a different approach to the detection problem – after detecting all abnormalities, if we can identify the actual lung fields (tumors inclusive), then we can differentiate lung tumors and abnormal lymph nodes based on the degree of overlap between the detected abnormality and the lung fields.[5] The main problem is how to estimate the original lung fields if the subject had been healthy. Limited studies exist in this area, and are mostly based on statistical shape model,[25,26] with time-consuming registration[25] or complex landmark detections.[26]

Since precise lung segmentation is not required for lesion detection, but a fair estimation of the overlap would suffice, we design a simpler atlas-based approach. Our design is similar to the approach[27] that obtains brain segmentation masks from multiple weak segmenters. Different from local-level computation,[28] the regression-based combination[27] minimizes the weighted difference for the whole image. However, its direct derivation of segmentation from other labeling outputs might impose a stringent requirement on the weight learning, which would be difficult to apply to the thoracic images due to the large variations of anatomical structures caused by lesions. This motivates us to opt for an indirect approach, with intermediate multi-atlas modeling of the feature space and a further classification for final labeling.

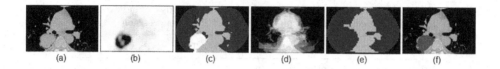

Fig. 3.   Method illustration.[5] (a) An axial CT slice (after preprocessing). (b) The co-registered
PET slice, where the dark region indicates a lung tumor with increased FDG uptake and a high
SUV. (c) Output of the initial abnormality detection, showing the lung fields, mediastinum and
abnormality with increasing grayscale values. (d) The appearance model generated with regression,
approximating the CT intensities if without the lung tumor. (e) Output of the graph-based
structure labeling for lung fields and medaistinum. (f) The detection output after tumor/lymph
node classification, with tumor highlighted in dark gray.

Our approach[5] consists of the following steps. All abnormalities are detected
via region-based classification. Then, the actual lung structure is estimated, with
regression and graph-based techniques. Thirdly, the detected abnormalities are
classified as tumors or abnormal lymph nodes based on contextual features. Fig. 3
illustrates the overall method.

1.4.1. *Initial Abnormality Detection*

The thoracic PET-CT images are first preprocessed to remove the background and
soft tissues outside of the lung and mediastinum with morphological operations. All
images are then aligned and rescaled to the same size. Next, the abnormalities are
detected by classifying the mean-shift clustered regions into lung fields (L), mediastinum (M) or abnormalities (O)[19] (Fig. 3c). The high-uptake in the myocardium
is masked-out based on its size, spatial location within the thorax and the shape of
the left lung field.

1.4.2. *Adaptive Structure Estimation*

To differentiate between lung tumors and abnormal lymph nodes, a general rule
is that lung tumors should be inside the lung fields, while lymph nodes are outside. However, as shown in Fig. 3c, due to the lung tumor, only a portion of the
right lung field is correctly identified, and the tumor then appears outside the lung
fields. Therefore, we need to estimate the actual lung fields before the tumor growth
(Fig. 3e). Given a 3D thoracic PET-CT volume I, our objective is to label each
voxel i to the lung field or mediastinum type. To do this, the thoracic appearance is
first modeled from a set of reference images, then the voxels are classified as L/M.

Regression-based Appearance Model:
   Although patient-specific conditions, such as body weights, introduce variational
factors, there is great similarity between images for the normal structures. It is thus
a fair assumption that one image can be approximated by a weighted combination

of multiple images. Therefore, we model the CT appearance of the original thoracic structures (Fig. 3d) based on other reference images.

We first introduce a basic formulation for the appearance model. Let $y \in \mathbb{R}^{n \times 1}$ be the n-dimensional feature vector (i.e. voxel-wise CT intensities) of I, and $D \in \mathbb{R}^{n \times K}$ be the matrix of K feature vectors from K reference images I_k $(n \gg K)$. The difference between y and the weighted combination of D should then be minimized: $\min_x \| y - Dx \|_2^2$, where $x \in \mathbb{R}^{K \times 1}$ is the weight vector; and Dx is the original appearance of I approximated.

With the derived x, each reference image I_k is assigned one weight x_k, and hence all voxels in I_k contribute equally to the approximated appearance. However, due to the non-rigid structure of the thorax and presence of the abnormalities, it is normal that only a portion of I_k is similar to I and the rest should take lower weights. Therefore, we incorporate a voxel-wise similarity-based weight vector for each I_k. For voxel i_k of image I_k, the weight $w_{i,k}$ is computed as:

$$w_{i,k} = \frac{1}{\alpha_i} \exp(-\frac{1}{\beta_i} \| i - i_k \|_2), \ \beta_i = \sum_{k=1}^{K} \| i - i_k \|_2 \tag{7}$$

where α_i is to normalize $\sum_k w_{i,k} = 1$. With the weight matrix $W = \{w_{i,k}\} \in \mathbb{R}^{n \times K}$, the regression formulation thus becomes: $\min_x \| y - (W \circ D)x \|_2^2$.

Furthermore, while the above formulation is sufficient to obtain a closely matching appearance model, the L/M labeling information is not utilized. Since the final objective is to achieve accurate structure labeling, it is natural to integrate the supervised information to enhance the discriminative power:

$$\min_x \| y - (W \circ D)x \|_2^2 + \| h - (W \circ A)x \|_2^2$$
$$= \min_x \| \begin{pmatrix} y \\ h \end{pmatrix} - \begin{pmatrix} W \circ D \\ W \circ A \end{pmatrix} x \|_2^2 \qquad = \min_x \| f - \Omega x \|_2^2 \tag{8}$$

where $h \in \{1, 2, 1.5\}^{n \times 1}$ is the label vector of I from the initial detection outputs (1=L, 2=M, and 1.5=O), and $A \in \{1, 2\}^{n \times K}$ for the reference images from the ground truth. The value 1.5 is chosen to have equal distance between O/L and between O/M, to assign no preference for matching such areas with L or M. Both h and A are normalized to the same range as y and D, and the approximated appearance model is then $(W \circ D)x$ and the labeling $(W \circ A)x$.

Finally, to avoid overfitting, we choose to not have all reference images contributing to the appearance approximation, with a sparse regularization:

$$\min_x \| f - \Omega x \|_2^2, \ s.t. \ \| x \|_0 \leq C \tag{9}$$

where C is the constant number of reference images we limit to. The OMP algorithm[29] is then used to solve x.

To compute the feature vector y, we divide I into multiple sections, each with three slices, and y is then derived for each section. To construct D, since the reference images also contain lung tumors or abnormal lymph nodes, rather than simply concatenating all voxels, the annotated tumor voxels are replaced with the average intensity of the lung fields labeled at the initial detection step.

Graph-based Structure Labeling:

Next, based on the appearance model (Fig. 3d), we classify the lung fields and mediastinum (Fig. 3e). A straightforward idea is to use the approximated labeling $(W \circ A)x$ as the classification output. However, such labelings can be erroneous especially for the boundary areas of tumors. Therefore, we design a further graph-based classification step for the structure labeling.

We first define a notation for the appearance model: $G = \{g_i\} = (W \circ D)x$, where g_i is the approximated intensity for voxel i. The problem is thus to derive a label set $V = \{v_i \in \{L, M\}\}$, to classify each voxel to category L or M.

We observe that the mislabeled parts usually appear lighter in G but still darker than the real mediastinum. This thus motivates us to encode contrast information for the labeling. To do this, from G, we first calculate the mean values (m) and the graylevel histograms (d) of the lung field and mediastinum (labeled during the initial abnormality detection). A 5-dimensional feature vector q_i is then computed for each voxel i: (i) g_i; (ii) g_i/m_L; (iii) g_i/m_M; (iv) $Pr[g_i \leq d_L \leq 256]$; and (v) $Pr[1 \leq d_M \leq g_i]$.

In addition to q_i, which incorporates the global-level information m and d, contrast information can also be described in a pairwise fashion. Specifically, for two voxels i and j, if g_i and g_j are similar and they are spatially close, they would likely take the same label. Hence we define the difference $s_{i,j}$ between i and j based on their intensity $|g_i - g_j|$ and spatial $\|i - j\|_2$ distances:

$$s_{i,j} = \log(\|i - j\|_2 + 1) \times \log(|g_i - g_j| + 1) \tag{10}$$

A lower $s_{i,j}$ would imply a higher probability of $v_i = v_j$.

We then design a CRF construct to integrate both q_i and $s_{i,j}$ to label G, with the following energy function:

$$E(V|G) = \sum_i \phi(v_i) + \sum_{i,j} \psi(v_i, v_j) \tag{11}$$

Here $\phi(v_i)$ represents the cost of i taking the label v_i, computed as $1 - p(v_i|q_i)$; and $p(.)$ is the probability estimate from a binary liner-kernel SVM classifier based on q_i. The pairwise term $\psi(v_i, v_j)$ penalizes the labeling difference between i and j.

Note that our pairwise term connects longer distance voxels to encourage consistent labelings for similar voxels, not limited to neighboring voxels as the traditional CRF construct. However, to ensure a sparse graph, a voxel i should be linked to a small number of other voxels only. Therefore, we introduce a constant threshold tr, so that $s_{i,j} = 0$, if $|g_i - g_j| > tr$. The labeling set V is then derived by minimizing $E(V|G)$ using graph cut.

Table 2. The detection recall and precision.

	Tumor	Node	Tumor[19]	Node[19]
Recall (%)	90.7	88.6	84.4	77.8
Precision (%)	89.1	88.6	83.8	76.9

1.4.3. *Feature Extraction and Classification*

Based on the estimated thoracic structure V (Fig. 3e), we then classify the detected abnormalities (O) into tumors (T) or abnormal lymph nodes (N) (Fig. 3f). A simple 4-dimensional feature vector is designed: (i) size of O; (ii) size of overlap between O and lung field labeled in V; (iii) size of overlap between O and mediastinum labeled in V; and (iv) size of overlap between O and the convex hull of lung field detected during initial abnormality detection. Features (ii)–(iv) are also normalized by the size of O. A binary linear-kernel SVM is then trained to classify O to T or N. To enhance the error tolerance, the classification is performed on a section basis as well, and the final T/N label is produced based on a weighted averaging of the probability estimates from each section. The weights are computed as $\exp(-d/\eta)$, where d is the distance between the section and center of O, and η is the maximum distance possible for O.

1.4.4. *Experimental Results*

The experiment was performed on 50 sets of 3D thoracic PET-CT images from patients with NSCLC. A total of 54 lung tumors and 35 abnormal lymph nodes were annotated as the ground truth. For each data set, the contour of lung field was also roughly delineated – we allowed some error margins in the delineation since we did not expect precise lung segmentation. Five images were selected as the training set for both structure labeling and classification between tumors and lymph nodes. The data sets were then randomly divided into five sets; and within each set, each image was used as the testing image, with the other nine as the reference images.

The usefulness of each components in the structure estimation was first analyzed. With the proposed graph-based structure labeling, we evaluated the appearance model with different constructs of the regression method. With the fixed regression-based appearance model, we then evaluated the structure labeling with different graphical constructs. The results clearly demonstrated the advantage of our proposed appearance model and the structure labeling. The overall detection recall and precision are shown in Table 2. The results exhibited marked improvement over our previous work,[19] especially for the abnormal lymph nodes; and it suggested the effectiveness of our approach for differentiating the two abnormalities, by mainly analyzing the degree of overlap between the detected abnormality and the estimated lung structures.

2. Thoracic Image Retrieval

In the past three decades, the volume of medical image data has rapidly expanded. Patient images are normally stored in the picture archiving and communication systems (PACS); and the vast amount of these data also opens an opportunity for case-based reasoning or evidence-based medicine support.[30] When a physician makes a diagnosis based on a patient scan, the physician may choose to browse through similar images in the database as a reference set to help reach the correct diagnosis. The ability to find images with similar content is thus important to facilitate diagnosis. In this section, we review the state-of-the-art in medical image retrieval, and describe our approaches[3,31] for the thoracic PET-CT.

2.1. Review of State-of-the-art

A typical content-based image retrieval (CBIR) system comprises three main components: feature extraction for image representation, similarity measure between feature descriptors, and image indexing for retrieval.[32] In the medical domain, since different disease patterns and imaging modalities (e.g. X-ray, CT, magnetic resonance imaging, PET-CT) are best characterized by different types of features, the majority of image retrieval studies focus on feature extractions,[33–39] designed for specific anatomical structures. The various types of features explored include intensity values,[35] textures describing the tissue appearances,[34,36,37,39,40] and shapes of anatomical structures.[38] Contextual features describing organ-related spatial information have also been recently incorporated.[36,39,41] However, most of these contextual features designed still largely resemble the standard feature descriptors, not optimized for the particular medical imaging problem. As a result, the retrieved images would still be mainly similar in their visual appearances, but not in terms of anatomical or pathological information.

In thoracic PET-CT, images representing similar pathological characteristics can be used as references to achieve accurate staging of NSCLC. The retrieved images are thus expected to exhibit a similar spatial extent for the lung tumor and disease spread in regional lymph nodes. Fig. 4 shows tumors in various locations. Studies in thoracic PET-CT image retrieval include design of overlapping[42] and graph-based features.[43] Both approaches rely on segmentation of thoracic structures and lesions, which however, might not error-prone with simple thresholding-based techniques. Our initial work[44] does not require precise segmentation, but it is designed for 2D image retrieval only. We have developed various learning-based similarity measure techniques,[19,45,46] which can be integrated with any feature representation.

2.2. Pathological Feature Description

In our work, we first proposed an image retrieval method,[3] which finds images exhibiting similar pathological features that are extracted based on the lesion

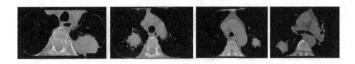

Fig. 4. Four examples of fused thoracic PET-CT images (transaxial slices). The images depict tumors at different locations in the lung fields, and in two images showing the tumors adjacent to the chest wall and the mediastinum.

detection results. As described in Section 1.2, tumors (T) and abnormal lymph nodes (N) are detected as 3D objects. The feature of a 3D T or N object F_{obj} is computed as a weighted combination of the feature vectors F_r of the comprising image slices. F_r is computed from the bounding box of the T/N region in the image slice. The weight of an image slice is adaptively assigned as its mean CT intensity and PET SUV, so that slices with more salient features would carry higher weights. A case is then represented by two feature vectors F_T and F_N, characterizing its tumor and lymph node appearances. The distance between the query case X and the reference case Y is then defined as the weighted intersection differences, with weights defined based on the volumes of the T or N objects.

2.3. *Spatial Feature Encoding*

The simple pathological feature description is usually insufficient to represent the large variations in spatial contexts of different cases, and would thus impact the retrieval performance. The most widely used spatial feature descriptor is the circular or square histogram.[36,47,48] The drawback of these feature descriptors is that they might not accommodate spatial variations well, due to the fixed grid structures. The hierarchical subdivision scheme, such as spatial pyramid matching (SPM),[49,50] are able to balance between the subdividing and disordering to a certain extent with a multi-scale design. We have designed spatial descriptors[51,52] based on the concept of SPM. However, such approaches might be still too rigid to handle the large inter-subject variations because of the even subdivision.

To better describe the pathological features, we then proposed a hierarchical contextual spatial descriptor,[31] with an adequate balance between its discriminative capability and geometric-transformation invariance suitable for the thoracic imaging domain. Fig. 5 gives an overview of the proposed method.

2.3.1. *Pathological Centroid Detection*

To build the spatial descriptor, we first detect the centroid of the pathology, which is the geometric center of a tumor. To do this, we first extract the maximally stable extremal regions (MSER)[53] from the image grid of feature words W_I. Next, the region of pathology is selected from the MSER outputs, by choosing the inner-most region that normally represents the center area of the tumor. The geometric center

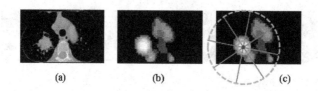

(a)   (b)   (c)

Fig. 5. Illustration of the proposed feature extraction and representation.[31] (a) A fused PET-CT slice, showing a primary lung tumor. (b) The feature-word grid, representing each image patch with its feature word value. (c) The hierarchical partition of the spatial contexts, showing only the level-2 structure for simplicity, with circles depicting the concentric circles, the dot at the center indicating the tumor centroid p_o, and ray lines dividing the radials.

of this detected region is thus the tumor centroid, and denoted by the patch index as p_o (example as illustrated in Fig. 5).

2.3.2. Context-based Partitioning Model

Based on the grid of feature words W_I and the pathological centroid p_o, we then formulate the spatial features using a context-based partitioning model. We incorporate the hierarchical partitioning concept similar to SPM; but rather than dividing a rectangle cell evenly into 4 sub-cells as in SPM, we design a hierarchical circular structure, as illustrated in Fig. 5. The circular model is more suitable here mainly because: (1) usually tumors are close to blob-like shapes; and (2) anatomical structures surrounding the tumors can be better fitted into radials rather than rectangles.

We define L as the total levels of hierarchy, with individual levels $l \in \{0, 1, ..., L-1\}$. At each level l, 4^l radials are created with the partitions of 2^{l-1} concentric circles while each circle is divided into 2^{l+1} radials. The overall spatial descriptor H_I of image I is concatenated from the feature vectors of individual levels: $H_I = \{H_I^l : l = 0, ..., L-1\}$, with a dimension of $K \sum_{l=0}^{L-1} 4^l$.

At level-0, there is actually no partitioning, and a circle O_I centered at p_o is created with radius r_I the largest distance between p_o and the image border. All feature words in O_I are accumulated into a weighted histogram $H_I^{l=0}$, with each feature word w_i Gaussian weighted according to its Chebyshev distance from p_o. At level-1, the circle O_I is evenly divided into $J = 4$ radials $O_I = \{R_{I,j} : j = 1, ..., J\}$ from the centroid p_o. The feature vector of each radial is then computed in the same way as level-0. At a higher level ($l \geq 2$), 4^l radials are then created from O_I in a similar way.

When creating the radials, rather than partitioning at fixed angles, our approach is to create a partition that minimizes the co-occurrences of multiple structure types within one radial, to reduce fragmented segments due to dividing in homogeneous regions. Denote the jth radial as $R_I(j, \theta)$ with θ representing the direction of the basis radial. The total variance $v_I(J, \theta)$ of such a partition is:

$$v_I(J, \theta) = \sum_{j=1}^{J} \sum_{i=1}^{N} (w_i - m_j)^2, \; s.t. \; p_i \in R_I(j, \theta) \tag{12}$$

where m_j is the mean of the feature words of radial $R_I(j, \theta)$. The best partition structure is thus the one resulting in the smallest variance: $\theta = argmin_\theta v_I(J, \theta)$, $\forall \theta = \{0, \frac{\pi}{2J}, \frac{\pi}{J}, \frac{3\pi}{2J}\}$. Here we choose to test four possible θ only, for convenient implementation and better efficiency.

2.3.3. *Similarity Measure*

To measure the degree of similarity between two images I (the query image) and J (the reference image), we compute the difference between feature descriptors H_I and H_J as a weighted histogram-intersection distance.[19] Images with smaller distances with the query image I are then retrieved as the searching results.

2.3.4. *Experimental Results*

For evaluation, a PET-CT database containing 50 sets of image scans from subjects diagnosed with NSCLC was used. We selected three key slices depicting the primary lung tumor from each patient scan, forming a database of 150 PET-CT slices. The ground truth indicating the similar or dissimilar relationships between each pair of slices were annotated. Two images were considered similar, if the tumors were in similar locations in the thorax (e.g. anterior or posterior), and showed similar spatial relationships relative to the chest wall and the mediastinum.

The retrieval performance was quantitatively compared with other methods, including two previous approaches proposed for tumor retrieval on PET-CT images,[19,52] and several techniques based on more standard algorithms (bag-of-words, SPM, and SIFT[54] features). Our proposed approach demonstrated clear performance improvements.

3. Summary

We have presented a brief review of our recent work on lesion detection and image retrieval for thoracic PET-CT imaging. For lesion detection, we described three different methods: region-based feature classification, multi-stage discriminative model, and data-adaptive structure estimation. While the second method is highly effective with its structural labeling and more discriminative features, the third approach requires only a simple feature set that is less empirical. For image retrieval, we described two different methods: pathological feature description, and spatial feature encoding. The second method presents a more discriminative hierarchical contextual spatial descriptor and improved the retrieval performance significantly. It is also worth noting that while some of the approaches, such as the region-based classification and multi-stage discriminative model, were customized towards the specific problem domain, the data adaptive structure estimation and spatial feature encoding are more general and can be extended to other imaging applications.

References

1. S. B. Edge, D. R. Byrd, C. C. Compton, A. G. Fritz, F. L. Greene, and A. Trotti (Eds.), *AJCC cancer staging handbook, 7th ed.* (Springer, 2010).
2. W. D. Wever, S. Stroobants, J. Coolen, and J. A. Verschakelen, Integrated PET/CT in the staging of nonsmall cell lung cancer: technical aspects and clinical integration, *Eur. Respir. J.* **33**, 201–212, (2009).
3. Y. Song, W. Cai, S. Eberl, M. J. Fulham, and D. Feng, Thoracic image case retrieval with spatial and contextual information, *in Proc. ISBI.* pp. 1885–1888, (2011).
4. Y. Song, W. Cai, J. Kim, and D. Feng, A multi-stage discriminative model for tumor and lymph node detection in thoracic images, *IEEE Trans. Med. Imag.* **31**(5), 1061–1075, (2012).
5. Y. Song, W. Cai, Y. Zhou, and D. Feng, Thoracic abnormality detection with data adaptive structure estimation, *in MICCAI, LNCS.* **7510**, 74–81, (2012).
6. I. Jafar, H. Ying, A. F. Shields, and O. Muzik, Computerized detection of lung tumors in PET/CT images, *in Proc. EMBC.* pp. 2320–2323, (2006).
7. Y. Cui, B. Zhao, T. J. Akhurst, J. Yan, and L. H. Schwartz, CT-guided automated detection of lung tumors on PET images, *in SPIE Med. Imaging.* **6915**, 69152N, (2008).
8. C. Ballangan, X. Wang, S. Eberl, M. Fulham, and D. Feng, Automated lung tumor segmentation for whole body PET volume based on novel downhill region growing, *in SPIE Med. Imaging.* **7623**, 76233O, (2010).
9. J. Gubbi, A. Kanakatte, T. Kron, D. Binns, B. Srinivasan, N. Mani, and M. Palaniswami, Automatic tumour volume delineation in respiratory-gated PET images, *J. Med. Imag. Radia. Oncol.* **55**, 65–76, (2011).
10. G. V. Saradhi, G. Gopalakrishnan, A. S. Roy, R. Mullick, R. Manjeshwar, K. Thielemans, and U. Patil, A framework for automated tumor detection in thoracic FDG PET images using texture-based features, *in Proc. ISBI.* pp. 97–100, (2009).
11. S. Renisch, R. Opfer, and R. Wiemker, Towards automatic determination of total tumor burden from PET images, *in SPIE Med. Imaging.* **7624**, 76241T, (2010).
12. H. Gutte, D. Jakobsson, F. Olofsson, M. Ohlsson, S. Valind, A. Loft, L. Edenbrandt, and A. Kjaer, Automated interpretation of PET/CT images in patients with lung cancer, *Nucl. Med. Commun.* **28**(2), 79–84, (2007).
13. Y. Song, W. Cai, S. Eberl, M. Fulham, and D. Feng, Automatic detection of lung tumor and abnormal regional lymph nodes in PET-CT images, *J. Nucl. Med. 52.* **52** (Supplement 1), 211, (2011).
14. Y. Song, W. Cai, and D. Feng, Global context inference for adaptive abnormality detection in PET-CT images, *in Proc. ISBI.* pp. 482–485, (2012).
15. Y. Song, W. Cai, H. Huang, Y. Wang, and D. Feng, Object localization in medical images based on graphical model with contrast and interest-region terms, *in Proc. CVPR Workshop.* pp. 1–7, (2012).
16. Y. Song, W. Cai, S. Eberl, M. J. Fulham, and D. Feng, Region and learning based retrieval for multi-modality medical images, *in Proc. Biomed.* pp. 723–063, (2011).
17. P. Perona and J. Malik, Scale-space and edge detection using anisotropic diffusion, *IEEE Trans. Pattern Anal. Mach. Intell.* **12**, 629–639, (1990).

18. C. Cortes and V. Vapnik, Support-vector networks, *Machine Learning.* **20**(3), 273–297, (1995).

19. Y. Song, W. Cai, S. Eberl, M. Fulham, and D. Feng, Discriminative pathological context detection in thoracic images based on multi-level inference, *in MICCAI, LNCS.* **6893**, 191–198, (2011).

20. Y. Song, W. Cai, S. Eberl, M. Fulham, and D. Feng, A content-based image retrieval framework for multi-modality lung images, *in Proc. CBMS.* pp. 285–290, (2010).

21. A. Vedaldi and S. Soatto, Quick shift and kernel methods for mode seeking, *in ECCV, LNCS.* **5305**, 705–718, (2008).

22. J. Lafferty, A. McCallum, and F. Pereira, Conditional random fields: probabilistic models for segmenting and labeling sequence data, *in Proc. ICML.* pp. 282–289, (2001).

23. V. Kolmogorov and R. Zabih, What energy functions can be minimized via graph cuts?, *IEEE Trans. Pattern Anal. Mach. Intell.* **26**(2), 147–159, (2004).

24. N. Dalal and B. Triggs, Histograms of oriented gradients for human detection, *in Proc. CVPR.* pp. 886–893, (2005).

25. I. Sluimer, M. Prokop, and B. van Ginneken, Toward automated segmentation of the pathological lung in CT, *IEEE Trans. Med. Imag.* **24**(8), 1025–1038, (2005).

26. M. Sofka, J. Wetzl, N. Birkbeck, J. Zhang, T. Kohlberger, J. Kaftan, J. Declerck, and S. K. Zhou, Multi-stage learning for robust lung segmentation in challenging CT volumes, *in MICCAI, LNCS.* pp. 667–674, (2011).

27. T. Chen, B. C. Vemuri, A. Rangarajan, and S. J. Eisenschenk, Mixture of segmenters with discriminative spatial regularization and sparse weight selection, *in MICCAI, LNCS.* pp. 595–602, (2011).

28. F. Rousseau, P. A. Habas, and C. Studholme, Human brain labeling using image similarities, *in Proc. CVPR.* pp. 1081–1088, (2011).

29. J. Tropp, Greed is good: Algorithmic results for sparse approximation, *IEEE Trans. Inform. Theory.* **50**, 2231–2242, (2004).

30. H. Muller, N. Michoux, D. Bandon, and A. Geissbuhler, A review of content-based image retrieval systems in medical applications - clinical benefits and future directions, *Int. J. Med. Inform.* **73**, 1–23, (2004).

31. Y. Song, W. Cai, Y. Zhou, L. Wen, and D. D. Feng, Hierarchical spatial matching for medical image retrieval, *in Proc. ISBI.* pp. 1–4, (2013).

32. W. Cai, J. Kim, and D. Feng, Content-based medical image retrieval, *Biomedical Information Technology, Chapter 4.* pp. 83–113, Edited by D. Feng, Elsevier, (2008).

33. W. Cai, D. Feng, and R. Fulton, Content-based retrieval of dynamic PET functional images, *IEEE Trans. Inf. Technol. Biomed.* **4**(2), 152–158, (2000).

34. W. Cai, S. Liu, L. Wen, S. Eberl, M. J. Fulham, and D. Feng, 3D neurological image retrieval with localized pathology-centric CMRGlc patterns, *in Proc. ICIP.* pp. 3201–3204, (2010).

35. B. Fischer, A. Brosig, P. Welter, C. Grouls, R. W. Gunther, and T. M. Deserno, Content-based image retrieval applied to bone age assessment, *in Proc. SPIE.* p. 762412, (2010).

36. D. Unay, A. Ekin, and R. S. Jasinschi, Local structure-based region-of-interest retrieval in brain MR images, *IEEE Trans. Inf. Technol. Biomed.* **14**(4), 897–903, (2010).

37. L. Sorensen, M. Loog, P. Lo, H. Ashraf, A. Dirksen, R. P. W. Duin, and M. D. Bruijne, Image dissimilarity-based quantification of lung disease from CT, *in MICCAI, LNCS.* **6361**, 37–44, (2010).

38. X. Qian, H. D. Tagare, R. K. Fulbright, R. Long, and S. Antani, Optimal embedding for shape indexing in medical image databases, *Med. Imag. Anal.* **14**, 243–254, (2010).

39. U. Avni, H. Greenspan, E. Konen, M. Sharon, and J. Goldberger, X-ray image categorization and retrieval on the organ and pathology level, using patch-based visual words, *IEEE Trans. Med. Imag.* **30**(3), 733–746, (2011).

40. A. Depeursinge, A. Vargas, A. Platon, A. Geissbuhler, P. A. Poletti, and H. Muller, Building a reference multimedia database for interstitial lung diseases, *Comput. Med. Imag. Graph. (2011)*. (2011).

41. S. Yu, C. Chiang, and C. Hsieh, A three-object model for the similarity searches of chest CT images, *Comput. Med. Imag. Graph.* **29**, 617–630, (2005).

42. J. Kim, L. Constantinescu, W. Cai, and D. Feng, Content-based dual-modality biomedical data retrieval using co-aligned functional and anatomical features, *in MICCAI Workshop, LNCS.* pp. 45–52, (2007).

43. A. Kumar, J. Kim, L. Wen, and D. Feng, A graph-based approach to the retrieval of volumetric PET-CT lung images, *in Proc. EMBC.* pp. 5408–5411, (2012).

44. Y. Song, W. Cai, S. Eberl, M. Fulham, and D. Feng, Structure-adaptive feature extraction and representation for multi-modality lung images retrieval, *in Proc. DICTA.* pp. 152–157, (2010).

45. Y. Song, W. Cai, and D. Feng, Disease-specific context modeling and retrieval with fast structure localization, *in MMBIA.* pp. 89–94, (2012).

46. W. Cai, Y. Song, and D. Feng, Regression and classification based distance metric learning for medical image retrieval, *in Proc. ISBI.* pp. 1775–1778, (2012).

47. S. Belongie, J. Malik, and J. Puzicha, Shape matching and object recognition using shape contexts, *IEEE Trans. Pattern Anal. Mach. Intell.* **24**(24), 509–522, (2002).

48. M. M. Rahman, S. K. Antani, and G. R. Thoma, A medical image retrieval framework in correlation enhanced visual concept feature space, *in Proc. CBMS.* pp. 1–4, (2009).

49. S. Lazebnik, C. Schmid, and J. Ponce, Beyond bags of features: spatial pyramid matching for recognizing natural scene categories, *in Proc. CVPR.* pp. 2169–2178, (2006).

50. J. Feulner, S. K. Zhou, E. Angelopoulou, S. Seifert, A. Cavallaro, J. Hornegger, and D. Comaniciu, Comparing axial CT slices in quantized N-dimensional SURF descriptor space to estimate the visible body region, *Comput. Med. Imag. Graph.* **35**(3), 227–236, (2011).

51. Y. Song, W. Cai, S. Eberl, M. Fulham, and D. Feng, Thoracic image matching with appearance and spatial distribution, *in Proc. EMBC.* pp. 4469–4472, (2011).

52. Y. Song, W. Cai, and D. D. Feng, Hierarchical spatial matching for medical image retrieval, *in Proc. ACM MM Workshop.* pp. 1–6, (2011).

53. J. Matas, O. Chum, M. Urban, and T. Pajdla, Robust wide baseline stereo from maximally stable extremal regions, *in Proc. BMVC.* pp. 384–396, (2002).

54. D. G. Lowe, Distinctive image features from scale-invariant keypoints, *Int. J. Comput. Vis.* **60**(2), 91–110, (2004).

CHAPTER 6

A NOVEL PARADIGM FOR QUANTITATION FROM MR PHASE

Joseph Dagher

Department of Electrical and Computer Engineering, University of Arizona, Tucson, AZ
E-mail: jdagher@email.arizona.edu

Numerous imaging methods require accurate quantitation from MR phase in order to extract important information about the underlying physiology or tissue property. Common to most emerging techniques is the need to unwrap and de-noise the measured phase. Whether the MR images are acquired at one or multiple echo time points, there exists inherent ambiguities about the underlying phase signal. A common class of "spatial phase regularization" algorithms, such as phase unwrapping and de-noising, attempt to resolve these ambiguities. Phase unwrapping attempts to recover ambiguities due to large phase build-up whereas de-noising methods attempt to recover those ambiguities due to small phase measurements. In this work, we rigorously formulate the problem of phase estimation. We quantitate the inherent ambiguities in the measured phase, for a given acquisition strategy. Next, we propose a solution which achieves robust estimates over large dynamic range of phase values, at very high spatial resolutions. Our in vivo results demonstrate substantially improved performance as compared to existing techniques. A key feature of our proposed method is that it does require the use of any spatial-domain processing, such as phase unwrapping or smoothing.

1. Introduction to Phase Mapping in MRI

Consider the measurement obtained using a spin-warp sequence at echo time TE [17,15,14]

$$g(x, y; \text{TE}) = \rho(x, y; \text{TE}) \exp \left\{ i2\pi \Delta B(x, y)\text{TE} \right\} + \mathbf{w}(x, y). \qquad (1)$$

In this equation, $\rho(x, y; \text{TE})$ is the spin density at TE and $\mathbf{w}(x, y)$ is the additive complex-valued Gaussian noise, $w(x, y) = w_R(x, y) + iw_I(x, y)$, with $w_R, w_I \sim \mathcal{N}(0, \sigma_w)$. We draw the reader's attention to the term $\Delta B(x, y)$ in the phase. This term (referred to as the "phase signal") represents any deviation from the magnetic field desired at location (x, y). This has traditionally been caused by hardware limitations (magnetic field/gradient imperfections). But, more recently, it has also been observed that $\Delta B(x, y)$ is introduced by any inherent variation in magnetic susceptibility, such as across different tissue interfaces. For example, in the brain, these inhomogeneities occur around the anterior-frontal regions, temporal lobes and around the sinuses. On a finer resolution scale, $\Delta B(x, y)$ is related to the presence of susceptibility-altering physiology, such as iron deposits, hemorrhages, blood de/oxygenation, fat content, etc. Accurate quantitation from phase maps is thus of critical importance in numerous MR applications, including quantitative susceptibility mapping, susceptibility weighted imaging, functional MRI, fat/water separation, MR thermometry, MR spectroscopy, and various quantitative MR methods [12,22,15,20,13,9]. More specifically, it is of clinical interest to be able to estimate $\Delta B(x, y)$, with high sensitivity, at very high spatial resolutions. Hereafter, we drop the pixel subscripts (x, y) with the understanding that the remaining analysis applies separately to each voxel in the image.

It is clear from Eq. 1 that we can compute ΔB from the slope of the phase of g as a function of TE. However, instead of the actual phase, we are restricted to work with the numerically computed angle, namely,

$$\psi_k = 2\pi\Delta B(\text{TE}_0 + k\Delta\text{TE}) + \mathbf{\Omega}_k + 2\pi\mathbf{r}_k, \tag{2}$$

where ΔTE is the echo spacing, k is the echo index, $k = 0, \ldots, K - 1$, TE_0 is the echo time at $k = 0$, and $\mathbf{\Omega}_k$ is the radian phase contribution of the additive noise term at time index k. Note that the phase noise Random Variable (RV) $\mathbf{\Omega}_k$ is a function of the echo time. The integer $\mathbf{r}_k$ in Eq. 2 is the phase wrapping term, which is non-zero when the sum of the first two terms on the right side of Eq. 2 falls outside $[-\pi, \pi)$. In that case, $\mathbf{r}_k$ forces the total phase back into the observed range $[-\pi, \pi)$.

It is clear from Eq. 2 that estimating the slope of ψ_k is affected by two sources of error: noise and phase wrapping. The contribution of each source to the overall error is determined by the value of ΔB with respect to a cutoff given by

$$\Delta B_{\text{cutoff}} = \frac{1}{2\Delta\text{TE}}. \tag{3}$$

The choice of ΔTE defines three regimes. It is well understood that whenever ΔB in a given voxel is larger than ΔB_{cutoff}, phase aliasing (wrapping) dominates the error in that voxel [6]. To avoid such a wrapping-limited regime (**Regime I**, hereafter), a small value of ΔTE is favored. On the other hand, in voxels where ΔB is small, noise dominates the error in Eq. 2 (**Regime II**) and a large value of ΔTE should be sought. Most phase mapping methods choose moderate values for ΔTE (**Regime III**) in an attempt to trade-off Regimes I and II. However, in addition to noise and phase-wrapping, Regime III is also amenable to noise-driven phase wrapping errors [7,5].

To overcome the resulting inaccuracies, a class of spatio-temporal post-processing algorithms, termed "phase unwrapping," has been proposed [16,7,2,11,23]. An inherent assumption with these methods imposes a smoothness constraint on the measured data. This reduces the spatial resolution of the measurements [6]. Furthermore, the efficiency of phase unwrapping algorithms often depends on the accuracy of the initial phase estimate [7], thus requiring expert user intervention. Finally, phase unwrapping methods are computationally expensive particularly in two-dimensions (2D) and higher where the unwrapping problem becomes NP hard [7,2]. Other existing methods adopt a more statistical approach but also rely on spatial regularization for robust mapping [6,17,23]. Such smoothness assumptions may not be realistic as they do not account for small or abrupt variations common in MR images. This is particularly important in quantitative imaging where physiological information is extracted from phase maps. Ultimately, the performance of all these methods is subject to the trade-off inherent in the choice of the echo time spacing [6]. Furthermore, we note that these trade-offs become even more challenging as the number of captured echoes K decreases. There, balancing between robustness and total scan time is obviously the limiting factor.

Three-echo methods have recently been proposed in the literature. Windischberger *et al.* [21] used irregular echo spacing of 0.5ms (Regime II) and 1.5ms (Regime I) at 3T to demonstrate phase maps over a limited dynamic range of ± 333Hz. Assuming a maximum of a single phase wrap between echo pairs, the authors in [21] applied linear fitting to determine the best fit (in least squares sense) from seven possible phase wrap scenarios. Then, median and Gaussian filtering was applied to average errors inherent in the linear fitting process. Aksit *et al.* [1] proposed another 3-echo method which computes an estimate of the phase twice, once using a very short ΔTE (Regime II) and another using a much longer ΔTE (Regime I). This method attempts to unwrap the long echo pair estimate using information from the short echo pair estimate. We will show that both of these approaches suffer from inherent ambiguities.

In this chapter, we quantify the ambiguity (error) space in a phase map estimate obtained with any given echo pair. Then, we show that by using an optimal choice of three echoes, the overall ambiguity space can be engineered to possess specific distinct features. We then design a simple estimation routine which takes advantage of such an engineered ambiguity space. We will show that this approach overcomes the trade-offs of Regimes I-III.

2. Theory

2.1. *Novel paradigm: Phase Ambiguity functions*

We propose first a novel paradigm for quantifying the uncertainty in the phase map estimate $\widehat{\Delta B}_{0,1}$ when computed from two echoes, TE_0 and TE_1. Namely,

$$\widehat{\Delta B}_{0,1} = \frac{\angle g(TE_1) - \angle g(TE_0)}{2\pi \Delta TE_{0,1}} \tag{4}$$

where $\Delta TE_{0,1} = TE_1 - TE_0$ is the echo spacing. In the absence of phase wrapping, it has been shown that $\widehat{\Delta B}_{0,1}$ is the Maximum Likelihood (ML) phase map estimate for methods utilizing 2 echo acquisitions [6]. We can easily show that the overall error in this estimate can be written as:

$$\mathcal{E}_{0,1} = \widehat{\Delta B}_{0,1} - \Delta B = \frac{\mathbf{n}_{0,1} + \Delta\Omega_{0,1}/2\pi}{\Delta TE_{0,1}} \tag{5}$$

where $\Delta\Omega_{0,1} = \Omega_1 - \Omega_0$ is the difference between the phase noise random variables in Eq. 2, and $\mathbf{n}_{0,1}$ denotes a phase wrapping integer which is non-zero whenever $2\pi \Delta B \Delta TE_{0,1} + \Delta\Omega_{0,1}$ falls outside $[-\pi, \pi)$. The probability density function (PDF) function of $\mathcal{E}_{0,1}$ completely describes the error in the estimate. This PDF gives rise to an uncertainty (ambiguity) about the original phase slope value, which we label as the Phase Ambiguity (PA) function.

Assuming that, over a range of phase map values of interest, all possible values for $n_{0,1}$ are equally likely, we can show that the PA function of $\mathcal{E}_{0,1}$ can be written as,

$$\chi_1 = \alpha_1 f_{\Omega_1}(2\pi\Delta TE_{0,1}\mathcal{E}) * f_{\Omega_0}(2\pi\Delta TE_{0,1}\mathcal{E}) * \sum_{\mathbf{p}} \delta(\mathcal{E} - \tfrac{p}{\Delta TE_{0,1}}) \tag{6}$$

where $\mathcal{E}$ is the observed error in Hz, $f_{\Omega_k}(\omega)$ is the PDF of $\mathbf{\Omega_k}$ and $*$ denotes the convolution operator. α_1 is a PDF scaling parameter over the domain of χ_1. Following derivations similar to [8], we can show that $f_{\Omega_k}(\omega)$ can be written as:

$$f_{\Omega_k}(\omega) = \frac{\exp\left(-\lambda_k^2/2\right)}{2\pi} \left\{ 1 + \lambda_k \sqrt{\frac{\pi}{2}} \cos\omega \exp\left(\lambda_k^2 \cos^2\omega/2\right) \left[1 + \mathrm{erf}\left(\frac{\lambda_k \cos\omega}{\sqrt{2}}\right) \right] \right\} \tag{7}$$

where

$$\lambda_k = 0.65 \mathrm{SNR}_0 \exp\left(-\frac{TE_k - TE_0}{T2^*}\right) \tag{8}$$

and SNR_0 is the magnitude-domain SNR at TE_0, $\mathrm{SNR}_0 = \rho(TE_0)/\sigma_{|w|}$. The 0.65 factor relates magnitude and complex domain SNRs. It is important to note that we are only interested in a limited sub-domain of the PA function corresponding to $[-2\delta B_{\max}, 2\delta B_{\max}]$, where $\delta B_{\max}$ is the maximum phase value expected over a region of interest. Hereafter we refer to the quantity $2\delta B_{\max}$ as the dynamic range of the phase map.

Figures 1(a)-1(c) show example PA functions for acquisitions at an echo spacing $\Delta TE_{0,1}$ of 1.5ms, 0.5ms and 1.0ms, respectively. The PA functions are plotted on a log scale. The horizontal axis denotes the error in the phase map estimate ($\mathcal{E}_{0,1}$ in Hz), while the vertical axis represents the likelihood of observing that error. The dynamic range of interest here is $2\delta B_{\max} = 900$Hz with a noise level corresponding to $\mathrm{SNR}_0 = 10$. The minimum decay constant $T2^*$ is set to 12ms. We clearly see that the PA function in Figure 1(a) is dominated by wrapping errors, as can be seen from the multiple peaks. This is expected in Regime I where phase values are larger than the cutoff $\Delta B_{\mathrm{cutoff}}$. On the other extreme, a very wide single lobe in Figure 1(b) implies a noise-limited performance, characteristic of Regime II. Finally, a moderate choice of $\Delta TE_{0,1}$ in Figure 1(c) displays a PA function with error contributions from both phase wrapping and noise, as well as noise-induced phase wrapping.

2.2. *Proposed solution: MAGPI*

The trade-offs in phase mapping Regimes I-III can be overcome using the Phase Ambiguity paradigm introduced above. Specifically, we show here that the underlying ambiguity can be resolved by using a careful choice of three echoes.

Repeating the same analysis above using echo pairs 0 and 2, we obtain Phase Ambiguity χ_2 where,

$$\mathcal{E}_{0,2} \triangleq \widehat{\Delta B}_{0,2} - \Delta B = \frac{n_{0,2} + \Delta\Omega_{0,2}/2\pi}{\Delta TE_{0,2}} \tag{9}$$

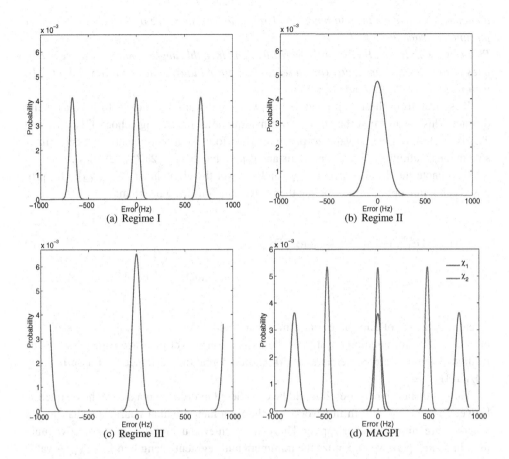

Fig. 1. Phase Ambiguity functions for the prescribed echo time spacings of (a) 1.5ms (b) 0.5ms and (c) 1.0ms over the dynamic range of interest, $[-2 \times 450 : 2 \times 450]$Hz, in a voxel with an SNR_0 of 10 and a decay constant $T2^*$ of 12ms. Regime I is limited by phase aliasing, as can be seen from the multiple peaks. Regime II has a wide single lobe, thus implying a noise-limited performance. Regime III attempts to trade-off Regime I and Regime II. (d) Phase Ambiguity functions at the echo time differences chosen by MAGPI: χ_1 for $\Delta TE_1 = 1.24$ms, and χ_2 for $\Delta TE_2 = 2.05$ms.

and

$$\chi_2 = \alpha_2 f_{\Omega_2}(2\pi \Delta TE_{0,2}\mathcal{E}) * f_{\Omega_0}(2\pi \Delta TE_{0,2}\mathcal{E}) * \sum_{\mathbf{q}} \delta\left(\mathcal{E} - \frac{q}{\Delta TE_{0,2}}\right) \qquad (10)$$

where $\mathcal{E}$ is the error variable in Hz, $f_{\Omega_k}(\omega)$ is as given in Eq. 7, $\mathbf{\Delta\Omega_{0,2}} \triangleq \Omega_2 - \Omega_0$, $\Delta TE_{0,2} \triangleq TE_2 - TE_0$, $\mathbf{n}_{0,2} = 0, \pm 1, \pm 2, \ldots$, and α_2 is a PDF scaling parameter over the range $[-2\delta B_{\max}, 2\delta B_{\max}]$.

We immediately point out two important properties from Eqs. 6 and 10:

Property PA-1: *Irrespective of the choice of echo times, the Phase Ambiguity functions will always have a non-zero peak at $\mathcal{E}_{0,1} = \mathcal{E}_{0,2} = 0$. That is, the original true solution is* *a common occurrence in both functions, irrespective of the value of the echoes and other parameters, such as SNR, T2*, etc.*

Property PA-2: *If both PA functions were identical, then this implies that knowledge of $\mathcal{E}_{0,2}$ does not reduce the ambiguity (or increase the information) about the true value of ΔB, with respect to $\mathcal{E}_{0,1}$. And vice versa.*

It is clear from these 2 properties that we would want χ_1 and χ_2 to be maximally distinct. This ensures that the ambiguity remaining after measuring echoes TE_0, TE_1 and TE_2 is as close to the real value as possible. Therefore, we advocate choosing echo times so that the resulting χ_1 and χ_2 are as distant as possible, over $[-2\delta B_{max}, 2\delta B_{max}]$.

We denote the distance between χ_1 and χ_2 over this domain as $\mathcal{D}(\chi_1, \chi_2)$. Our proposed echo time optimization routine then solves the following problem:

$$[TE_0^{opt}, TE_1^{opt}, TE_2^{opt}] = \underset{[TE_0, TE_1, TE_2]}{\arg\max} \ \mathcal{D}(\chi_1, \chi_2) \tag{11}$$

$$\text{such that,} \quad [TE_0, TE_1, TE_2] \in \mathcal{C},$$

where $\mathcal{C}$ is the set of allowable echo times that could be utilized with the pulse sequence of choice. This formulation constitutes the basis of our novel joint acquisition/estimation method, which we refer to hereafter as, **M**aximum **A**mbi**G**uity distance for **P**hase **I**maging (MAGPI).

Various distance measures $\mathcal{D}$ could be considered in order to maximize the distinction between χ_1 and χ_2 [3,19]. In this work, we choose a metric which guarantees that the PA functions are minimally overlapping. This can be achieved using a two-part objective function. In its first part, we maximize the minimum null segment's length in $\chi_1 + \chi_2$. A value in $\chi_1 + \chi_2$ is declared "null" if it falls below a threshold, chosen low enough to account for 99.9% of the noise PDFs, $f_{\Omega_k}(\omega)$. This step alone would increase the distance between peaks. However, this also inherently broadens the peaks, as we have seen. This is undesirable as we aim to minimize the overlap between the center peak of χ_1 and that of χ_2, corresponding to the "noisy" true solution. The overall objective function $\mathcal{D}$ thus combines these two geometrical metrics, namely, $\mathcal{D} = \{$minimum null segment length in $\chi_1 + \chi_2\} - \{$total length of central peaks$\}$.

We apply MAGPI, with our choice of $\mathcal{D}$, to our acquisition scenario of Figure 1. We optimize echo times to operate over a dynamic range of 900Hz, a worst case SNR_0 of 10 and T2* values as low as 12ms. The resulting optimal echo times were: $TE_0 = 2ms$, $TE_1 = 3.24ms$ and $TE_2 = 4.05ms$ ($\Delta TE_{0,1} = 1.24ms$ and $\Delta TE_{0,2} = 2.05ms$). The corresponding PA functions are shown in Figure 1(d). We note that both echo pairs have a large spacing with respect to $1/2\times900$, thus operating in a wrap-dominated regime (Regime I). Nevertheless, the overlap pattern of the two error distributions is engineered to disambiguate phase wrapping (due to minimal overlap of peaks) and reduce noise variance (due to large echo time spacings). Note that, out of three echoes, optimizing two PAs uniquely determines the overall ambiguity space.

2.3. *Corresponding estimation method: CL2D*

The echoes optimized by Eq. 11 guarantee that the resulting PA functions are maximally distinct, in the sense defined by the metric $\mathcal{D}$ above. We present here a corresponding estimation method which takes advantage of the designed ambiguity space in order to recover the original phase map value.

Similar to the distance metric $\mathcal{D}$, the estimation algorithm proposed here is based on an intuitive geometrical approach. Specifically, we first point out that the angle given by Eq. 4 corresponds simply to one sample realization from the PA function χ_1. We illustrate this in Figure 2 with the magenta "x" marker, where the horizontal axis denotes all possible phase map values. This sample could have resulted from any one of the periodic peaks in χ_1. Thus, replicating this sample by the inherent period of $1/\Delta_{TE_{0,1}}$ results in the set of all possible solutions to Eq. 5 (magenta "o" marker), for this particular noise realization. Any one of these replicated values could in fact belong to the wrap-free peak of χ_1. This ambiguity is readily resolved using the second echo pair (TE_0, TE_2): we repeat the same steps for $\widehat{\Delta B}_{0,2}$ and its corresponding χ_2 and obtain another set of values, as shown in Figure 2 in "x" and "o" markers. Given that the designed PA functions are maximally distant, we know that the two values from these two sets that are closest to one another (in $\mathcal{L}2$-distance sense) correspond to the two wrap-free peaks from χ_1 and χ_2. This is illustrated in Figure 2. Finally, a phase map estimate can be easily recovered by, for example, averaging these two closest values. We summarize this Closest-L2 Distance (CL2D) estimation method in Table 1 below. This proposed CL2D estimation method is applied **independently one voxel at a time**.

Note that other estimation methods could be proposed at the final step. In this work, we use a straightforward weighted averaging procedure thereby highlighting the advantages of our novel MAGPI echo optimization, in spite of using a simple estimation method.

3. Results

3.1. *Simulation results*

The optimization routine of Eq. 11 is run offline, once. We can see from Eqs. 7, 8 and 11 that the only prior information needed to compute the optimal echo times with MAGPI are the maximum dynamic range of interest $2\delta B_{max}$, the minimum SNR_0 and the minimum expected T2* in the regions of interest. We solve the optimization problem using an Adaptive Simulated Annealing (ASA) routine [10,18].

We illustrate in Figure 3 a basic numerical example highlighting the properties of each of the acquisitions discussed in Figure 1. The example simulates GRE measurements taken at three echo times in two voxels with phase offset values of 400Hz (Figure 3(a)) and 10Hz (Figure 3(b)). The noise level corresponds to an initial SNR of $SNR_0 = 10$ and T2*of 12ms. We first simulate 3 echoes acquired at an echo spacing of 1.5ms ($\Delta B_{cutoff} \approx 333$Hz), 0.5ms ($\Delta B_{cutoff} = 1$KHz) and 1.0ms ($\Delta B_{cutoff} = 500$Hz). We then compute the angle at each echo time and perform a phase unwrapping operation across the three time samples. The solid lines are the Least Squares (LS) linear fit to the unwrapped angle data.

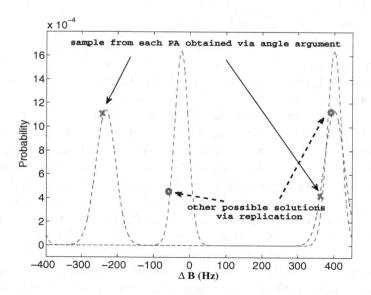

Fig. 2.   A demonstration of the estimation algorithm described in Table 1. Note that the horizontal axis correspond to the possible phase map values $[-\delta B_{\max} : \delta B_{\max}]$, and not the error. The estimation method takes advantage of the prior-information that the optimizer guarantees maximum separation between the peaks. The closest solutions would inherently belong to the peaks corresponding to the true phase value, in this example 400Hz.

Algorithm Table 1. Closest L2-Distance (CL2D) Estimation

Step 1: For echo pair $(0, 1)$, compute the angle at location (x, y). The result yields $\widehat{\Delta B}_{0,1}(x, y)$ in Eq. 4. As shown with the magenta "x" marker in Figure 2, the resulting value constitutes one realization from χ_1. Repeat the same procedure for echo pair $(0, 2)$ ("x" marker in Figure 2).

Step 2: Replicate $\widehat{\Delta B}_{0,1}$ and $\widehat{\Delta B}_{0,2}$ by $1/\Delta\text{TE}_{0,1}$ and $1/\Delta\text{TE}_{0,2}$, respectively, over the dynamic range of interest. This is shown with the "o" markers in Figure 2. The x and o samples thus constitute a set of values from each PA function that would solve each of Eqs. 5 and 9, respectively.

Step 3: The solutions that are closest, in the $\mathcal{L}^2$ sense, to one another correspond to samples from the lobes centered around the original phase value. This utilizes the important prior information that all the lobes are guaranteed by the optimizer to be maximally distant.

Step 4: Finally, we estimate the phase map as the weighted average of these closest 2 samples. The weighting would take into account the respective echo times (later echoes would have a lower weight, to account for T2* effects).

The trade-offs in each of the regimes are consistent with the trade-offs discussed earlier. Our proposed method samples the phase irregularly at large echo time spacings of 1.24ms ($\Delta B_{\text{cutoff}} \approx 403\text{Hz}$) and 2.05ms ($\Delta B_{\text{cutoff}} \approx 244\text{Hz}$), as optimized by MAGPI for

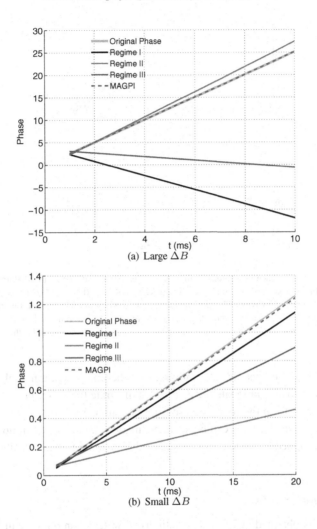

(a) Large ΔB

(b) Small ΔB

Fig. 3. Example illustrating the trade-off in the choice of the echo time steps, as represented by Regime I (ΔTE = 1.5ms), Regime II (ΔTE = 0.5ms) and Regime III (ΔTE = 1.0ms). The original linear phase (green line) has a slope of (a) 400Hz and (b) 10Hz. In each of these traditional regimes, data is sampled regularly at 3 time intervals. The slope is estimated using a Least Squares fit. Regime I achieves the best results when the original slope is low, while Regime II produces a good estimate for large slope values. In Regime III, attempts to balance both regimes. Our proposed method MAGPI (red) samples the phase irregularly at 1.24ms and 2.05ms. With a simple estimation procedure (CL2D), MAGPI achieves in this example the best performance for both the large and small slope values.

$2\delta B_{max} = 900$Hz, a worst case SNR_0 of 10 and minimum T2* of 12ms (Figure 1(d)). The dashed line shows the result of the simple estimation procedure CL2D. As we can see, our method consistently achieves the correct estimate in this example, for both large and small values of ΔB.

In addition to our proposed CL2D method, there exists multiple estimation algorithms that could recover the original phase map value from the optimized MAGPI acquisitions.

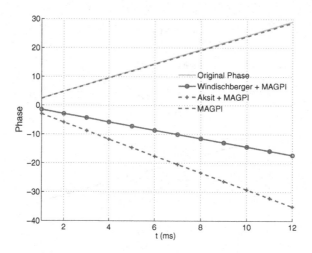

Fig. 4. Estimation performance of methods from the literature when used along with MAGPI echoes. The original phase (green line) has a slope of 380Hz, in a voxel with SNR_0 of 10 and T2* of 12ms. Methods "Windischberger+MAGPI" and "Aksit+MAGPI" use the 3 echoes proposed by our optimizer in Figure 1(d), along with the estimation algorithm proposed in [1] and [25], respectively. In this case, our proposed simple estimation routine (CL2D) is the only method which takes into account the designed ambiguity space, and is thus able to recover the correct phase.

Such methods, however, should take into account the unique pattern of the designed PA functions in order to disambiguate the errors. We illustrate this in Figure 4 where different estimation methods from the literature are used in conjunction with echoes optimized for the scenario of Figure 1(d). As can be seen, estimation methods which did not utilize the feature of the designed PA functions still suffered from ambiguities, despite using optimal MAGPI echoes.

3.2. Real phantom results

We report results obtained at 7T with a cylindrical water phantom containing oil and air running in tubes along its long axis. The data was acquired on a 7T Siemens Trio scanner (Siemens Medical Solutions, Erlangen, Germany). The acquisition parameters were as follows: Field of View (FOV) = $120 \times 120mm^2$, slice thickness 1.5mm, matrix size 256×256, flip angle $45°$, 8 slices, TR= 185ms, with fat saturation turned off, and automatic shimming turned on. The acquisition thus generates images with high spatial resolution, corresponding to $0.46 \times 0.46 \times 1.5mm^3$ voxels.

Since we did not suppress fat signals with the GRE sequence, we expect the phase (field) map to contain offsets due to both, chemical shifts and B0 field inhomogeneity. At 7T, fat is offset by about 980Hz, thereby implying a dynamic range of 1960Hz. This requires sampling at echo spacings less than 0.51 ms. Figures 5(b) and 5(c) show the phase map obtained with 16 regularly spaced echoes, with $\Delta TE = 0.25ms$. The method in Figure 5(b), labeled DFT-16, estimates the slope in each voxel using the Discrete Fourier Transform (DFT) along with temporal zero-padding, while in Figure 5(c) the slope is estimated directly in temporal domain using an LS fit (LS-16) [4]. We also show a phase map obtained using the traditional 2-echo method in Figure 5(d) (labeled ML-2), computed according to Eq. 4, with $\Delta TE = 0.25$ms. For further comparison, we present in Figure 5(e) the phase map obtained using the 3-point method proposed by Aksit *et al.* [1]. This Long Echo/Short Echo (LeSe-3) method attempts to balance the advantages of each regime. A short echo spacing, ΔTE_{se} (Regime II) is used to unwrap the phase from the long echo spacing, ΔTE_{le} (Regime I). Here we used $\Delta TE_{se} = 0.25$ms and $\Delta TE_{le} = 15 \times \Delta TE_{se}$, as suggested in [1]. Finally, we show the result obtained with our method, using the 3 echoes $TE_0 = 5$ms, $TE_1 = 6.32$ms, $TE_2 = 6.76$ms (or $\Delta TE_1 = 1.32$ms and $\Delta TE_2 = 1.76$ms), as prescribed by the optimizer in Eq. 11. MAGPI picked these optimal echo times for a worst case SNR_0 of 20, a minimum expected $T2^*$ of 15ms, and a maximum expected dynamic range of 2200Hz.

We used the 16-point methods of DFT-16 (Figure 5(b)) and LS-16 (Figure 5(c)) as a "gold standard" in this case. Despite the fact that these phase maps were obtained from the noise-limited Regime II, we expect improved robustness with 16 echoes in static phantoms with long $T2^*$ decay. Obviously, such long acquisitions are sub-optimal in practical applications, due to subject motion, $T2^*$ decay effects, and long acquisition times. In comparison, the commonly used two-point method (Figure 5(d)), suffers from severe noise amplification. This behavior is justified by the acquisition's Phase Ambiguity function, shown in Figure 6(a). We immediately observe its single peak with a wide lobe extending over hundreds of Hertz, characteristic of a noise-limited regime. The LeSe-3 method (Figure 5(e)) also exhibits large variations, despite using 3 echoes. To understand its performance, we also refer to the PA functions of LeSe-3, shown in Figure 6(b). We note the significant overlap between the PA function of the short echo spacing pair ΔTE_{se} and the PA function of the long echo spacing pair ΔTE_{le}. As explained in *Property PA-2* in Theory, such an acquisition strategy leads to an inherent ambiguity about the true phase value. Irrespective of the estimation algorithm used, such ambiguity could not be resolved without making additional assumptions about the spatial behavior of the phase map (smoothing or regularization). MAGPI, on the other hand, uses echo times which result in maximally distant PA functions, as shown in Figure 6(c). The resulting high-resolution phase map in Figure 5(f) looks very similar to those obtained with DFT-16 and LS-16, displaying robust and large dynamic range estimates.

We inspect these phantom results numerically in Figure 7 by considering profiles along 2 different rows. The location of the rows is indicated by the dotted lines in Figure 5(a). The profile in Figure 7(a) plots the phase map through 2 oil rings and the water background, while the profile in Figure 7(b) shows the phase map in water only. Figure 7(c) is a magnified profile through one oil ring. These plots demonstrate the efficiency and robustness of the MAGPI phase estimates and their similarity to phase maps obtained with 16 point methods. In comparison, LeSe-3 and ML-2 struggle to achieve the desired phase map values, especially in water (Figure 7(b)) where the performance of MAGPI is particularly impressive. The fact that MAGPI produces high resolution ($0.46 \times 0.46 \times 1.5$mm^3) phase maps comparable to those obtained with 16-point methods, at 18% of the acquisition time, is noteworthy.

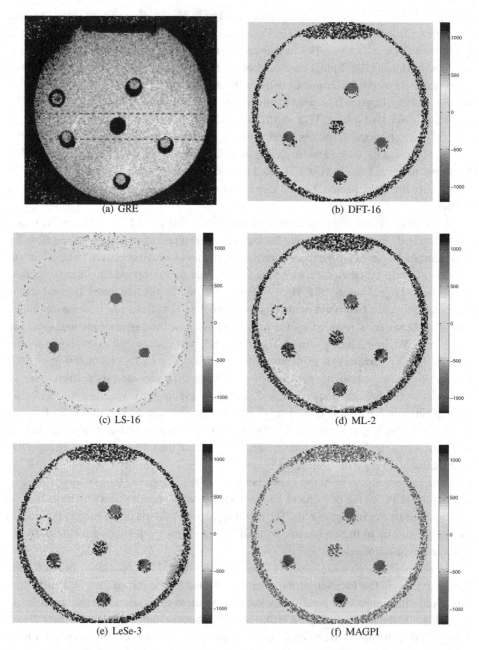

Fig. 5.   (a) Axial GRE image of a water/oil/air phantom. The tubes containing oil (yellow arrows) are expected to yield a phase offset value around 980Hz at 7T. Phase maps as estimated using (b) 16 point DFT method (c) 16-point Least Squares fitting method (d) the well-known 2-point method (e) a 3-point method proposed by Aksit *et al.* and (f) MAGPI. Our method used $TE_0 = 5ms$, $TE_1 = 6.32ms$, $TE_2 = 6.76ms$ (or $\Delta TE_1 = 1.32ms$ and $\Delta TE_2 = 1.76ms$), as prescribed by the optimizer in Eq. 11. MAGPI optimized the echo times for a worst case SNR_0 of 20, a minimum expected $T2^*$ of 15ms, and a maximum expected dynamic range of 2200Hz.

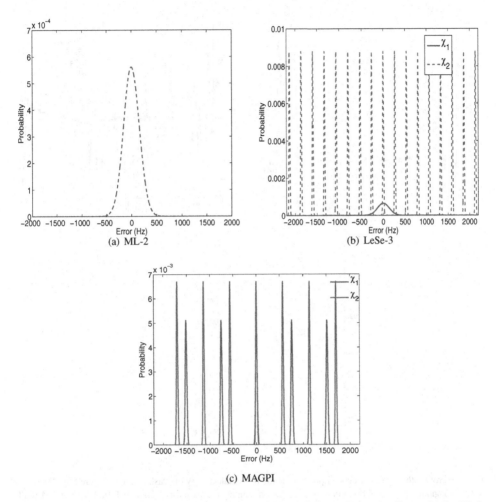

Fig. 6. Phase Ambiguity functions for the phantom acquisitions of Figure 5 corresponding to (a) the ML-2 echoes with $\Delta TE = 0.25$ms, (b) the LeSe echoes with $\Delta TE_{se} = 0.25$ms and $\Delta TE_{le} = 3.75$ms, (c) MAGPI with $\Delta TE_1 = 1.32$ms and $\Delta TE_2 = 1.76$ms.

We also should emphasize that the smallest echo time spacing used with MAGPI in our phantom experiment would traditionally have caused aliasing for phase values larger than $\Delta B_{cutoff} \approx 379$Hz. Our method was able to disambiguate phase values up to a maximum value of 1100Hz using the engineered structure of the PA functions. This implies an impressive gain in dynamic range by a factor of 2.9.

3.3. *In Vivo results*

We also demonstrate the utility of our method in vivo. The brain of healthy volunteers were imaged after approval was obtained from our Institutional Review Board (IRB) and informed consent was given by the subjects.

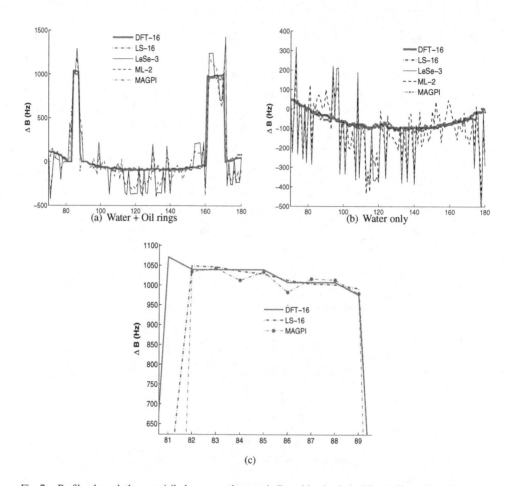

Fig. 7.   Profiles through the water/oil phantom at the rows indicated by the dashed line in Figure 5(a). We show in (c) a magnified portion of the profile in (a), which highlights the similarity of the DFT-16, LS-16 and MAGPI methods. Note also the drastically improved robustness with MAGPI from the profile through water (b), as compared to ML-2 and LeSe-3. This challenging high resolution ($0.46 \times 0.46mm^2$) mapping shows that we are able to obtain robust, large dynamic range phase maps at a fraction (18%) of the time needed by 16 echo methods. The gain in dynamic range compared to methods using the same minimum echo time spacing as MAGPI is a factor of 2.9.

We acquire phase maps in a volunteer's brain using a 7T Siemens Trio. We use both, GRE acquisitions as well as Multi-Echo Gradient-Echo (MEGE) acquisitions. Both sequences acquire high resolution images, corresponding to approximately $0.33 \times 0.33 \times 1.5mm^3$ voxels. The parameters for the GRE acquisitions were: FOV = $210 \times 210mm^2$, slice thickness 1.5mm, matrix size 640×640, flip angle $45°$, 8 slices, TR= 180ms, with both fat saturation and automatic shimming turned on. The parameters for the MEGE acquisitions were: FOV = $146 \times 210mm^2$, read out axis set along the shorter dimension, slice thickness 1.5mm, matrix size 420×640, flip angle $55°$, 8 slices, TR= 100ms, with both fat saturation and automatic shimming turned on.

Figures 8(a) and 8(b) show two GRE axial images in two different slices. All phase map methods here use only 3 echoes, with either GRE or MEGE sequences.

Figures 8(c) and 8(e) display the phase maps estimated with the GRE sequences. Figure 8(c) uses the Least-Squares fit method (LS-3) with echoes captured regularly at $4, 4.5$, and 5ms. Figure 8(e) shows the result obtained with our proposed method. MAGPI used the echo times of $4, 5, 6.5$ms, or $\Delta TE_1 = 1$ms and $\Delta TE_2 = 2.5$ms, optimized for a minimum SNR_0 of 18, a maximum expected $2\delta B_{max}$ of 1700Hz and a minimum $T2^*$ of 15ms.

Phase maps generated using the MEGE sequence are shown in Figure 8(d) (LS-3) and Figure 8(f) (MAGPI). MEGE sequences are often preferred in phase map imaging over GRE sequences for being faster at acquiring the same number echoes with similar parameters. However, MEGE sequences have an inherent constraint on the minimum echo spacing that could be accommodated. With our sequence parameters here, this minimum possible echo spacing is 1.2ms. Therefore, regularly spaced echo time methods, such as LS-3 would use echoes $4, 5.2$, and 6.4ms. The resulting phase map is shown in Figure 8(d). The phase map obtained with our MAGPI method is shown in Figure 8(f). The MAGPI echoes used were optimized to yield optimal phase maps over a dynamic range of 1600Hz in regions with minimum SNR_0 of 18, and minimum $T2^*$ of 15ms. Furthermore, the set $\mathcal{C}$ in Eq. 11 constrained consecutive echoes to be separated by at least 1.2ms, resulting in $TE_1 = 4$ms, $TE_0 = 5.2$ms, $TE_2 = 7$ms.

We can clearly see from Figure 8(e) that our proposed method achieves more robust estimates as compared to methods with the same amount of acquisition time, such as LS-3 (Figure 8(c)). The phase map obtained with MAGPI displays high resolution features at a markedly reduced noise variance, as we can clearly see from the magnified image section. Our method also exhibits robust estimation for both large and low phase map values across the brain.

The second 7T experiment consisted of extracting phase maps from a 3-echo MEGE sequence, often used for its faster acquisition time. The 1.2ms minimum echo spacing constraint of this sequence imposes a maximum dynamic range of ± 417Hz in phase maps obtained with regularly spaced echoes. This is seen in Figure 8(d) where LS-3 suffers from wrapping artifacts (white arrow and sinus areas). The long echo spacings with MEGE and LS-3 reduced noise contributions as compared with GRE and LS-3 (Figure 8(c)), but this significantly increased wrapping errors.

On the other hand, our imaging paradigm is readily suited for this large echo time spacing constraint, which is incorporated in $\mathcal{C}$ Eq. 11. The optimal echo times $TE_1 = 4$ms, $TE_0 = 5.2$ms, and $TE_2 = 7$ms are designed to disambiguate phase maps over a dynamic range of 1600Hz and a worst case SNR of 18. We note the location of the reference echo, TE_0. Our optimizer automatically determines that this arrangement is optimal here as it reduces the value of the last echo time TE_2, and in turn $T2^*$ decay effects. The resulting phase map in Figure 8(f) displays properties similar to what we observed and validated in the phantom study: low variance in smooth regions and large dynamic range mapping up to ± 780Hz. This is a significant 91% gain in dynamic range, as compared to sequences

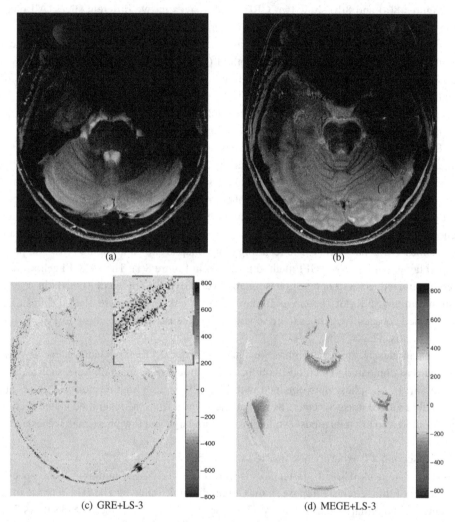

(c) GRE+LS-3   (d) MEGE+LS-3

Fig. 8.   Results from the 7T brain scan, where we estimate phase maps at a spatial resolution of $0.33 \times 0.33 \times 1.5$ (mm^3). Two example GRE slices are shown in (a) and (b), both taken at TE $= 5$ms. The second row displays phase maps obtained with a Least-Squares fitting method (LS-3), using 3 echoes. In the third row we show the phase maps obtained with our method, MAGPI. In (c) and (e) we estimate phase maps from GRE acquisitions, taken at 3 different echo times. The echoes used by LS-3 in (c) were $4, 4.5, 5$ms while MAGPI used the optimized echo times of $4, 5, 6.5$ms, corresponding to $\Delta TE_1 = 1.0$ms and $\Delta TE_2 = 2.5$ms. Note the impressive noise performance of MAGPI, without the use of any spatial smoothing. This is particularly apparent in the enlarged section of the phase maps, where the map is scaled between $[-300, 300]$Hz for better visualization. In (d) and (f), we generate phase maps from a MEGE sequence with 3 echoes. The MEGE sequence has an inherent constraint on the minimum echo time spacing of 1.2ms. Thus, we see that in (d) the LS-3 method, with echoes captured at $4, 5.2, 6.4$ms, suffers from phase wrapping in regions where phase map values exceed ± 417Hz. On the other hand, MAGPI in (f) produced phase maps without any wrapping artifacts, using the optimized echo times $TE_1 = 4$ms, $TE_0 = 5.2$ms, $TE_2 = 7$ms. The high resolution phase map obtained with MAGPI (f) has a dynamic range that is 91% larger than methods with similar echo spacing constraint (d).

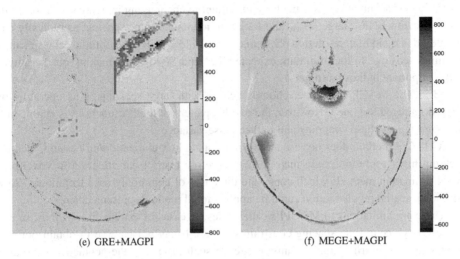

(e) GRE+MAGPI   (f) MEGE+MAGPI

Fig. 8. (*Continued*)

limited by the 1.2ms minimum echo spacing constraint. In this example, hardware limitations constrain the dynamic range achievable even with 16-point methods. MAGPI is immune to this constraint and becomes an essential tool in such applications.

4. Discussion and Conclusions

We presented phantom data as well as in vivo results showing robust high-resolution phase maps obtained without the traditional trade-offs of Regimes I-III. It is important to emphasize the salient aspects of our proposed method which consist of:

A. quantifying the ambiguity in the phase map estimate (PA function) for a given echo time spacing (Eqs. 6, 7 and 10),
B. optimizing 3 echo times (2 echo spacings) for a given SNR_0, $T2^*$ and δB_{max} of interest, so that the two resulting PA functions are maximally distinct Eq. 11,
C. designing a corresponding estimation routine which takes advantage of the engineered ambiguity space above in order to recover the original phase map value.

We make the following important observations about each of the points above:

(A.1) We have validated the theoretical noise PDF in Eq. 7, and PA functions of Eqs. 6, 10 using numerical simulations and phantom data. The histograms perfectly match our theoretical predictions for various scenarios. We skip this demonstration here for space constraints.

(B.1) Our optimizer chooses the echo times based on worst case imaging scenarios, corresponding to a maximum dynamic range and minimum SNR_0 and $T2^*$ of interest. In our work, we simply picked these values based on prior knowledge of the magnetic field strength, the sequence parameters and the material of interest.

(B.2) Our formulation is particularly important in challenging imaging scenarios, with short T2*, low SNR_0, large δB_{max} and long minimum echo time spacing, as typically encountered in rapid high resolution phase mapping. At low SNRs, the optimal echo spacings are more sensitive to the minimum expected T2* and SNR_0, thus making our paradigm really important in those settings.

(B.3) The MAGPI optimizer chooses echoes with large spacings, thus operating in wrap-dominated Regime I. However, the overlap pattern of the PA functions is engineered to disambiguate phase wrapping and reduce noise variance.

(C.1) Our method does not use any form of spatial regularization/processing, thereby yielding high resolution phase maps [6]. We therefore restrict our attention to voxel-per-voxel estimation methods which constitute the bases of commonly used techniques. Any additional spatial regularization could be applied to all methods presented here.

There are limitations to MAGPI's capabilities. In cases of extremely low SNR, or extremely large echo time spacing constraints, MAGPI may not be able to obtain optimal echoes over arbitrarily large dynamic range. In such instances, the geometrical distance measure employed here may not be able to attain a robust solution. The onus then is placed on the pulse sequence to alleviate one of the constraints. Nevertheless, we should mention that we have not yet explored the theoretical limit of our method, as it may be possible to use more suitable distance measures $\mathcal{D}$ under such extreme conditions. Additional future work includes investigating statistical distance measures, instead of our proposed geometrical measure, and corresponding statistical estimation algorithms, in lieu of the simple weighted averaging procedure.

In conclusion, we demonstrated here a new paradigm for estimating off-resonance maps using 3 echoes only. Our proposed echo time optimizer is able to explore search spaces corresponding to large echo time spacing, which was never considered before to the best of the author's knowledge. Our proposed method is able to simultaneously combine in 3 echoes the advantages of large echo spacings without their inhibiting wrapping constraints. The MAGPI scheme selects the echo times and characterizes the resulting phase errors so as to be maximally disambiguated in estimation. MAGPI overcomes many of the traditional constraints on phase maps, as demonstrated throughout this work. Specifically, in our proposed paradigm: (i) reducing ΔTE is not required to increase the dynamic range, (ii) using large ΔTE is no longer limited by wrapping artifacts and, (iii) no spatial regularization or phase unwrapping are needed.

References

1. Aksit, P., Derbyshire, J., Prince, J.: Three-point method for fast and robust field mapping for EPI geometric distortion correction. 4th IEEE International Symposium on Biomedical Imaging pp. 141–144 (2007)
2. Bioucas-Dias, J., Valadao, G.: Phase Unwrapping via Graph Cuts. IEEE Transactions on Image Processing 16(3), 698–709 (2007)
3. Cha, S.H.: Comprehensive survey on distance/similarity measures between probability density functions. International Journal of Mathematical Models and Methods in Applied Sciences 1(4), pp. 300–307 (2007)

4. Chen, N., Wyrwicz, A.: Correction for EPI distortions using multi-echo gradient-echo imaging. Magnetic Resonance In Medicine 41(6), 1206–1213 (1999)

5. Frey, B., Koetter, R., Petrovic, N.: Very loopy belief propagation for unwrapping phase images. Neural Information Processing Systems pp. 737–743 (2001)

6. Funai, A., Fessler, J., Yeo, D., Olafsson, V., Noll, D.: Regularized field map estimation in MRI. IEEE Transactions on Medical Imaging 27(10), 1484–1494 (2008)

7. Ghiglia, D.C., Pritt, M.D.: Two-Dimensional Phase Unwrapping: Theory, Algorithms, and Software. Wiley-Interscience (1998)

8. Hagmann, W., Habermann, J.: On the phase error distribution of an open loop phase estimator. IEEE International Conference on Communications 2, 1031–1037 (1988)

9. Holland, D., Kuperman, J.M., Dale, A.M.: Efficient correction of inhomogeneous static magnetic field-induced distortion in Echo Planar Imaging. NeuroImage 50(1), 175–183 (Mar 2010)

10. Ingber, A.L.: Adaptive simulated annealing (asa): Lessons learned. Control and Cybernetics 25(1), 33–54 (1996)

11. Jenkinson, M.: Fast, automated, N-dimensional phase-unwrapping algorithm. Magnetic Resonance In Medicine 49(1), 193–197 (2003)

12. Jezzard, P., Balaban, R.: Correction for Geometric Distortion in Echo Planar Images from B0 Field Variations. Magnetic Resonance In Medicine 34(1), 65–73 (July 1995)

13. Kressler, B., de Rochefort, L., Liu, T., Spincemaille, P., Jiang, Q., Wang, Y.: Nonlinear regularization for per voxel estimation of magnetic susceptibility distributions from MRI field maps. IEEE Transactions on Medical Imaging 29(2), 273–281 (2010)

14. Liang, Z.P., Lauterbur, P.C.: Principles of Magnetic Resonance Imaging: A Signal Processing Perspective. Wiley-IEEE Press (2000)

15. Liu, G., Ogawa, S.: EPI image reconstruction with correction of distortion and signal losses. Journal of Magnetic Resonance Imaging 24(3), 683–689 (2006)

16. Moon-Ho Song, S., Napel, S., Pelc, N., Glover, G.: Phase unwrapping of MR phase images using Poisson equation. IEEE Transactions on Image Processing 4(5), 667–676 (1995)

17. Nguyen, H., Sutton, B., Morrison Jr, R., Do, M.: Joint Estimation and Correction of Geometric Distortions for EPI functional MRI using Harmonic Retrieval. IEEE Transactions on Medical Imaging 28(3), 423–434 (2009)

18. Oliveira, H.A., Ingber, L., Petraglia, A., Petraglia, M.R., Machado, M.A.S.: Stochastic Global Optimization and Its Applications with Fuzzy Adaptive Simulated Annealing, chap. 4. Springer (2012)

19. Papoulis, A.: Probability, Random Variables and Stochastic Processes. Mcgraw-Hill College (1991)

20. Rieke, V., Butts Pauly, K.: MR thermometry. Journal of Magnetic Resonance Imaging 27(2), 376–390 (2008)

21. Windischberger, C., Robinson, S., Rauscher, A., Barth, M., Moser, E.: Robust field map generation using a triple-echo acquisition. Journal of Magnetic Resonance Imaging 20(4), 730–734 (Oct 2004)

22. Yu, H., Reeder, S., Shimakawa, A., Brittain, J., Pelc, N.: Robust field map estimation in a Dixon water-fat separation algorithm with short echo time increments. International Society for Magnetic Resonance in Medicine 11, 345 (2004)

23. Zhou, K., Zaitsev, M., Bao, S.: Reliable two-dimensional phase unwrapping method using region growing and local linear estimation. Magnetic Resonance In Medicine 62(4), 1085–1090 (2009)

CHAPTER 7

A MULTI-RESOLUTION ACTIVE CONTOUR FRAMEWORK FOR ULTRASOUND IMAGE SEGMENTATION

Weiming Wang, Jing Qin, Pheng-Ann Heng, Yim-Pan Chui

Department of Computer Sci. and Eng., The Chinese University of Hong Kong
Hong Kong SAR, China
Shenzhen Institutes of Advanced Technology, Chinese Academy of Sciences
Shenzhen, China

Liang Li

The First Affiliated Hospital, Anhui Medical University, Hefei, China

Bing Nan Li

Department of Biomedical Engineering, Hefei University of Technology
P.O. Box 112, Hefei 230009, China
E-mail: bingoon@ieee.org

A novel multi-resolution framework for ultrasound image segmentation is presented. The framework is based on active contours and exploits both local intensity and local phase features to deal with degradations of ultrasound images such as low signal-to-noise, intensity inhomogeneity and speckle noise. We first build a Gaussian pyramid for each input image and employ a local statistics guided active contour model to delineate initial boundaries of interested objects in the coarsest pyramid level. Both means and variances of local intensities are utilized to handle local intensity inhomogeneity. In addition, as speckle noise is greatly reduced in the coarsest pyramid level, the contours can avoid trapping in local minima during the evolution. A phase-based geodesic active contour (GAC) is implemented to refine the boundaries in finer pyramid levels. Compared to traditional gradient-based GAC methods, the phase-based model is more suitable for ultrasound images with low contrast and weak boundaries. We employed the proposed framework for left ventricle, liver and kidney segmentation in echocardiographic images; comparative experiments demonstrate the advantages of the proposed segmentation framework.

1. Introduction

Ultrasound imaging has become one of the most widely used diagnostic and therapeutic tools in a lot of modern medical applications, especially image-guided interventions and therapy. Compared with other medical imaging modalities, such as computer tomography (CT) and magnetic resonance imaging (MRI), it is more portable and versatile, and does not produce any harmful radiation. In order to improve diagnosis and treatment performance, reliable automatic or semi-automatic segmentation methods are usually needed to detect interested organs in ultrasound images. However, accurate segmentation of interested structures from an ultrasound image is still a challenging task due to the poor image quality caused by some characteristic artifacts including low signal-to-noise, intensity inhomogeneity and speckle noise.

A lot of efforts have been devoted to enhancing the ultrasound image quality and improving the segmentation results.[1] In early investigations, statistical analysis of speckle noise was studied and filtering techniques for noise reduction were presented.[2-4] To handle intensity distortion of ultrasound images, Xiao *et al.* proposed an expectation-maximization method that simultaneously estimates the intensity distortion and segments the image into different regions based on the assumption that the image distortion follows a multiplicative model.[5] Shape knowledge is also incorporated for more accurate segmentation. For example, Johan *et al.* applied active appearance motion model to detect endocardial contour over the full heart cycle.[6] However, inclusion of *a priori* shape information may lead to erroneous segmentation when interested organs are deformed due to pathological changes.

Active contour models[7] have been widely used for image segmentation for many years and can be broadly categorized into two classes: edge-based models and region-based models. Both models have been incorporated into level set formulations for ultrasound image segmentation.[8-10] While edge-based models utilize image gradient to guide curve evolution,[11] region-based models tend to rely on statistical intensity information to deform the curve.[12] However, only gradient and statistic intensity information is usually insufficient for ultrasound image segmentation.[13,14] On the other hand, phase-based methods have been shown to perform well in feature detection of ultrasound images. Mulet-Parada and Noble[15] first successfully used local phase information to detect boundaries on echocardiographic sequences, which was later extended for feature detection[16] by using local phase computed from monogenic signal.[17] Recently, Belaid *et al.* employed both local phase and local orientation derived from monogenic signal to capture the boundaries of left ventricle.[13] However, these phase-based methods may be sensitive to initial contours due to limited capture range as they do not include any region term. In this paper, we aim at improving the performance of active contour models for ultrasound image segmentation by comprehensively exploiting both local intensity and local phase features.

Multi-resolution scheme has been demonstrated to be an efficient technique for ultrasound image segmentation.[18] It relies on the conversion of ultrasound images with Rayleigh statistics to subsampled images with Gaussian statistics by using a Gaussian pyramid.[8] Due to Gaussian smoothing and subsampling, high-frequency noise is smoothed out in coarser levels of the pyramid and neighboring pixels in these levels are more likely to be independent as subsampling reduces their correlation. According to Central Limit Theorem, the gray values of these pixels can be approximated as Gaussian distribution, which is far more mathematically tractable and separable than the Rayleigh distribution that actually characterizes ultrasound images. Lin *et al.* presented a multi-scale framework that combines region and edge information for echocardiographic image segmentation.[19] However, their method is based on Chan-Vese model which assumes the regions to be segmented are homogeneous, and thus has limit ability for ultrasound images with intensity inhomogeneity.[20]

We present a novel multi-resolution scheme in a variational level set formulation for ultrasound image segmentation. First, multi-resolution scheme is employed to build a Gaussian pyramid from the input image which corresponds to the finest level of the pyramid. Local Gaussian distribution (LGD) is adopted to model intensity statistics in the coarsest level and drive contours to object boundaries. Here both intensity means and variances of the local Gaussian distribution are modeled as spatially varying parameters. Three advantages come with the multi-resolution scheme: (1) speckle noise is highly reduced in the coarsest level of the pyramid due to Gaussian smoothing and subsampling, which assists the contour to pass through many local minima during the evolution; (2) local intensity statistics has been found to be useful to handle images with intensity inhomogeneity;[21, 22] and (3) it helps to improve the overall performance by transferring most of the computation to the coarsest level with relatively small image resolution. Second, a phase based edge stop function is defined and incorporated into the traditional geodesic active contours to further evolve and refine the boundaries in finer levels.[23] This modified phase-based geodesic active contours work well for images with low contrast and weak boundaries since the local phase information is theoretically intensity invariant. Furthermore, we use Gaussian derivative filters, as a better alternative to the commonly used log-Gabor filters, to extract local phase information from monogenic signal. We employ the proposed framework for left ventricle segmentation on echocardiographic images; preliminary comparative experiments demonstrate the advantages of the proposed segmentation framework.

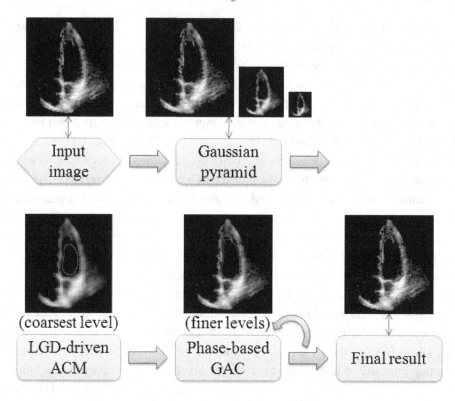

Fig. 1. Overview of the multi-resolution framework.

2. Methods

The pipeline of the proposed multi-resolution framework is shown in Fig. 1. The segmentation process is performed in a coarse-to-fine manner. After the Gaussian pyramid is built from the input image, we first employ the LGD-driven active contour model to extract the object boundaries in the coarsest level. Then the boundaries are passed to the next finer level as initial contour, and phase-based geodesic active contour is applied to further deform the boundaries until convergence is reached.

2.1. *LGD-driven Active Contour Models*

Let us consider an image I defined in the image domain $\Omega \subset \Re^2$, image segmentation is to find a contour C that separates the image domain into different regions Ω_i, such that $\Omega = \bigcup_{i=1}^{n} \Omega_i$, $\Omega_i \bigcap \Omega_j = \varnothing$, $\forall i \neq j$, where n refers to the number of regions. We denote $P_i = \Pi_{\Omega_i} p(I(y))$ to be the probability of the random field of region Ω_i, where $p(I(y))$ refers to the probability density function

(PDF) of image intensity at point y. Assuming the gray levels of pixels are uncorrelated and independently distributed, to segment the image domain corresponds to look for a C that maximizes the likelihood function $\Pi_{i=1}^{n} P_i$, given by the product of probability of each region. By taking the negative logarithm operation, the maximization is turned to the following minimization problem

$$\sum_{i=1}^{n} -\log(P_i) = \sum_{i=1}^{n} \int_{\Omega_i} -\log(p(I(y)))dy \qquad (1)$$

For dissociative recombination of polyatomic molecular ions it has so far been possible in storage rings to measure only the branching ratios into neutral products, but not their state of excitation. The technique used for doing these measurements will be described in Section 2.

As stated in the previous section, local energy model works as a better alternative to global energy model for images with intensity inhomogeneity. To achieve this property, a kernel function with a scale parameter α is introduced to define a local region

$$K_\alpha(d) = \frac{1}{\sqrt{2\pi}\alpha} \exp(-\frac{|d|^2}{2\alpha^2}) \qquad (2)$$

This kernel function has a localization property that $K_\alpha(d)$ decreases and approaches to zero as $|d|$ increases. Hence, the local version of (1) within the neighborhood of a center point x is given by

$$E_x(I,C) = \sum_{i=1}^{n} \int_{\Omega_i} -K_\alpha(x-y)\log(p(I(y)))dy. \qquad (3)$$

In order to segment the whole image, we need to minimize the integral of (3) over the image domain Ω:

$$E(I,C) = \int_\Omega \left(\sum_{i=1}^{n} \int_{\Omega_i} -K_\alpha(x-y)\log(p(I(y)))dy \right)dx. \qquad (4)$$

In our multi-resolution framework, the probability density function of intensity distribution in the coarsest level of the pyramid can be approximated as Gaussian distribution as explained previously. Thus we adopt the following local Gaussian distribution to model the probability density function $p(I(y))$ within the neighborhood of x:

$$p_x(I(y)) = \frac{1}{\sqrt{2\pi}\sigma(x)} \exp(-\frac{(\mu(x)-I(y))^2}{2\sigma^2(x)}) \qquad (5)$$

Here both local intensity means $\mu(x)$ and standard deviations $\sigma(x)$ are modeled as spatially varying parameters to control the influence from neighboring pixels. This local Gaussian distribution has also be used in[24,25] to model pixel intensity distribution and its performance on images with intensity inhomogeneity is shown to be better than the global region model.

Without loss of generality, we assume the image domain is partitioned into foreground and background for simplicity. To take advantage of level set methods, these two regions are represented as outside and inside of zero level set of the level set function ϕ. By using the Heaviside function H, we introduce the following energy function to be minimized

$$E(I,\phi) = \sum_{i=1}^{2} \int\int - K_\alpha(x-y)\log(p(I(y)))M_i(\phi(y))dydx$$

$$+ \mu \int \frac{1}{2}(|\nabla\phi(x)-1|)^2 dx + \lambda \int |\nabla H(\phi(x))|dx \qquad . \qquad (6)$$

where $M_1(\phi) = H(\phi)$, $M_2(\phi) = 1 - H(\phi)$ and the subscript Ω is deleted for simplification. The second part of the energy function is a penalizing term used to penalize the deviation of the level set function from a signed distance function, which is common in level set diffusion for image enhancement,[26] and the third part corresponds to the length of the contour, which is used to smooth the contour during the evolution.[20] These two terms are weighted by two scale parameters μ and λ, respectively. Finally, by calculus of variations, we obtain the gradient descent flow that minimizing (6) as

$$\frac{\partial\phi}{\partial t} = -\delta(\phi)(e_1-e_2) + \mu\left(\nabla^2\phi - \mathrm{div}\frac{\nabla\phi}{|\nabla\phi|}\right) + \lambda\delta(\phi)\mathrm{div}\frac{\nabla\phi}{|\nabla\phi|}, \qquad (7)$$

where

$$e_i(x) = \int_\Omega K_\alpha(x-y)\left[\log(\sigma_i(y)) + \frac{(\mu(y)-I(x))^2}{2\sigma^2(y)}\right]dy, i \in \{1, 2\}, \qquad (8)$$

and δ is the derivative of H.

2.2. Phase-based Geodesic Active Contours

Geodesic active contours is originally proposed in [23] and its level set formulation is given by

$$\frac{\partial\phi}{\partial t} = g|\nabla\phi|\mathrm{div}\frac{\nabla\phi}{|\nabla\phi|} + \nabla g \cdot \nabla\phi + vg|\nabla\phi|, \qquad (9)$$

Here v is a constant and acts like the balloon force to inflate or deflate the contour depending on its sign.[27] The edge stop function g, generally taken as

$$g = \frac{1}{1+\left|\nabla G_\sigma * I\right|^2},$$
(10)

is used to stop the contour at object boundaries with high gradient. There are two shortcomings in the traditional GAC.[11,14] First, a careful initial contour is needed due to its limited capture range. In our method, this problem is solved by setting the result from the coarsest level, which is quite closed to the object boundaries, as the initial contour. Second, gradient-based operators usually do not work well for ultrasound images with low contrast and weak boundaries. We solve the problem by using local phase information derived from monogenic signal, which is theoretically intensity invariant.

2.2.1. *Monogenic Signal*

To perform local analysis (local phase and local amplitude) of one-dimensional signal, one usually needs to construct a complex analytic signal, which is formed by taking the original signal f and its Hilbert transform f_H (90 degree phase shift of f) as the real part and imaginary part, respectively. That is, $f_A = f + jf_H$, and local phase is computed as $\phi = \arctan(f_H / f)$. However, since the Hilbert transform is only restricted for one-dimensional function, the extension to two-dimensional local analysis is usually performed by applying one-dimensional analysis over several orientations and combining the results in some way, which is very complicated. Recently, Felsberg and Sommer proposed a two-dimensional generalization of the analytic signal based on the Riesz transform instead of the Hilbert transform: monogenic signal.[17] The monogenic signal preserves the core properties of the one-dimensional analytic signal that decompose a signal into local phase and local amplitude, and is defined by combining the original two-dimensional signal with its Riesz transform f_R to form a three-dimensional vector

$$f_M = (f, f_R) = (f, h_1 * f, h_2 * f).$$
(11)

In spatial domain, the Riesz filters are represented as

$$\begin{cases} h_1(x, y) = -\dfrac{x}{2\pi(x^2 + y^2)^{3/2}} \\[4mm] h_2(x, y) = -\dfrac{y}{2\pi(x^2 + y^2)^{3/2}} \end{cases}.$$
(12)

In practical applications, the local properties are estimated via a bank of quadrature filters tuned to various spatial frequencies because real images usually consist of a wide range of frequencies. Therefore a set of bandpass filters are combined with the monogenic signal, which now becomes

$$f_M = (g * f, \ g * h_1 * f, \ g * h_2 * f).$$ (13)

Then the monogenic signal can be represented by scalar-valued even and vector-valued odd filtered responses as even $= g * f$ and odd $= (g * h_1 * f, g * h_2 * f)$, respectively. Here g is the spatial representation of an isotropic bandpass filter. Previously, several works use the log-Gabor filter to detect features. However, it has been shown that Gaussian derivative filter could be a better alternative to log-Gabor filter in the case of feature detection.[27] In frequency domain, the two-dimensional isotropic bandpass Gaussian derivative filter is defined as

$$G(\omega) = n_c |\omega|^\alpha \exp(-s^2 |\omega|^2).$$ (14)

where $\alpha \geqslant 1$, $\omega = (u, v)$, s is the scale parameter, and n_c is a normalization constant. Please refer to[28] for more details.

2.2.2. FA-based Edge Stop Function

Phase congruency model assumes that features are perceived at points in the image, where the Fourier components are maximally in phase, rather than points with maximal intensity gradient.[29] Various feature types give rise to points of high phase congruency, including step edges, line and roof edges. The detection of step edges, which are our focus, corresponds to find points that have phase responses near to 0 or π. However, previous phase-based methods are sensitive to noise and may provide inaccurate localization. Kovesi proposed to detect step edges using feature asymmetry to improve the localization. Our edge stop function is also based on feature asymmetry.[30] However, the feature asymmetry in our case is derived from the monogenic signal, which is expected to work better as it is the natural extension of the one-dimensional analytic signal. Moreover, as suggested by Kovesi to use feature asymmetry over a number of scales for step edge feature detection, we define the following multi-scale monogenic feature asymmetry

$$FA_{ms} = \frac{1}{N} \sum_{s=1}^{N} \frac{\lfloor |odd_s| - |even_s| - T_s \rfloor}{\sqrt{odd_s^2 + even_s^2} + \varepsilon}.$$ (15)

where N is the number of scales, ε is a small constant to avoid division by zero, T_s is the scale specific noise threshold and $\lfloor \cdot \rfloor$ denotes zeroing of negative values.

For each scale, the feature asymmetry takes value close to zero in smooth regions and close to one near boundaries. Finally, the multi-scale feature asymmetry is used to define the local phase-based edge stop function, which will be incorporated into the geodesic active contours to replace the previous gradient-based edge stop function, as following

$$g = \frac{1}{1 + FA_{ms}^{\beta}},$$
(16)

where β is the parameter to control the influence of FA_{ms}. This new edge stop function plays an important role for feature detection of images with low contrast and weak boundaries since the feature asymmetry is independent of intensity variation.

3. Experiments and Results

We demonstrate the effectiveness of the proposed method on the segmentation of left ventricle from echocardiographic images with high speckle noise and low contrast. We use the following parameters for all the experiments: time step $\Delta t = 0.1$, $\mu = 1.0$, $\lambda = 0.0001 \times 255 \times 255$, $\alpha = 3$, $\beta = 0.3$, $N = 3$, $a = 1.58$ (bandwidth 2 octaves), wavelengths $s = (12, 15, 18)$, and the size of the kernel function K_{α} is set as $(4\alpha + 1) \times (4\alpha + 1)$. Parameter v in (9) depends on the content of the images and is set separately. The Heaviside function H and its derivative δ are regularized as

$$\begin{cases} H_{\varepsilon}(x) = \frac{1}{2}\left[1 + \frac{2}{\pi}\arctan(\frac{x}{\varepsilon})\right] \\ \delta_{\varepsilon}(x) = \frac{1}{\pi}\frac{\varepsilon}{\varepsilon^2 + x^2} \end{cases},$$
(17)

where ε was simply taken as 1 in all experiments unless stated. Lastly, the level set function ϕ is initialized to be a binary function, taking constant value -1 for region inside and 1 for region outside.

In order to validate the advantages of our method, we compare our results with those from two classical segmentation methods. The first one is LGDFE model,[25] and the second one is the GAC model.[23] For the two classical methods, we use the parameters that produce best results. Fig. 2 compares the segmentation results of different methods on four echocardiographic images.[15] The first row shows the original images overlaid with circular initial contour and the results segmented by an expert are presented in second row. As can be seen from these figures, high speckle noise exits in Figs. 2(a) and 2(b), and Figs. 2(c)

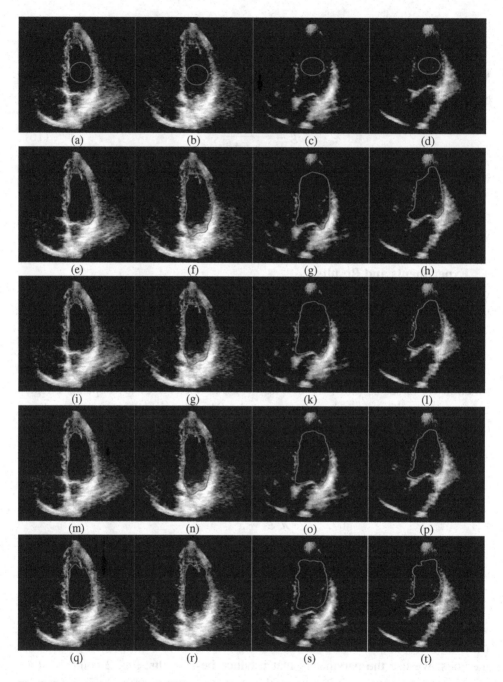

Fig. 2. Segmentation results of different methods on echocardiographic images. First row: original images overlaid with initial contours; second row: results of manual segmentation; third row: results of our method; fourth row: results of LGDFE model; fifth row: results of GAC model.

Table 1. Quantitative comparisons of the three segmentation methods.

Methods/Figures	Fig. 2 (a)	Fig. 2 (b)	Fig. 2 (c)	Fig. 2 (d)
Our method	0.9600	0.9530	0.9696	0.9581
LGDFE model	0.9111	0.8071	0.8922	0.8696
GAC model	0.8569	0.8751	0.8874	0.8864

and 2(d) reveal low contrast and weak boundaries. The segmentation results of our method are shown in third row and the parameter v for the four images is set as -0.8, -1.0, -0.6 and -0.8, respectively. Here we can see that our method captures well the boundaries of left ventricle, and the results are almost the same as the ones presented in the second row. The segmentation results of LGDFE model and GAC model are shown in fourth and fifth row, respectively. The LGDFE model can only detect partial region of the left ventricle as it uses Gaussian statistics to model the image intensity distribution. Different from the LGDFE model, our method only assumes the Gaussian statistics to be held in the coarsest level of the pyramid, which is true due to Gaussian smoothing and subsampling. Hence our method can accurately extract the object boundaries in the coarsest level and pass them to finer level for further evolution. The GAC also cannot handle well the speckle noise, as shown in Figs. 2(q) and 2(r). Furthermore, edge leakage is also exhibited in the GAC model for images with low contrast and weak boundaries, seeing Figs. 2(s) and 2(t). This is mainly due to the use of gradient-based edge stop function, which cannot stop the contour on weak boundaries. With the local phase-base edge stop function, our methods can successfully stop the contour on the right position.

Table 1 shows the quantitative comparisons of the three segmentation methods using Dice similarity coefficient, which is defined as

$$dice = 2 \times \frac{|S_m \cap S_c|}{|S_m| + |S_c|}, \tag{18}$$

where S_m and S_c are manual and computer generated segmentation. The closer the disc value is to 1, the better the segmentation is. The number in Table 1 represents the *dice* values of the three methods on the four echocardiographic images shown in Fig. 2. It can be seen that the *dice* values of our method are much higher than the ones of LGDFE model and GAC model, which implies that our method performs better than the other two methods.

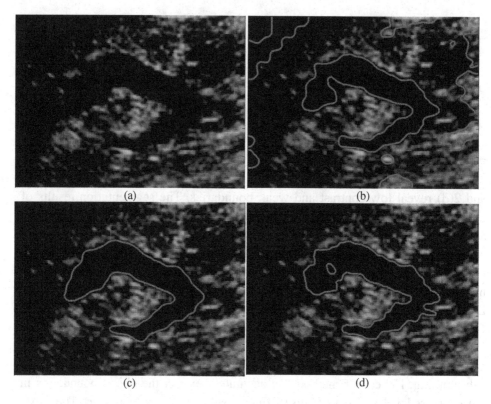

Fig. 3. Comparison of the result of our method with that of single level implementation and the RSF model on a kidney image: (a) original image, (b) result of single level implementation, (c) result of our multi-level method and (d) result of the RSF model.

In Fig. 3, we compare the segmentation result of our method with that of single level implementation and the RSF model[21] on a kidney image. Intensity inhomogeneities and speckle noise are obvious in the original image (Fig. 3(a)). Fig. 3(b) is the result of directly using the local statistic driven active contour model on the original image while Fig. 3(c) presents the result of our multi-level implementation. A lot of redundant contours emerge in Fig. 3(b) due to the speckle noise. This problem is eliminated in our multi-level implementation since the algorithm works from the coarsest level where the speckle noise has been smoothed. Fig. 3(d) shows the result of RSF model. To be fair, instead of directly using RSF on the original image, we implemented the original RSF model on our multi-level framework. It is observed that our result is much better than that of RSF model. In addition, thanks to the Gaussian filter based regularization, our resultant boundary is much smoother than that of RSF model.

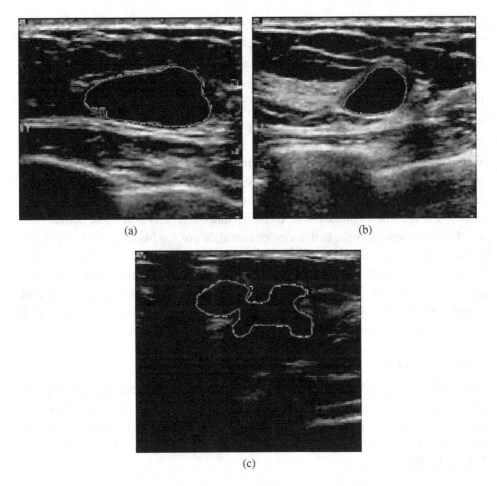

(a)   (b)

(c)

Fig. 4. Segmentation of ultrasound breast lesion images: Manual segmentation results (green dash line) and our results (red solid line).

To further validate the proposed method, comparison between manual segmentation results by a doctor and our results is illustrated in Fig. 4. We use three ultrasound breast lesion images for this experiment. Green lines represent manual segmentation results and red lines refer to our results. As can be seen in the figures, our results are visually the same with manual segmentation results. For quantitative comparison, we measure the mismatch ratio between manual segmentation results and our results as

$$\tau = 1 - \frac{2 \times Area(\Omega_{C_1} \cap \Omega_{C_2})}{Area(\Omega_{C_1}) + Area(\Omega_{C_2})}, \tag{19}$$

where Ω_C represents the region inside contour C. The mismatch ratios for Figs. 4(a), 4(b) and 4(c) are 0.0252, 0.0122 and 0.0284, respectively. All the mismatch ratios are below 0.03, which verifies the accuracy of our method.

4. Conclusions

Active contour models are a kind of general-purpose mathematical tools for partial differential equation problems. It is possible to adapt them for dynamic wave simulation, image denoising and enhancement, and shape recovery from unorganized samples, etc. In this study, we aim at inventing some active contour models for ultrasound image segmentation. However, the latter is technically challenging because of spike noise, intensity inhomogeneity and weak boundaries, which makes conventional active contour models not readily applicable. A series of innovative measures have been proposed to improve active contour models, including filtering-based multi-resolution framework, combinational intensity and phase analysis. We evaluated their performance on different ultrasound images from clinics by comparing with the classical LGDFE, GAC and RSF models. The results are pretty supportive for further investigation.

Acknowledgments

This work was supported partially by the National Natural Science Foundation of China under Grants 61271123 and 61233012, a grant from the Research Grants Council of Hong Kong (Project No. CUHK412510), and in part by the Fundamental Research Funds for the Central Universities with Grant 2013HGCH0009.

References

1. J. A. Noble, D. Boukerroui, Ultrasound image segmentation: a survey. IEEE Trans. Med. Imag. 25(8) (2006) 987–1010
2. R. Wagner, S. Smith, J. Sandrik, H. Lopez, Statistics of speckle in ultrasound B-scans. IEEE Trans. Sonics Ultrason. 30(3) (1983) 156–163
3. V. Dutt, J. Greenleaf, Adaptive speckle reduction filter for log-compressed B-scan images. IEEE Trans. Med. Imag. 15(6) (1996) 802–813
4. A. Evans, M. Nixon, Biased motion-adaptive temporal filtering for speckle reduction in echocardiography. IEEE Trans. Med. Imag. 15(1) (1996) 39–50
5. G. Xiao, M. Brady, J. A. Noble, Y. Zhang, Segmentation of ultrasound B-mode images with intensity inhomogeneity correction. IEEE Trans. Med. Imag. 21(1) (2002) 48–57
6. J. G. Bosch, S. C. Mitchell, B. P. F. Lelieveldt, F. Nijland, O. Kamp, M. Sonka, J. H. C. Reiber, Automatic segmentation of echocardiographic sequences by active appearance motion models. IEEE Trans. Med. Imag. 21(11) (2002) 1374–1383
7. M. Kass, A. P. Witkin, D. Terzopoulos, Snakes: Active contour models. International Journal of Computer Vision 1(4) (1988) 321–331
8. A. Sarti, C. Corsi, E. Mazzini, C. Lamberti, Maximum likelihood segmentation of ultrasound images with rayleigh distribution. IEEE Trans. Ultrason. 52(6) (2005) 974–960

9. Z. Tao, H. D. Tagare, Tunneling descent for m.a.p. active contours in ultrasound segmentation. Medical Image Analysis 11(3) (2007) 266–281

10. Y. Zhu, X. Papademetris, A. J. Sinusas, J. S. Duncan, A coupled deformable model for tracking myocardial borders from real-time echocardiography using an incompressibility constraint. Medical Image Analysis 14(3) (2010) 429–448

11. B. N. Li, C. K. Chui, S. Chang, S. H. Ong, Integrating spatial fuzzy clustering with level set methods for automated medical image segmentation. Computers in Biology and Medicine 41 (1) (2011) 1–10

12. B. N. Li, C. K. Chui, S. H. Ong, T. Numano, T. Washio, K. Homma, S. Chang, S. Venkatesh, E. Kobayashi, Modeling shear modulus distribution in magnetic resonance elastography with piecewise constant level sets. Magnetic Resonance Imaging 30(3) (2012) 390

13. A. Belaid, D. Boukerroui, Y. Maingourd, J. F. Lerallut, Phase-based level set segmentation of ultrasound images. IEEE Transactions on Information Technology in Biomedicine 15(1) (2011) 138–147

14. B. N. Li, C. K. Chui, S. Chang, S. H. Ong, A new unified level set method for semi-automatic liver tumor segmentation on contrast-enhanced CT images. Expert Systems with Applications 39(10) (2012) 9661–9668

15. M. Mulet-Parada, J. A. Noble, 2D+T acoustic boundary detection in echocardiography. Medical Image Analysis 4(1) (2000) 21–30

16. K. Rajpoot, A. Noble, V. Grau, N. Rajpoot, Feature detection from echocardiography images using local phase information. In: Proceedings 12th Medical Image Understanding and Analysis (MIUA'2008). (2008)

17. M. Felsberg, G. Sommer, The monogenic signal. IEEE Transactions on Signal Processing 49(12) (2001) 3136–3144

18. E. Ashton, K. Parker, Multiple resolution Bayesian segmentation of ultrasound images. Ultrason. Imag. 17(4) (1995) 291–304

19. N. Lin, W. Yu, J. S. Duncan, Combinative multi-scale level set framework for echocardiographic image segmentation. Medical Image Analysis 7(4) (2003) 529–537

20. T. F. Chan, L. A. Vese, Active contours without edges. IEEE Trans. Imag. Proc. 10(2) (2001) 266–277

21. C. Li, C. Y. Kao, J. C. Gore, Z. Ding, Minimization of region-scalable fitting energy for image segmentation. IEEE Trans. Imag. Proc. 17(10) (2008) 1940–1949

22. T. Brox, D. Cremers, On local region models and a statistical interpretation of the piecewise smooth mumford-shah functional. International Journal of Computer Vision 84(2) (2009) 184–193

23. V. Caselles, R. Kimmel, G. Sapiro, Geodesic active contours. International Journal of Computer Vision 22(1) (1997) 61–79

24. T. Brox, D. Cremers, On the statistical interpretation of the piecewise smooth mumford-shah functional. In Sgallari, F., Murli, A., Paragios, N., eds.: SSVM. Volume 4485 of Lecture Notes in Computer Science., Springer (2007) 203–213

25. L. Wang, L. He, A. Mishra, C. Li, Active contours driven by local Gaussian distribution fitting energy. Signal Processing 89(12) (2009) 2435–2447

26. B. N. Li, C. K. Chui, S. H. Ong, S. Chang, E. Kobayashi, Level set diffusion for MRE image enhancement. Lecture Notes in Computer Science 6326 (2010) 305–313

27. L. D. Cohen, On active contour models and balloons. CVGIP: Image Underst. 53(2) (1991) 211–218

28. D. Boukerroui, J. A. Noble, M. Brady, On the choice of band-pass quadrature filters. Journal of Mathematical Imaging and Vision 21(1-2) (2004) 53–80

29. M. C. Morrone, R. A. Owens, Feature detection from local energy. Pattern Recogn. Lett. 6(5) (1987) 303–313

30. P. Kovesi, Image features from phase congruency. Videre: Journal of Computer Vision Research 1(3) (1999)

Part 2

2D, 3D, Reconstructions/Imaging Algorithms, Systems & Sensor Fusion

CHAPTER 8

MODEL-BASED IMAGE RECONSTRUCTION IN OPTOACOUSTIC TOMOGRAPHY

Amir Rosenthal[*], Daniel Razansky, and Vasilis Ntziachristos

Institute for Biological and Medical Imaging (IBMI)
Technische Universität München and Helmholtz Zentrum München
Ingoldstädter Landstraße 1, 85764 Neuherberg, Germany
[*]E-mail: eeamir@tum.de

Optoacoustic tomography is a powerful hybrid bioimaging method which retains rich optical contrast and diffraction-limited ultrasonic resolution at depths of varying from millimeters to several centimeters in biological tissue irrespective of photon scattering. Optoacoustic imaging is commonly performed with high power optical pulses whose absorption leads to instantaneous temperature increase, thermal expansion and, subsequently, to the generation of a pressure field proportional to the distribution of the absorbed energy. For tomographic data acquisition, the optoacoustically generated waves are detected on a surface surrounding the imaged region. Recovery of the initially generated pressure distribution from the detected tomographic projections, and hence of the optical energy deposition in the tissue, constitutes the inverse problem of optoacoustic tomography, which is often solved using closed-form inversion formulae. However, those closed-form solutions are only exact for ideal detection geometries, which often do not accurately represent the experimental conditions. Model-based image-reconstruction techniques represent an alternative approach to solving the inverse problem that can significantly reduce image artifacts associated with approximated analytical formulae and significantly enhance image quality in non-ideal imaging scenarios. In the model-based reconstruction, a linear forward model is constructed to accurately describe the experimental conditions of the imaging setup. Inversion is performed numerically and may include regularization when the projection data is insufficient. This chapter demonstrates the benefits of the model-based reconstruction approach and describes numerically efficient methods for its implementation.

1. Introduction

Optoacoustic tomography enables visualization of optical contrast in optically turbid medium, retaining high resolution independent from photon scattering. In its most common form, the technique is based on excitation of the imaged object with short light pulses and subsequent detection of the optoacoustically generated responses. Biological and medical applications of optoacoustic tomography have experienced exponential growth in the last decade, mostly due to tremendous progress in hardware development that enabled rapid data acquisition [1-4]. As optoacoustic tomography develops into a viable imaging tool for medical research and clinical use, the importance of efficient optoacoustic image-formation techniques has equally increased.

Although a great variety of optoacoustic-based techniques exists for imaging and sensing of biological tissue, e.g. optical resolution microscopy [4] or flow cytometry [5], our focus is on tomographic imaging scenarios that use stationary illumination of the imaged region while the projection data relates to the ultrasound signals collected at different positions around this region. Exact (closed-form) solutions to the inverse problem usually require that the detection of the optoacoustic responses be performed by an ideal point detector, which has isotropic sensitivity, continuously scanned over a closed surface surrounding the imaged object [6]. For a few specific detection surfaces, explicit inversion formulae are known, which are commonly known as back-projection algorithms [7, 8].

In practice, the solution to the inverse problem cannot be exact under realistic experimental conditions. First, as always true for experimental measurements, the projection data is contaminated by noise. Second, the projection data that can be experimentally collected is always limited, whereas the exact mathematical solutions assume that the projection data is defined over continuous variable and is therefore infinite. If the measured projection data is too sparse, it may lead to streak artifacts in the reconstructed images when back-projection algorithms are used [9, 10]. Third, when the aperture of the detector is greater than the size of features in the reconstructed image, the assumption of an ideal point detector loses its accuracy. In such cases, the use of exact reconstruction algorithms unavoidably leads to loss of image resolution [11, 12]. Finally, in many cases, the imaged object is not accessible from all angles, leading to the so-called limited view scenario, in which the detection surface does not fully surround the object [13]. In such cases, in addition to inevitable loss of image resolution, the use of back-projection algorithms would lead to additional streak artifacts.

Model-based reconstruction constitutes an alternative approach to tomographic reconstruction that is based on a discrete reformulation of the inverse problem. The first step of model-based techniques is therefore accurate discretization of the forward problem, leading to the best possible description of the experimental setup by a numerical model. Since optoacoustic imaging is generally governed by linear equations, the forward model may be represented by a matrix. Once a matrix relation between the image and projection data is established, image reconstruction is performed by solving a set of linear equations. In the following sections we present different approaches for constructing the model matrix and performing the inversion.

2. The model matrix

In an acoustically homogenous medium, under the condition of thermal confinement, the optoacoustically induced pressure wave $p(r, t)$ obeys the following differential equation [12]:

$$\frac{\partial^2 p(r,t)}{\partial t^2} - v^2 \nabla^2 p(r,t) = \Gamma H_r(r) \frac{\partial H_t(t)}{\partial t}, \tag{1}$$

where v and ρ are velocity of sound in tissue and its density, Γ is the Grüneisen parameter, and $H(r,t) = H_r(r) H_t(t)$ is the amount of energy absorbed in the tissue per unit volume and per unit time.

We start our treatment by using the solution to Eq. (1) for a delta-function source, i.e. the right-hand side of the equation is substituted with $\delta(r)\delta(t)$. Its solution in that case consists of a spherical delta function [12]:

$$p_\delta(r,t) = \frac{\delta(|r| - vt)}{4\pi |r|}. \tag{2}$$

Due to the linearity of Eq. (1), any solution can be represented as a superposition of the fundamental solution given in Eq. (2), i.e.

$$p(r,t) = \frac{\Gamma}{4\pi} \int \frac{\delta(|r - r'| - v(t - t'))}{|r - r'|} H_r(r') \frac{\partial}{\partial t} H_t(t') dr' dt'. \tag{3}$$

Assuming that the laser pulse is significantly shorter than the temporal resolution of the detectors, the function $H_t(t)$ can be substituted by a temporal delta function, yielding:

$$p(r,t) = \frac{\Gamma}{4\pi} \int \frac{\delta'(|r - r'| - vt)}{|r - r'|} H_r(r') dr', \tag{4}$$

where δ' is the derivative of Dirac's delta function. Further simplification leads to

$$p(r,t) = \frac{\Gamma}{4\pi v} \frac{\partial}{\partial t} \int_{|r - r'| = vt} \frac{H_r(r')}{|r - r'|} dr', \tag{5}$$

where the integration is performed on the sphere defined by $|r - r'| = vt$. When the problem is reduced to two-dimensional (2D) space, the optoacoustic sources are assumed to be located on a plane, i.e. $H_r(r) = H_{xy}(x, y)\delta(z)$; in which case the integration is performed on an arc.

Eq. (5) constitutes a continuous representation of the optoacoustic forward problem, in which the image is a continuous function of the space variables. In a discrete model, the image is represented by a finite set of pixels or voxels. Discretization of Eq. (5) thus involves approximating $H_r(r)$ by a finite sum of a priori defined interpolation functions:

$$H_r(r) \approx \sum_{n=1}^{N} h_n f_n(r),$$ (6)

where h_n are the values of $H_r(r)$ on the image grid. The choice of interpolation functions in Eq. (6) is crucial to the accuracy of the discrete model. Specifically, if the image is approximated by a piece-wise constant function [14], discontinuities in the interpolation functions may lead to spurious spike-artifacts in the calculated acoustic signal owing to the derivative term in Eq. (5). More accurate discretization of Eq. (5) may be achieved when $H_r(r)$ is approximated by smooth interpolation functions [9, 10 15], as shown in Fig. 1. Substituting Eq. (6) into Eq. (5) and performing the integral, a matrix relation between the acoustic signal and optoacoustic image is obtained:

$$\mathbf{p} = \mathbf{Mh}$$ (7)

where $\mathbf{p}$ is a column vector representing the acoustic fields measured at a set of positions and time instants; $\mathbf{h}$ is a column vector representing the values of the optoacoustic image on the grid; and $\mathbf{M}$ is the model matrix discretely representing the integral operation in Eq. (5).

Eq. (7) may be used for reconstructing the optoacoustic image from measurements of the optoacoustic responses at a set of positions. However, in reality ultrasound transducers are often designed to operate in a specific frequency band, thus possess a non-flat frequency response which may distort the acoustic signals. This response, referred to herein as the transducer electric response, is a result of acoustic and electric impedance mismatches and may be measured experimentally [16]. An additional effect which needs to be taken into consideration in practice is the geometric (spatial) response of the detector. Since ultrasound transducers have a finite aperture, they do not measure the pressure wave at a point, but rather over a finite surface, or, more generally, a finite volume. This may be mathematically described as

$$P_{\text{detect}}(t) = \int p(r,t)D(r)dr,$$ (8)

where

$$D(r) = \begin{cases} 1 & r \in \text{detected area} \\ 0 & \text{else} \end{cases}.$$ (9)

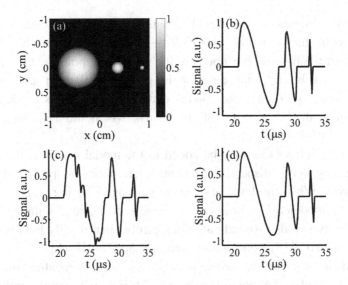

Fig. 1. The importance of interpolation on the accuracy of the optoacoustic model: (a) an optoacoustic image containing three parabolic objects. (b) The analytically calculated optoacoustic signals detected by a sensor at (-4,0) cm. (c) The optoacoustic signals calculated using the model of Ref. [14] where piecewise-constant interpolation was used. (d) The optoacoustic signals calculated using the model of Ref. [9] which uses smooth interpolation.

As a result of the electric and geometric responses of the detector, the measured signals often significantly deviate from the actual pressure profiles.

Both the electric and geometric responses of the detector may be incorporated into the model matrix. First, the response of the detector should be either measured or simulated [12, 16, 17]. In analogy to Eq. (4), the pressure wave detected by the finite-aperture transducer is given by

$$p(t) = \frac{\Gamma}{4\pi v} \frac{\partial}{\partial t} \int R(t,r')H_r(r')dr', \qquad (10)$$

where $R(t,r')$ is the spatially dependent response of the transducer. We note that for each time point, the integration is performed over all values of r' and not only along a single arc or sphere. In order to discretize Eq. (9), we first bring it to the form of Eq. (4):

$$p(t) = \frac{\Gamma}{4\pi} \int |r-r'| R\left(t+\frac{|r-r'|}{v},r'\right) * \frac{\delta'(|r-r'|-vt)}{|r-r'|} H_r(r')dr', \quad (11)$$

where convolution is performed in the time domain. Thus, in order to obtain the signal measured by a finite-size detector, for each value of r' contribution of the optoacoustic source to the signal measured by a point detector should be convolved with the function $|r-r'|R(t+|r-r'|/v,r')$. In the discretized equations, contribution of the optoacoustic source at point r_j to the acoustic signal measured by a point detector is given by the jth column of the matrix $\mathbf{M}$. Thus, to obtain the model matrix for a finite-size detector, for all values of j, the jth column of the matrix $\mathbf{M}$ should be convolved with $|r-r_j|R\left(t+|r-r_j|/v,r_j\right)$.

An additional effect that may be added to the model matrix is the impact of acoustic heterogeneity, dispersion, and attenuation on the propagation of the acoustic waves. When the level of acoustic heterogeneity is relatively small, its effect may be modeled by variations in the speed of sound within the imaged object. Arbitrary speed-of-sound variations can be then readily incorporated into the model matrix [18], but would require additional experiments to first determine their distribution. Acoustic dispersion and attenuation may also be modeled and added to the model matrix [19-21]. However, since both effects are frequency dependent, their modeling so far has been restricted to frequency-domain formulations. Additionally, since both acoustic dispersion and attenuation generally depend on the particular tissue being imaged, more measurements may become necessary in order to accurately model their effect.

3. Image formation

Within the model-based framework, image formation is performed by inverting the matrix relation in Eq. (7). When the inverse problem is well-posed, i.e. the projection data is sufficient for forming an image, the inversion of Eq. (7) may be performed by solving the following least-square problem [9]:

$$\mathbf{h}_{\text{sol}} = \arg\min_{\mathbf{h}} \|\mathbf{p} - \mathbf{Mh}\|^2, \tag{12}$$

where $\|\cdot\|$ is the ℓ_2 norm. The solution to Eq. (12) is given by the Moore–Penrose pseudo-inverse:

$$\mathbf{h}_{\text{sol}} = \mathbf{M}^{\dagger}\mathbf{p}, \tag{13}$$

where $\mathbf{M}^{\dagger}$ is the pseudo-inverse and is given by $\mathbf{M}^{\dagger} = \left(\mathbf{M}^T\mathbf{M}\right)^{-1}\mathbf{M}^T$, and T denotes the conjugate transpose operator. The advantage of using the pseudo-inverse approach is that it is determined only by the experimental setup, e.g., positions of the detectors, their electric and geometric responses, etc., and not by the measured data. Thus, the pseudo-inverse $\mathbf{M}^{\dagger}$ may be calculated once for every measurement configuration with inversion reduced to multiplying it by the measured values of $\mathbf{p}$ – a process that can be realistically performed in real time.

The disadvantage of the pseudo-inverse approach is that its calculation might involve multiplication and inversion of very large matrices, which may turn impractical.

When the model matrix is too large to be inverted directly, iterative algorithms may be used instead to solve Eq. (12), e.g. gradient descent or conjugate gradient. In the iterative process, matrix-matrix multiplications are avoided, and matrix-vector multiplications are performed instead. Thus, the calculation of each iteration may be performed with high numerical efficiency. Generally, the conjugate-gradient method is a preferred method as it is characterized by a fast convergence rate. Further increase in efficiency may be achieved by using LSQR [22] – an implementation of the conjugate-gradient method which is exceptionally efficient in the case of sparse matrices. Indeed, model matrices in optoacoustic tomography are generally sparse because acoustic signals measured at a specific projection angle and time instant are not affected by the entire image, but rather by a small portion of it, which in the case of ideal detection withers into an arc or a sphere (Eq. (5)).

In many cases, the inversion problem is either ill-conditioned or ill-posed, i.e. the acquired projection data is insufficient to both uniquely and accurately determine the image over the prescribed grid. In other words, a large number of inherently different images may all produce a projection dataset that is very close to the measured data. To effectively perform inversion, it thus becomes necessary to impose constraints on the image by means of regularization. Many regularization techniques have been demonstrated for optoacoustic tomography, including Tikhonov regularization [10, 23], singular value decomposition (SVD) [13, 24], limited-iteration LSQR [13], multi-scale techniques [23, 25, 26], and total-variation (TV) regularization [27].

Theoretically, the inversion problem is well-posed when the projection data corresponds to full tomographic view, the detectors are ideal, the density of projections is sufficient, and the measurements are performed with sufficient signal-to-noise ratio (SNR) and bandwidth. In practice, fulfilling all these conditions in a single system is a highly challenging task and often trade-offs exist between the different constraints. For instance, if only a finite number of detectors is given, a trade-off exist between the tomographic coverage and density of projections. Also, in detection based on piezoelectric elements, reduction in size to achieve a point-like transducer often leads to reduction in SNR. Another example is detectors having their sensitivity increased by means of acoustically resonating designs, which are usually characterized by reduced bandwidth.

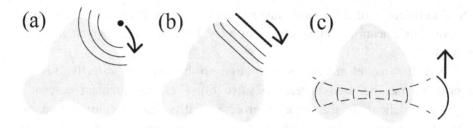

Fig. 2. Three common scenarios for optoacoustic tomography schematically presented in 2D.

Fig. 2 schematically shows three detection geometries commonly used in optoacoustic tomography: (a) point detectors, (b) flat detectors, and (c) focused detectors. For simplicity, the drawing is shown in 2D, though the concepts are generally applicable to 3D, e.g. cylindrically focused transducers are flat in one of their dimensions and focused in the other whereas spherically focused transducers are focused in both dimensions. The figure further illustrates the different detection patterns characterizing these three geometries. In the case of a point detector, the sensitivity is isotropic while the signals detected at a given time instant are assumed to originate from sources located on an arc (Eq. (5)). In the case of flat detectors, the sensitivity is anisotropic and generally higher for regions directly facing the detector. In contrast to the point detector, sources whose detection delay is the same (i.e. the duration of time it takes for the acoustic signals they generate to be detected) generally lie on a line (2D) or a plane (3D). Naturally, sensitivity is also anisotropic in the case of focused detectors and is significantly higher within the focal region.

Fig. 3 shows a reconstruction of a mouse head from experimental data obtained with a system whose geometry may be approximated in 2D by the one shown in Fig. 2a. The reconstructions were performed using (a) back-projection and (b) model-based inversion using the LSQR algorithm [28]. The imaging system consisted of an ultrasound detector cylindrically focused in the imaging plane and rotated around the mouse head for the acquisition of tomographic data. Illumination was restricted to a thin layer which coincided with the transducer's focal plane. Although light diffusion prevented maintaining a thin sheet illumination within the mouse, the combination of the illumination pattern and acoustic focusing has effectively led to an approximately 2D tomographic imaging scenario, for which a 2D model matrix can be constructed. Clearly, the image reconstructed using the model-based approach suffered from less artifacts and was able to visualize more precisely its boundary and various anatomical features [28].

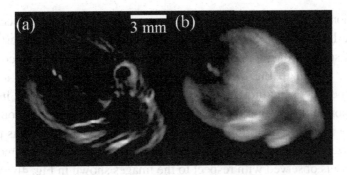

Fig. 3. A comparison between (a) backprojection and (b) model-based reconstruction in an image of a mouse head [28].

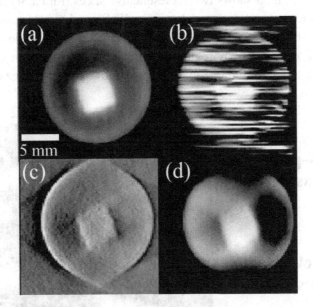

Fig. 4. The effect of limited tomographic coverage on the quality of the reconstructed image [13]. (a) A reconstruction of a cylindrical phantom with a square inclusion from full-view experimental data. (b) Model-based reconstruction with no regularizarion when only 130° of the projection data is used. (c) Back-projection reconstruction of the phantom in the limited-view scenario. (d) Regularized model-based reconstruction of the phantom in the limited-view scenario.

In geometries which relate to the case presented in Fig. 2a, regularization is often used to overcome limited tomographic coverage, or limited view. In these cases, spatial frequencies which correspond to the orientation of the missing projections cannot be accurately recovered [13]. Fig. 4a shows an image of a tissue-mimicking cylindrical phantom imaged with a system similar to that used in Fig. 3 and reconstructed without regularization [13]. In Fig. 4b, the same reconstruction is performed, but with using only 130° of the projection data. Clearly, the lack of projection data has unavoidably led to image artifacts and smearing of some of the phantom's boundary. The back-projection reconstruction in this case, shown in Fig. 4c, also exhibited artifacts in addition to a higher level of superfluous texture observed also in the full view case in Fig. 3a. Regularization in this example was performed using a modified version of LSQR in which the image gradient in the direction of the stripe artifacts was penalized; the regularized result is shown in Fig. 4d. A significant improvement in the image quality is observed with respect to the images shown in Fig. 4b and 4c.

The relatively good image quality obtained by regularized model-based inversion as compared to back-projection reconstructions has been also observed in 3D geometries. Fig. 5 shows two representative slices from a 3D reconstruction of an excised mouse heart performed using a 3D limited-view optoacoustic setup [10]. The reconstructions on the top were obtained using back-projection, whereas for the bottom ones Tikhonov-regularized model-based inversion was used. As can be seen, the model-based reconstructions exhibited better image quality.

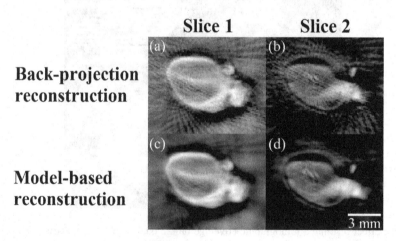

Fig. 5. A comparison between back-projection and model-based reconstructions of a mouse heart in a 3D limited view scenario [10]. The reduction of streak aritifacts in the model-based reconstruction is readily seen in the images.

The major disadvantage of using ultrasound detectors that are sufficiently small to be considered as point detectors (Fig. 2a) is that sensitivity often scales with the size of the detector. Thus, larger detectors (Fig. 2b) may achieve higher sensitivity. However, the higher sensitivity comes at a price of signal distortion with higher frequencies suppressed in the detection [12]. This bias is spatially variant, i.e. it depends on the location of the optoacoustic source, whereas increasing the offset of the source's location from the central axis of the detector, which is perpendicular to its surface, leads to stronger suppression of high frequency components in the detected signals. When this bias is not taken into account in the reconstruction, smearing effects in the tangential direction are expected in the images [12], as demonstrated in Fig. 6. The images in Fig. 6 were obtained using the optoacoustic setup used in Fig. 3, i.e. the cylindrically focused transducer scanned to attain full tomographic view in 2D. The length of the detector in the imaged plane was 1.3 cm, sufficiently large to create significant distortions in the detected signals. Figs. 6a and 6b respectively show reconstructions of a dark hair with an approximate diameter of 100 μm using model matrices with assumed point detector versus a flat 1.3 cm wide detector. Clearly, proper modelling of the transducer's geometry led to higher resolution image. Although the restoration of the high-frequency components in the optoacoustic image is a task which would usually require regularization, owing to the relatively simple geometry of the imaged object and good SNR in the measured data, no regularization was required. Figs. 6c and 6d respectively show the corresponding reconstructions of a mouse head using the same experimental setup and the two modelling approaches. In this case, owing to the complexity of the image and lower SNR, Tikhonov regularization was used for the reconstruction in Fig. 6d. As can be readily seen, incorporating the detector's geometric response in the model has again resulted in an image with more defined anatomical details.

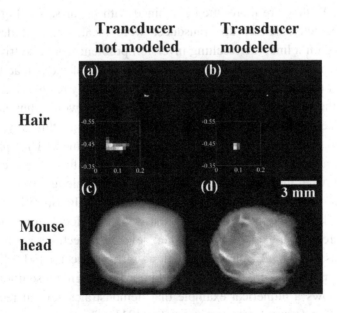

Fig. 6. Resolution enhancement for a large flat detector due to modelling the shape of the transducer achieved for a cross-section of a dark hair and mouse head [12].

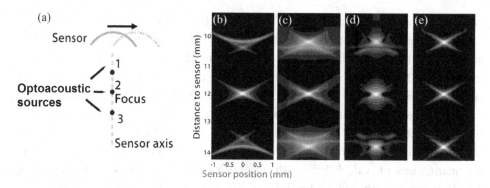

Fig. 7. (a) Simulation of a linear scan with a spherically focused detector [31]. The detector is scanned along the top of the image. (b) reconstruction using the ideal-focus assumption. (c) VD reconstruction. (d) Filtered VD reconstruction. (e) Reconstruction with IMMI. The images are represented in a linear color scale and normalized to their respective maxima.

In many applications, focused detectors are used to improve detection sensitivity and thus increase the speed of image acquisition. One of the advantages of focused detectors is that optoacoustic sources in the focus may be detected without significant suppression of their high frequencies. Therefore, in high-resolution imaging applications, e.g. optoacoustic microscopy, focused detectors are a common geometry for achieving both high sensitivity and high resolution. Although focused detector may be used in a tomographic scanning geometry [29], they are more often combined with linear scans (Fig. 2c). If the focusing characteristics of the transducer were ideal, i.e. if it detected only sources lying on a line, the resulting inversion problem would be trivial, namely the integral in Eq. (5) would be replaced by the value of the optoacoustic image at a point on the detection line whose distance is directly related to the detection instant via the time-of-flight principle. Reconstruction would thus mean simply projecting the measured signal over the detection line. In this way, by linearly scanning the detector, an entire image may be formed. This procedure is extremely simple as each projection is separately used to reconstruct a separate part of the image. In practice, however, ideal focusing along a line is impossible owing to the laws of diffraction. Thus, the suggested algorithm is valid only to regions of the image located within the so-called focal zone. In order to reconstruct regions outside the focal zone, several projections are required. For these regions, analytical techniques, such as virtual detector (VD) [30] may be used to pre-process the projection data and improve imaging resolution.

Fig. 7 shows a numerical example that demonstrates several reconstruction approaches for focused-detector geometry [31]. The response of a focused detector with a focal length of 12 mm was simulated for an image that included three identical sources at distances of 10.7 mm, 12 mm, and 13.3 mm from the sensor (Fig. 7a). Fig. 7b shows the reconstruction obtained by using the ideal-focus assumption. Clearly, the source at the sensor's focus was reconstructed well, whereas outside the focal region significant smearing is observed. Fig. 7c shows the reconstruction obtained using the VD method. Although significant improvement is attained in the high-frequency content of the image (recovery of small features), the reconstruction still suffers from significant low-frequency-related artifacts. If the projection signals are first high-pass-filtered before applying the VD method, the low-frequency errors are reduced, but the amplitude of the out-of-focus sources remains lower than the one of sources in the focus (Fig. 7d). The reason for the reduced amplitude is that the signals generated from out-of-focus sources are effectively low-passed filtered by the detector's geometrical response and are thus more attenuated by the high-pass filter used in the reconstruction. Finally, Fig. 7e shows the model-based reconstruction obtained when the geometric response of the detector is included in the model matrix. Since the model is accurate at low as well as high frequencies, the amplitude of the sources is accurately reconstructed. Limited-iteration-LSQR regularization was used in the model-based reconstruction owing to the limited-view projection data. Despite regularization, the limited-view problem led to x-shaped artifacts even in the model-based reconstruction.

4. Wavelet-packet formulation

Although model-based techniques are indeed able to achieve superior reconstruction quality than analytical solutions, their use may turn impractical owing to the high computational cost. In particular, inverting the matrix relation in Eq. (7) becomes increasingly more time consuming as the matrix size grows. Furthermore, the computational challenge increases nonlinearly with image resolution. For instance, in the 2D case, every time the image resolution is doubled, the number of pixels increases by a factor of 4. Since the amount of information in the projection data should follow that of the image, 4 times more data is thus required for the inversion. This readily results in a factor of 16 increase in the size of the model matrix for the 2D case, and correspondingly a factor of 64 increase in the case of 3D imaging. Finally, many inversion algorithms scale non-linearly with matrix size, leading to even greater effective increase in the computational load.

While the trend in required computational resources seems prohibitive, it is often the case that when a problem becomes too complex to be solved directly, an alternative solution is sought in which the problem is separated into a set of simpler problems. One of the better known examples of this approach in tomography is the projection-slice theorem, which is a representation of the Radon transform in Fourier space. According to the theorem, each spatial frequency component in the image generates only a single non-zero projection. Thus, when reconstructing in Fourier space, each projection may be used separately to reconstruct a single spectral component in the image.

While the projection-slice theorem applies only to the Radon transform, it may be generalized to the case of optoacoustic tomography by replacing its global analysis by a local one [32]. Specifically, in the Radon transform both the projections, which are calculated by integrating over lines, and the Fourier transform are global functions of the image. A local version of the Radon transform, i.e. integration over line segments, may approximately describe the projections in optoacoustic tomography for sufficiently small objects, i.e. objects for which the curvature in the projection arcs (Fig. 2a) is sufficiently small. Small objects, however, cannot by definition contain a single spatial frequency and are rather characterized by a relatively broad spatial frequency band. As a result, such objects cannot be characterized well by a single non-zero (or numerically significant) projection, but rather by a projection band. Fig. 8 illustrates the connection between a localized-cosine object and its projection data in 2D. The sinogram, which is the 2D data representation of the projection data, is presented over the projection angle (θ) and the radius (r) of the curve over which the integration in Eq. (5) is performed. The figure shows that the frequencies in the vertical and horizontal slices of the sinogram follow the actual spatial frequencies of the objects, i.e. the bottom object with double the spatial frequency creates corresponding projections with double the frequency in each direction. This property suggests that different frequency bands in the image may be separately reconstructed from a small set of frequency bands in the sinogram.

In Ref. [32], the details of constructing a separable model matrix are discussed. Wavelet packets were used as the function base to describe both the images and sinograms. Similarly to the objects shown in Fig. 8, wavelet packets are localized in both space and frequency. Additionally, wavelet packets constitute an orthogonal base, and therefore the images may be readily restored from their wavelet-packet representation. The algorithm described in Ref. [32] is thus composed of four major steps: (a) represent Eq. (5) in wavelet-packet domain; (b) separate the resulting model matrix into a set of matrices each corresponding to a unique frequency band in the image; (c) independently invert the resulting matrices; (d) transform the solution obtained in the wavelet-packet domain back to standard space.

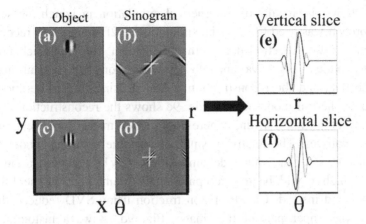

Fig. 8. The effect of an object's spatial-frequency content on its corresponding sinogram [32]. (a) The object with the lower spatial frequency content creates (b) a sinogram characterized by low frequencies in comparison to (c) a higher frequency object and its corresponding sinogram. (e) vertical and (f) horizontal slices of the two sinogram readily show the difference between the projections of the low-frequency object (solid curve) and high-frequency object (dashed-curve).

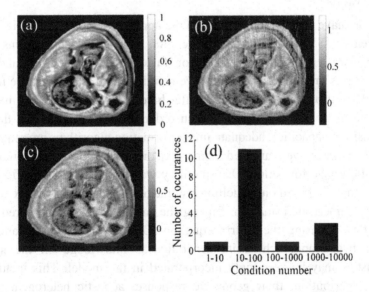

Fig. 9. A limited-view simulation demonstrating the advantages of a wavelet-packet based approach for tomographic model-based reconstruction [32]. (a) The originating image. (b) Model-based reconstruction performed on the entire model matrix with limited-LSQR-iteration regularization. (c) Model-based reconstruction performed with the wavelet-packet approach and SVD regularization. The use of SVD was possible only owing to the smaller size of the matrices in the wavelet-packet approach and led to a more precise reconstruction. (d) The condition-number distribution for the model-matrices of the different wavelet packets, which reveals that only a few spatial frequencies are responsible for the ill-conditioned nature of the inverse problem.

Fig. 9 shows the results of a numerical simulation in which the separable-model approach was used [32]. In the simulation, a 2D image was reconstructed from limited-view projection data with coverage of 180° to which noise was numerically added. Figs. 9a and 9b show the original optical absorption distribution data and the reconstruction obtained using limited-iteration LSQR performed on the full model matrix. Fig. 9c shows the reconstruction performed in the wavelet-packet domain, where the model matrix was separated into 16 smaller matrices. The relatively small size of the resulting model matrices enabled using singular value decomposition (SVD) regularization in the inversion, which would be too computationally demanding if the full model matrix was used instead. Clearly, reconstruction using SVD reduced the stripe artifacts in the upper part of the image. Fig. 9d shows a histogram of the condition numbers obtained for the 16 reduced model matrices. It can be seen that reconstruction instability was dominated by only 4 of the wavelet packets – an expected result since image artifacts in limited-view scenarios exhibit distinct spatial frequencies, as can be seen also in Fig. 4b.

5. Conclusions

Recent years have seen a rapid growth in the application of optoacoustic imaging in the fields of biology and medicine. As many new applications of the technology are emerging, the need for faster image rendering and better quantification is growing as well. Improvement in imaging performance has been mainly achieved by new designs and better hardware, which can acquire higher quality data in less time. Nonetheless, in order to fully benefit from the better data-acquisition capacities, adequate image-formation algorithms are required.

In this chapter we surveyed some existing algorithms for tomographic optoacoustic image formation. Our summary was focused on a specific class of algorithms that are based on modelling the imaging system via a matrix equation. Under this numerical formalism, finding the image from the measured data is equivalent to inverting the matrix equation. One of the major advantages of the model-based approach is its generality as knowledge on the system's characteristics may be seemingly incorporated in the model. This includes the detectors' distribution, their geometric response, acoustic heterogeneities and attenuation of the medium, etc. Due to the availability of numerous numerical techniques for solving algebraic equations, the model-based approach further allows incorporating prior knowledge or imposing constraints on the image. With the steady improvement in the efficiency and sophistication of algorithms and the exponential growth of computing power, model-based reconstruction methods are expected to play an increasing role in optoacoustic tomography.

References

[1] D. Razansky, M. Distel, C. Vinegoni, R. Ma, N. Perrimon, R. W. Köster, and V. Ntziachristos, "Multispectral opto-acoustic tomography of deep-seated fluorescent proteins in vivo," *Nature Photonics*, vol. 3, pp. 412–417, 2009.

[2] D. Razansky, A. Buehler, and V. Ntziachristos, "Volumetric real-time multispectral optoacoustic tomography of biomarkers," *Nature Protocols*, vol. 6, pp. 1121–1129, 2011.

[3] B. Cox, J. G. Laufer, S. R. Arridge, and P. C. Beard, "Quantitative spectroscopic photoacoustic imaging: a review," *Journal of Biomedical Optics*, vol. 17, 061202, 2012.

[4] L. V. Wang, "Multiscale photoacoustic microscopy and computed tomography," *Nature Photonics*, vol. 3, pp. 503–509, 2009.

[5] V. P. Zharov, E. I. Galanzha, E. V. Shashkov, N. G. Khlebtsov, and V. V. Tuchin, "In vivo photoacoustic flow cytometry for monitoring of circulating single cancer cells and contrast agents," *Optics Letters*, vol. 31, pp. 3623–3625, 2006.

[6] P. Burgholzer, G. J. Matt, M. Haltmeier, and G. Paltauf, "Exact and approximate imaging methods for photoacoustic tomography using an arbitrary detection surface," *Physical Review E*, vol. 75, 046706, 2007.

[7] L. A. Kunyansky, "Explicit inversion formulae for the spherical mean Radon transform," *Inverse Problems*, vol. 23, pp. 373–383, 2007.

[8] M. Xu and L. V. Wang, "Universal back-projection algorithm for photoacoustic computed tomography," *Physical Review E*, vol. 71, 016706, 2005.

[9] A. Rosenthal, D. Razansky, and V. Ntziachristos, "Fast semi-analytical model-based acoustic inversion for quantitative optoacoustic tomography," *IEEE Transactions on Medical Imaging*, vol. 29, pp. 1275–1285, 2010.

[10] X. L. Dean-Ben, A. Buehler, V. Ntziachristos, and D. Razansky, "Accurate model-based reconstruction algorithm for three-dimensional optoacoustic tomography," *IEEE Transactions on Medical Imaging*, vol. 31, pp. 1922–1928, 2012.

[11] M. Xu and L. V. Wang, "Analytic explanation of spatial resolution related to bandwidth and detector aperture size in thermoacoustic or photoacoustic reconstruction," *Physical Review E*, vol. 67, 056605, 2003.

[12] A. Rosenthal, D. Razansky, and V. Ntziachristos, "Model-based optoacoustic inversion with arbitrary-shape detectors," *Medical Physics*, vol. 38, pp. 4285–4295, 2011.

[13] A. Buehler, A. Rosenthal, T. Jetzfellner, A. Dima, D. Razansky, and V. Ntziachristos, "Model-based optoacoustic inversions with incomplete projection data," *Medical Physics*, vol. 38, pp. 1694–1704, 2011.

[14] G. Paltauf, J. A. Viator, S. A. Prahl, and S. L. Jacques, "Iterative reconstruction algorithm for optoacoustic imaging," *Journal of Acoustical Society of America*, vol. 112, pp. 1536–1544, 2002.

[15] X. L. Dean-Ben, V. Ntziachristos, and D. Razansky, "Acceleration of optoacoustic model-based reconstruction using angular image discretization," *IEEE Transactions on Medical Imaging*, vol. 31, pp. 1154–1162, 2012.

[16] A. Rosenthal, V. Ntziachristos, and D. Razansky, "Optoacoustic methods for frequency calibration of ultrasonic sensors", *IEEE Transactions on Ultrasonics Ferroelectrics and Frequency Control*, vol. 58, pp. 316–326, 2011.

[17] A. Rosenthal, M. Á. A. Caballero, S. Kellnberger, D. Razansky, and V. Ntziachristos, "Spatial characterization of the response of a silica optical fiber to wideband ultrasound," *Optics Letters*, vol. 37, pp. 3174–3176, 2012.

[18] J. Jose, R. G. H. Willemink, W. Steenbergen, C. H. Slump, T. G. van Leeuwen, and S. Manohar, "Speed-of-sound compensated photoacoustic tomography for accurate imaging," *Medical Physics*, vol. 39, pp. 7262–7271, 2012.

[19] X. L. Dean-Ben, D. Razansky, and V. Ntziachristos, "The effects of acoustic attenuation in optoacoustic signals," *Physics in Medicine and Biology*, vol. 56, pp. 6129–6148, 2011.

[20] B. E. Treeby, J. G. Laufer, E. Z. Zhang, F. C. Norris, M. F. Lythgoe, P. C. Beard, and B. T. Cox, "Acoustic attenuation compensation in photoacoustic tomography: Application to high-resolution 3D imaging of vascular networks in mice," *Protocols of SPIE*, vol. 7899, paper 78992Y, 2011.

[21] C. Huang, L. Nie, R. W. Schoonover, L. V. Wang, and M. A. Anastasio, "Photoacoustic computed tomography correcting for heterogeneity and attenuation," *Journal of Biomedical Optics*, vol. 17, 061211 (2012).

[22] C. C. Paige and M. A. Saunders, "LSQR: An algorithm for sparse linear equations and sparse least squares," ACM *Transactions on Mathematical Software*, vol. 8, pp. 43–71, 1982.

[23] J. Provost and F. Lesage, "The application of compressed sensing for photo-acoustic tomography," *IEEE Transactions on Medical Imaging*, vol. 28, pp. 585–594, 2009.

[24] M. Roumeliotis, R. Z. Stodilka, M. A. Anastasio, G. Chaudhary, H. Al-Aabed, E. Ng, A. Immucci, and J. J. L. Carson, "Analysis of a photoacoustic imaging system by the crosstalk matrix and singular value decomposition," *Optics Express*, vol. 18, pp. 11406–11417, 2010.

[25] X. Liu, D. Peng, W. Guo, X. Ma, X. Yang, and Jie Tian, "Compressed sensing photoacoustic imaging based on fast alternating direction algorithm," *International Journal of Biomedical Imaging*, vol. 2012, 206214, 2012.

[26] Z. Guo, C. Li, L. Song, and L. V. Wang, "Compressed sensing in photoacoustic tomography in vivo," *Journal of Biomedical Optics*, vol. 15, 021311, 2010.

[27] K. Wang, R. Su, A. A. Oraevsky, and M. A. Anastasio, "Investigation of iterative image reconstruction in three-dimensional optoacoustic tomography," *Physics in Medicine and Biology*, vol. 57, pp. 5399–5423, 2012.

[28] T. Jetzfellner, A. Rosenthal, K. H. Englmeier, A. Dima, M. A. A. Caballero, D. Razansky, and V. Ntziachristos, "Interpolated model-matrix optoacoustic tomography of the mouse brain," *Applied Physics Letters*, vol. 98, pp. 163701, 2011.

[29] J. Gateau, M. Á. A. Caballero, A. Dima, and V. Ntziachristos, "Three-dimensional optoacoustic tomography using a conventional ultrasound linear detector array: Whole-body tomographic system for small animals," *Medical Physics*, vol. 40, 3302, 2013.

[30] M. L. Li, H. E. Zhang, K. Maslov, G. Stoica, and L. V. Wang, "Improved in vivo photoacoustic microscopy based on a virtual-detector concept," *Optics Letters*, vol. 31, pp. 474–176, 2006.

[31] M. A. A. Caballero, A. Rosenthal, J. Gateau, D. Razansky, and V. Ntziachristos, "Model-based optoacoustic imaging using focused detector scanning," *Optics Letters*, vol. 37, pp. 4080–4082, 2012.

[32] A. Rosenthal, T. Jetzfellner, D. Razansky, and V. Ntziachristos, "Efficient framework for model-based tomographic image reconstruction using wavelet packets," *IEEE Transactions on Medical Imaging*, vol. 31, pp. 1346–1357, 2012.

CHAPTER 9

THE FUSION OF THREE-DIMENSIONAL QUANTITATIVE CORONARY ANGIOGRAPHY AND INTRACORONARY IMAGING FOR CORONARY INTERVENTIONS

Shengxian Tu[1,*], Niels R. Holm[2], Johannes P. Janssen[1], and Johan H. C. Reiber[1]

[1]*Division of Image Processing, Department of Radiology*
Leiden University Medical Center, Leiden, The Netherlands
Albinusdreef 2, 2333 ZA, Leiden, The Netherlands
[2]*Department of Cardiology, Aarhus University Hospital, Skejby, Aarhus, Denmark*
E-mail: Sanventu@gmail.com

Coronary imaging is essential for stent selection and treatment optimization during revascularization procedures. X-ray angiography and intracoronary imaging such as intravascular ultrasound (IVUS) and optical coherence tomography (OCT) document coronary anatomy from different perspectives. Thus, the fusion of these imaging modalities can help the interventionalist in the anatomical interpretation, which may aid tailoring the treatment of individual patients. In this book chapter a novel system for the fusion of X-ray angiography and intracoronary imaging devices combined with three-dimensional (3D) quantitative assessments is presented, as well as its potential clinical applications. Two validation studies addressing the accuracy of the co-registration and the discrepancy in assessing arterial lumen size by co-registered X-ray angiography and IVUS or OCT are presented, followed by the discussions of our findings.

1. Introduction

Coronary artery disease (CAD) is the leading cause of mortality and morbidity in industrialized countries. The main disease process is located in the blood vessel supplying the heart muscle. The fatty plaques built-up within the wall of the coronary arteries might rupture and create a thrombus, thereby blocking the entire flow through the vessel, which is followed by the symptoms of a heart attack. Patients who suffer from a heart attack are immediately or within three days referred to a catheterization laboratory for an invasive procedure called PCI (Percutaneous Coronary Intervention) to open the vessel. This is done by introducing and dilating a small balloon at the site of occlusion and subsequent deploying a "stent" as a scaffolding device to keep the vessel open. This procedure has undergone a remarkable evolution over the past decades. It is now regarded as one of the primary treatments of established ischemic heart disease. The efficacy of PCI merits from both stent manufacturing and stenting techniques. Suboptimal stent sizing and positioning may result in stent malapposition or incomplete lesion coverage; as a result, the risk of target vessel revascularization and thrombus formation can significantly increase [1].

For decades, X-ray angiography has been the standard imaging modality in the catheterization laboratories used for diagnosis and for guiding PCI. The coronary anatomy of the arteries and thus the narrowings of the lumen can be visualized well from this conventional two-dimensional (2D) technique. However, the purely visual assessment of vessel size and disease is subjective, and therefore suffers from significant inter- and intra-observer variations [2]. There has been a continuing interest in developing robust and automated segmentation techniques to obtain objective and reproducible data. This leads to the development of quantitative coronary angiography (QCA), an automatic analysis and quantification system of the X-ray-images, which has evolved substantially since late 1970's [2-4]. So far it has been applied worldwide for on-line vessel sizing to aid selecting the proper size of interventional treatment devices and to assess the efficacy of individual procedures. The paramount use of QCA has been and is still in core laboratories and clinical research sites to study the efficacy of PCI procedures and related devices. The recent developments in 3D angiographic reconstruction further extends its capability by resolving some of the well-known limitations of 2D QCA, e.g., foreshortening and overlap thereby enabling more accurate vessel measurements and the calculation of optimal viewing angles [5-7] for the subsequent interventional procedures. By using 3D QCA and based on such more accurate 3D data, clinical decision making can be affected, thus possibly leading to a more efficient and economic usage of contrast, stents and other devices [8]. This may have significant impact in today's cost-constrained health care systems.

Despite the fact that 3D QCA has great potential in supporting clinical decision making, X-ray angiography is inherently limited by imaging only the lumen and it is impossible to assess the presence and extent of vessel wall thickening where the actual disease occurs. In other words, 3D QCA remains as a lumenogram, though with better 3D quantification capabilities. Thus, early stages of plaque formation may not be evident with X-ray angiography due to the occurrence of vessel remodelling [9], and the vulnerable plaques [10] cannot be recognized which may be clinical relevant for possible implementations of measures to prevent these from rupturing.

The limitations of angiography are well addressed by intracoronary imaging techniques, such as intravascular ultrasound (IVUS) and optical coherence tomography (OCT) which have been increasingly used. IVUS and OCT provide a wealth of information including dimensions, disease processes in the vessel wall, and how implanted stents are apposed to the vessel wall. However, the fact that these intracoronary imaging devices do not preserve the natural 3D vascular shape could lead to erroneous interpretations. Although a longitudinal view (L-View) is available in most IVUS/OCT consoles to provide an overview of the pullback series, the presentation of the L-View by stacking the cross-sectional images along a straightened version of the catheter pullback trajectory is a very unnatural way of conceptualization. As a result, the interpretation and mental mapping between different imaging modalities can be quite challenging. The modern treatment approach requires the combination of multiple imaging modalities to be able to objectively assess coronary disease and to effectively guide the intervention, especially for complex PCI procedures.

Given the different but complementary perspectives provided by X-ray angiography and IVUS/OCT, the fusion of these imaging modalities using 3D angiographic reconstruction as a roadmap while exploiting detailed vessel wall information from IVUS/OCT will provide a complete picture of vessel morphology and hence, help the interventional cardiologist in on-line decision making and PCI optimization.

2. Three-dimensional Angiographic Reconstruction and QCA

Accurate and robust 3D angiographic reconstruction is the foremost important step in 3D QCA and the subsequent image fusion. Early research on 3D reconstruction can be traced back to decades ago [11, 12]. However, approved clinical systems were announced only recently and there is still no widespread acceptance of such systems in routine clinical practice. One of the reasons is the fact that mechanical distortions in X-ray systems and noisy angiographic images in routine clinical acquisitions could significantly affect the accuracy and reproducibility of the 3D reconstruction. For monoplane X-ray angiographic acquisitions, the shift of the whole coronary tree due to the patient's respiration or the non-isocentric condition could greatly deteriorate the system's reliability. Such system distortions should be corrected before or during the 3D angiographic reconstruction.

A number of approaches [11-13] have been proposed to correct for these angiographic system distortions. Ideally, a couple of reliable landmarks, e.g., the catheter tip or bifurcations, should be identified on the both angiographic views as reference points in order to correct the system distortions. However, the practical applicability of such approaches in on-line applications has been hampered by the efforts in identifying many reliable landmarks, which turned out to be too time consuming or even impossible to find such reliable landmarks on the two angiographic views, especially when significant vessel overlap is present. To guarantee the reliability in the identification of reference landmarks has already proven to be a non-trivial task.

To come up with a practical and attractive workflow, we have developed a new approach by using only one to three reference points to correct the system distortions. In case of small perspective viewing angles [14] for noisy angiographic images, the reliability and robustness of the angiographic reconstruction is further improved by constructing a distance transformation matrix and by searching for the optimal corresponding path in the matrix to refine the correspondence between the two angiographic views [15]. The approach has been validated with high accuracy in both phantom and in-vivo datasets [14, 16, 17]. In short, the 3D angiographic reconstruction consisted of only a few major steps: 1) two image sequences acquired at two arbitrary angiographic views with projection angles at least 25° apart were loaded; 2) properly contrast-filled frames of these angiographic image sequences were selected; 3) one to three anatomical markers, e.g., bifurcations, were identified as reference points in the two angiographic views for the automated correction of angiographic system distortions; 4) the target straight vessel or bifurcation was defined and automated 2D lumen edge detection was performed using our extensively validated QCA algorithms [3, 18, 19]; 5) the lumen and reference surface, i.e., the normal lumen as if there was no obstruction, was reconstructed in 3D after refining the correspondence between the two projections. The resulting lumen surface colored by the extent of lesion severity was presented. A red color indicates a narrowing while a white color represents the normal/healthy situation.

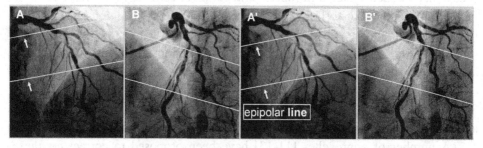

Figure 1. Automated correction of system distortions in the image geometry for the 3D angiographic reconstruction: A and B were the two angiographic views (15 RAO, 33 Cranial and 31 LAO, 31 Cranial) used for the 3D reconstruction. The two epipolar lines did not go through their corresponding reference points (proximal and distal landmarks at the bifurcations), indicating that system distortions were present. A' and B' show the results after the automated correction of the system distortions: The two epipolar lines now goes right through their corresponding red and blue reference points in both angiographic views.

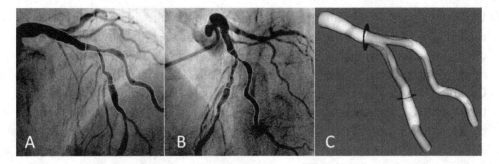

Figure 2. 3D bifurcation reconstruction and QCA: A and B shows the two angiographic views with lumen contours superimposed on the LAD/D1 bifurcation. C shows the reconstructed bifurcation lumen and the reference surface in the optimal viewing angle, being 17 RAO, 40 Cranial.

An example of correcting system distortions in the image geometry for the 3D angiographic reconstruction is given in Figure 1. The two bifurcations in the left anterior descending artery (LAD) were identified as reference points and their epipolar lines, being the projection of the X-ray beam directed towards a particular point on one of the projections onto the second projection [11], were superimposed on the two angiographic views by Figures 1A and 1B. Due to the system distortions, the epipolar lines did not go through their corresponding reference points. Figures 1A' and 1B' show the results after the automated correction of system distortions: The epipolar lines now go right through their corresponding reference points in both angiographic views, demonstrating the success of this automated procedure.

Figure 2 shows the 3D bifurcation reconstruction and QCA. Figures 2A and 2B show the two angiographic views (15 RAO, 33 Cranial and 31 LAO, 31 Cranial) with the detected lumen contours superimposed on the LAD and the first diagonal bifurcation (LAD/D1). Figure 2C shows the reconstructed LAD/D1 bifurcation lumen and the reference surface in 3D. The lesion was automatically detected and the three markers corresponding to the lesion borders and the minimum lumen diameter (MLD) position were synchronized in both 2D and 3D views. In this case, the lesion defined by the two green markers in the LAD had a length of 16.6 mm, a MLD of 1.13 mm, and a diameter stenosis of 51%. The distal bifurcation angle, i.e, carina angle, between the LAD and the D1 was 51°.

3. Fusion of 3D QCA and IVUS/OCT

Upon completing the 3D angiographic reconstruction, the fusion of X-ray angiography and intracoronary imaging devices requires two further steps, i.e., the co-registration/alignment and the merging of the two imaging modalities.

Under the condition that a motorized transducer pullback with constant speed is used in the IVUS/OCT image acquisition, the rationale for the co-registration of X-ray angiography and IVUS/OCT pullback series is to use the spatial relationship between vessel segment and the IVUS/OCT pullback trajectory. Conventional registration approaches [20-22] would require the reconstruction of the IVUS/OCT imaging catheter from two angiographic views, and assume it to be the pullback trajectory so that the IVUS/OCT cross-sectional images can be aligned along the trajectory. This is not a trivial task due to the difficulty in segmenting both the IVUS/OCT catheter and the lumen, and the requirement of a second angiographic view for the IVUS/OCT catheter, which is not always included in the current workflow. The assumption that the IVUS/OCT transducer path forms the exact pullback trajectory could also be jeopardized by the fact that spatial displacement of the catheter could occur inside the vessel after the pullback machine is switched on, in order to reach the state of minimum bending energy. It has been reported that there was significant delay from the moment the IVUS pullback machine was switched on to the moment the transducer tip really started to move [22].

In order to have a rapid and straightforward on-line solution that could assist coronary interventions and would fit most into the current workflow in catheterization laboratories, we have taken a different approach by estimating the corresponding IVUS/OCT cross-sectional image frames from the reconstructed vessel centerline, based on the curvature data and therefore, skipping the reconstruction of the pullback trajectory. The approach only requires the operator to reconstruct the vessel centerline in 3D (which is a standard step in 3D angiographic reconstruction) and register it with IVUS/OCT pullback series by indicating a baseline position. Such baseline positions can be found in anatomical or mechanical landmarks visible in both angiographic and IVUS/OCT images, such as bifurcations or stent borders.

After the registration, the markers superimposed on the angiographic views and the IVUS/OCT L-View are synchronized. The interpretation of vessel dimensions becomes more comprehensive and the interventionalist now knows exactly where to position the stent under the guiding of X-ray images. An example of combining 3D QCA and IVUS is given by Figure 3. In the registered dataset, the same lesion is identified in both the X-ray and the IVUS images. The quantifications from these two imaging modalities are seamlessly integrated. In this example, the target vessel in the LAD has a MLD and minimum lumen area of 1.5 mm and 2.1 mm^2 as assessed by 3D QCA, while the IVUS measurements at the same position (P2) are 1.8 mm and 2.8 mm^2, respectively.

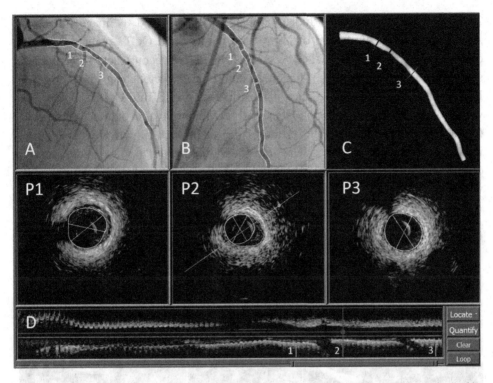

Figure 3. The co-registration of 3D QCA and IVUS pullback. (A) and (B) Two X-ray angiographic projections demonstrating a moderately diseased lesion in the LAD. (C) The reconstructed lumen in 3D with the automatically detected lesion borders and MLD position. (D) The longitudinal view of the IVUS pullback acquired in the LAD. Numbered line markers correspond to the same markers in Panel A, B, and C. (P1-P3) The transversal IVUS images corresponding to the three numbered line markers in D.

In order to merge X-ray angiography and IVUS/OCT in 3D, the IVUS/OCT image frames are re-angulated using the common bifurcation carina visualized in both imaging modalities, followed by image resampling and rendering in 3D. Thus, the geometric distortion of the IVUS/OCT pullback, i.e., losing the natural vascular shape, can be corrected using the "roadmap" from 3D angiography. In particular, subsequent assessments on IVUS/OCT can be automatically guided by the 3D angiographic centerlines. Figure 4 shows an example of centerline-guided assessment of sidebranch ostium on a main vessel OCT pullback [23]. A 76 year old male with stable angina due to a LAD/diagonal lesion was treated with the simple stenting technique of just stenting across the offspring of the sidebranch. The diagonal was dilated by a 2.5 mm Cutting Balloon (Boston Scientific) with subsequent predilatation and stenting of the LAD by an Abbott Xience V stent leaving the diagonal jailed behind the stent struts. Frequency domain OCT at

20 mm/sec (C7 system, St. Jude Medical) was performed to image the LAD. After carrying out the fusion of X-ray angiography and OCT, evaluation of the diagonal ostium (panel D1-D5) was performed by reconstructed OCT cross sections perpendicular to the diagonal centerline extracted from the 3D QCA. In this case the area of the diagonal ostium was 1.78 mm^2 by 3D QCA and was 1.67 mm^2 by OCT in the plane perpendicular to the diagonal centerline (panel D2). Thus full characterization of the sidebranch offspring was achieved without introducing the OCT wire into the sidebranch. This latter advantage is critical due to the risk of sidebranch dissection when introducing relatively stiff wires.

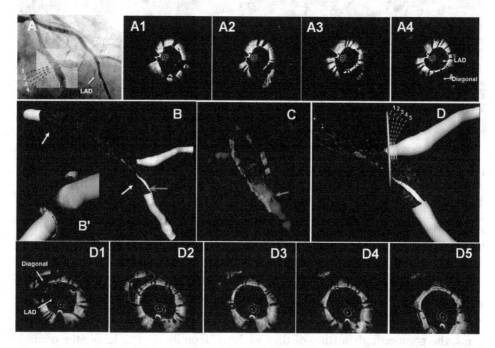

Figure 4. Three-dimensional assessment of a coronary bifurcation using QAngioOCT Advance Edition [23]. (A) X-ray angiography after implanting a 28 x 3.0 mm Xience V stent in the LAD. The four numbered lines indicate the corresponding positions where the four consecutive OCT image frames at top panels were acquired. (B) Fusion of X-ray angiography with OCT in naturally bent 3D shape. The two white arrows: stent edges. Guidewire artifact: orange arrow. (B') Distal-to-proximal view of the bifurcation demonstrating that 3D angiography corresponds well with 3D OCT at the carina. (C) Cut-through view showing the opening of the diagonal branch and the well-apposed struts; note the half-transparent angiographic lumen and the well-visualized guidewire (the most distal arrow). (D) Centerline-guided sidebranch assessment from OCT acquired in the main vessel. The five numbered lines correspond to the five OCT image frames at the bottom panels.

4. Validations

4.1. *Co-registration of X-ray angiography and IVUS/OCT*

Materials and methods

Phantoms

The accuracy of the registration was evaluated by acquiring a series of 12 different silicone phantoms (Via Biomedical, CA, USA) with coronary stents (Cypher Select+, Cordis, Johnson & Johnson, Miami Lakes, Fla., USA) placed by the culotte two-stent technique. Main branch intracoronary acquisitions were used for the registration with the 3D angiographic reconstruction. Stent borders were used as markers for the validation. While the proximal border was set as the baseline position for the co-registration, the distal border was used to evaluate the registration error. The registration error was defined by the following protocol: Move a marker that was superimposed in the IVUS/OCT L-View to the position to be evaluated (in this case, the distal stent border); Move a second marker that was superimposed in the IVUS/OCT L-View to the position that corresponds to the same position to be evaluated in the angiographic views; The signed distance from the first to the second marker in the L-View was defined as the registration error.

For each phantom, the angiographic acquisitions were performed at two projections 60 degrees apart by a monoplane X-ray system (AXIOM-Artis, Siemens, Germany). The phantoms were filled with iodinated contrast media (Visipaque 270, GE Healthcare, WI, USA) during the acquisitions. To obtain IVUS images, the phantoms were immersed in water and acquisitions were performed at a constant pullback speed of 0.5 mm/sec by using a 20 MHz transducer with a dedicated workstation (EagleEye Gold and s5, Volcano Corporation, Rancho Cordova, CA, USA) for 6 phantoms and a 40 MHz transducer with a dedicated workstation (Atlantis SR Pro and iLab, Boston Scientific, Boston, MA, USA) for the other 6 phantoms. IVUS images were recorded at 30 frames/sec. To obtain OCT images, Fourier domain-OCT pullbacks were performed at 20 mm/sec by non-occlusive flushing technique using Visipaque 270 iodinated contrast media, and an OCT imaging catheter with a dedicated workstation (C7 Dragonfly and C7-XR, Lightlab Imaging, Westford, MA, USA). OCT images were recorded at 100 frames/sec.

In-vivo

At the Department of Cardiology, Nanfang Hospital affiliated to the Southern Medical University in Guangzhou, China, 24 patients who underwent both angiographic and IVUS examinations of the LAD were retrospectively selected for the validation. Inclusion criteria were: 1) patients had no prior history of coronary artery bypass surgery; 2) motorized pullback was used during the IVUS image acquisition; 3) angiographic images were recorded by digital flat-panel X-ray acquisition systems.

Angiographic images were recorded by a monoplane X-ray system (AXIOM-Artis, Siemens, Germany). IVUS pullbacks were performed by using a motorized transducer pullback system (0.5 mm/sec) with a rotating 40 MHz transducer catheter and 2.6 F imaging sheath (Boston Scientific, Boston, MA, USA). The sheath prevents direct contact of the imaging core with the vessel wall and increases the stability of the pullback procedure. All parameters required by the 3D angiographic reconstruction and the co-registration were stored in DICOM files.

Reliable anatomical landmarks in the LAD, e.g., ostia of diagonal or septal branches, were identified from both angiographic and IVUS images and used as reference markers for the validation study. When IVUS pullbacks covered the left main bifurcation and the ostium of the left circumflex artery (LCx) was well visualized in angiographic images (no significant overlap with the proximal LAD), the left main bifurcation point (carina) was included as a reference marker. The LAD (including the left main if applicable) was reconstructed from two angiographic views and registered with IVUS pullback series by the distance mapping algorithm. While the most proximal reference marker was set as the baseline position for the distance mapping, the subsequent markers were used to evaluate the registration error. The registration error was defined using the same protocol as used in the phantom validation. The correlation between the registration error and the distance from the evaluated marker to the baseline position was analyzed.

Statistics

Quantitative data are presented as mean ± standard deviation and the correlations were assessed by using Pearson's correlation coefficient. A 2-sided p-value of <0.05 was considered to be significant. All statistical analyses were carried out by using a statistical software package (SPSS, version 16.0; SPSS Inc; Chicago, IL, USA).

Results

Phantoms

The lengths of the 12 stents in the main branches ranged from 12.00 mm to 32.00 mm, with an average value of 22.92 ± 7.26 mm. The registration error for the 12 IVUS pullbacks ranged from -0.33 mm to 0.57 mm, with an average value of 0.03 ± 0.32 mm ($p = 0.75$). For the OCT data, one pullback series was excluded from the study, since the pullback did not cover the distal stent border. The registration error for the remaining 11 OCT pullbacks ranged from -0.20 mm to 0.40 mm, with an average value of 0.05 ± 0.25 mm ($p = 0.49$).

In-vivo

From the 24 patients selected for the study, 2 patients were excluded due to insufficient image quality for the 3D angiographic reconstruction and the subsequent analysis. Baseline characteristics for the remaining 22 patients include age (60.5 ± 13.2), male (17), and diameter stenosis (48.66 ± 17.82%). 13 (59%), 7 (32%), and 2 (9%) patients had lesions in 1, 2, and 3 vessels, respectively. A total of 78 reliable reference markers were identified from both angiographic and IVUS images. While the 22 most proximal markers were used as baseline positions for the distance mapping algorithm, the registration error was evaluated on the remaining 56 markers. The registration error ranges from -1.33 mm to 1.13 mm, with an average value of 0.03 ± 0.45 mm ($p = 0.67$). A scatter plot of the registration error is presented by Figure 5. The error is not correlated to the distance between the evaluated marker and the baseline position ($p = 0.73$).

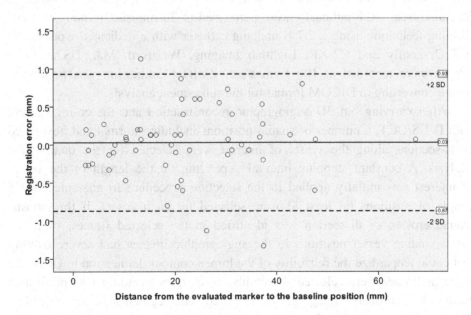

Figure 5. The registration error for the co-registration of X-ray angiography and IVUS pullbacks.

4.2. *Comparison of lumen dimensions by 3D QCA and IVUS/OCT*

Materials and methods

At the Catheterization Lab, National Center for Cardiovascular Diseases of China and Fu Wai Hospital in Beijing, China, and the Department of Cardiology, ErasmusMC in Rotterdam, the Netherlands, a total of 74 patients with indication for cardiac catheterization were retrospectively included in this study. Inclusion criteria were: 1) X-ray angiographic images were acquired by digital image intensifiers (flat-panel systems). 2) Two angiographic projections at least 25 degrees apart with lumen well filled with contrast dye agent were recorded. 3) The vessel of interest was imaged with motorized IVUS or OCT pullbacks at constant pullback speeds. 4) The vessel of interest was not totally occluded and had no history of coronary bypass surgery. 5) If stents were present in the vessel of interest, the entire IVUS/OCT pullback series completely imaged another non-stented lesion.

Angiographic images were recorded by different X-ray systems (AXIOM-Artis, Siemens, Erlangen, Germany; AlluraXper, Philips, Best, the Netherlands; and Safair, Shimadzu, Kyoto, Japan). The angiographic images used for 3D QCA were acquired prior to inserting the guidewire and intracoronary imaging catheter. Grayscale IVUS imaging was carried out using a 40 MHz transducer and a 2.9 F imaging sheath with a dedicated workstation (Atlantis SR Pro and Galaxy, Boston Scientific, Boston, MA, USA). Images were recorded at 30 frames/sec. OCT pullbacks were performed at 20 mm/sec by non-occlusive flushing technique using a 2.7 F imaging catheter with a dedicated workstation (C7 Dragonfly and C7-XR, Lightlab Imaging, Westford, MA, USA). OCT images were recorded at 100 frames/sec. Z-offset calibration was performed before converting to DICOM format for the subsequent analysis.

After carrying out 3D angiographic reconstruction and the co-registration with IVUS/OCT, a number of spatial positions including normal and obstructed cross-sections along the vessel of interest were selected for the quantitative analysis. A constant stepping interval depending on the length of the vessel of interest was initially applied in the selection procedure to guarantee that a couple of positions (at least 8) were selected for each vessel. If thrombosis, plaque erosion or dissection was identified in the selected frames, or if the corresponding vessel positions in the angiographic images had severe overlap that could jeopardize the reliability of the lumen contour delineation in QCA, the adjacent frames were selected. If predilation or thrombectomy was performed before intracoronary imaging, the injured sub-segments were excluded. Bifurcations were excluded as well since there was no well-established standard to compare bifurcation dimensions between 3D QCA and IVUS or OCT. In such a way a couple of reliably co-registered positions were analyzed for each vessel and the variability introduced by the analysis methodology itself was reduced. As a result, the comparisons reflected the systematic difference between 3D QCA and IVUS or OCT. For IVUS images, only frames that corresponded to the end-diastolic phase in the cardiac cycle were considered, since 3D QCA was also performed at the end-diastolic phase. A well validated algorithm integrated in a commercial software package (QIvus 2.1, Medis medical imaging systems bv, Leiden, the Netherlands) [24] was used for the IVUS segmentation and quantitative analysis. For quantitative OCT analysis, a new mincost algorithm was directly integrated in the registration software to automatically detect the lumen-intima interface from OCT images. The algorithm used the asymmetric sticks [25] to construct a matrix with each cell representing the edge strength/probability for the corresponding position. In a next step, a global optimization algorithm, the so-called mincost algorithm, was applied to find the optimal path (lumen-intima interface) with the strongest edge strength.

Frame-based comparison between 3D QCA and IVUS or OCT was performed on all the selected positions. The mean lumen size calculated from all the selected positions for each vessel was used to represent the lumen size for that specific vessel and used for the vessel-based comparison.

Quantitative IVUS/OCT analysis was performed on the selected corresponding positions by an analyst, who was unaware of the 3D QCA results. The measurements in the first 10 vessels were repeated by the same analyst one month later, and by a second analyst, both blinded to the earlier results. From these measurements, intra- and inter-observer variabilities were derived.

Statistics

3D QCA was compared to IVUS or OCT by using paired t-test, while the differences were evaluated by Bland-Altman plots. Quantitative data were presented as mean difference $\pm$ standard deviation and the correlations were assessed by using Pearson's correlation coefficient, providing the correlation coefficient (r) and the regression line. A 2-sided p-value of <0.05 was considered to be significant. Confounders independently influencing the vessel-based discrepancy between 3D QCA and IVUS or OCT were analyzed using a stepwise multiple linear regression. The intra- and interobserver variabilities were reported as mean difference $\pm$ standard deviation. All statistical analyses were carried out using SPSS software (PASW version 18.0.0, 2009; SPSS Inc, Chicago, IL).

Results

The baseline characteristics for the included patients and assessed vessels are given in Table 1. A total of 40 vessels (LAD = 35, LCx = 5, Diagonal = 1, RCA = 1) from 37 patients were included to compare lumen size by 3D QCA and by IVUS. In 4 of these vessels, manual calibration had to be performed in the 3D angiographic reconstruction. For the remaining 36 vessels, automated calibration was applied. The segment of interest had a mean diameter stenosis of 45.5% as assessed from 3D QCA. 24 vessels were revascularized after the examinations. A total of 40 vessels (LAD = 22, LCx = 5, OM = 1, RCA = 11, Ramus Intermedius = 1) from the other 37 patients were included to compare 3D QCA and OCT. Automated calibration was applied for all the vessels in the 3D angiographic reconstruction. The assessed segments of interest had a mean diameter stenosis of 45.4% as assessed from 3D QCA. 25 vessels were revascularized after the examinations.

A total of 519 distinct positions were selected for the comparison between 3D QCA and IVUS in measuring short diameter (SD), long diameter (LD) and lumen area. Scatter plots of the comparison are presented in Figure 6. There were good correlations between 3D QCA and IVUS: SD ($r = 0.761$, $p < 0.001$); LD ($r = 0.790$, $p < 0.001$); Area ($r = 0.799$, $p < 0.001$). Bland-Altman plots in Figure 6B' and 6C' show that there was an increasing bias towards larger lumen size by IVUS, which was more pronounced in larger vessels. Quantitative data are presented in Table 2. Lumen sizes were larger by IVUS than by 3D QCA: SD 2.51 ± 0.58 mm vs 2.34 ± 0.56 mm ($p < 0.001$); LD 3.02 ± 0.62 mm vs 2.63 ± 0.58 mm ($p < 0.001$); Area 6.29 ± 2.77 mm^2 vs 5.08 ± 2.34 mm^2 ($p < 0.001$) in frame-based analysis. The difference was 0.16 mm (6.6%) in SD, 0.39 mm (13.8%) in LD, and 1.21 mm2 (21.3%) in area. Vessel-based analysis showed similar discrepancies: SD 2.53 ± 0.39 mm vs 2.35 ± 0.37 mm ($p < 0.001$); LD 3.05 ± 0.43 mm vs 2.64 ± 0.36 mm ($p < 0.001$); Area 6.41 ± 1.92 mm^2 vs 5.12 ± 1.45 mm^2 ($p < 0.001$).

Table1. Baseline Characteristics

	IVUS	OCT
Patient	n = 37	n = 37
Age	55.8 (41-75)	60 (44-78)
Male/Female	26/11	21/16
Imaged vessel:	n = 40	n = 40
LAD/Diagonal/LCx/OM/RCA/RI	35/1/5/1/0/0	22/0/5/1/11/1
Stents in subsegment	19	1
Assessed lesion:		
Predilatated before intracoronary imaging	6	3
Ostial or bifurcation lesion	23	13
Diffused lesion	18	11
Calcified lesion	13	23
Diameter stenosis*	45.5($\pm$12.5)%	45.4($\pm$17.0)%
Lesion treated later by revascularization	24	25

*Assessments based on 3D QCA. LAD = Left Anterior Descending; LCx = Left Circumflex Artery; OM = Obtuse Marginal; RCA = Right Coronary Artery; RI = Ramus Intermedius.

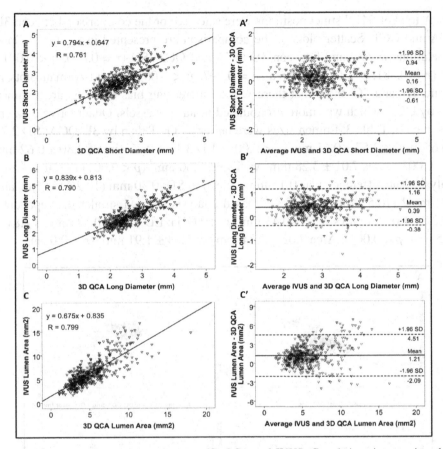

Figure 6. Frame-based comparison between 3D QCA and IVUS. Correlations in assessing short diameter (A), long diameter (B), and area (C). Bland-Altman plots show the differences of the measurements in short diameter (A'), long diameter (B'), and area (C'). There is an increasing bias towards larger discrepancy in long diameter and area at larger vessels. n = 519 in 40 vessels.

Table 2. Comparison between 3D QCA and IVUS in Assessing Lumen Size

	IVUS	3D QCA	Difference (95% CI)	Intra-observer variability*	Inter-observer variability*
Positions, n = 519					
Short diameter (mm)	2.51±0.58	2.34±0.56	0.16 (0.13-0.20) [†]	0.022±0.131	0.025±0.097
Long diameter (mm)	3.02±0.62	2.63±0.58	0.39 (0.36-0.42) [†]	0.039±0.162	0.042±0.092
Lumen area (mm²)	6.29±2.77	5.08±2.34	1.21 (1.07-1.35) [†]	0.124±0.534	0.134±0.356
Vessels, n = 40					
Short diameter (mm)	2.53±0.39	2.35±0.37	0.18 (0.10-0.26) [†]	-	-
Long diameter (mm)	3.05±0.43	2.64±0.36	0.41 (0.34-0.48) [†]	-	-
Lumen area (mm²)	6.41±1.92	5.12±1.45	1.29 (0.95-1.63) [†]	-	-

*Observer variability was calculated from 136 positions from the first 10 vessels. CI = confidence interval; [†]$p < 0.001$.

A total of 541 distinct positions were selected for the comparison between 3D QCA and OCT. Scatter plots of the comparison are presented in Figure 7. Good correlations were found between 3D QCA and OCT: SD ($r = 0.880$, $p < 0.001$); LD ($r = 0.881$, $p < 0.001$); Area ($r = 0.897$, $p < 0.001$). Bland-Altman plots in Figure 7B' and 7C' show that there was an increasing bias towards larger lumen size by OCT, which was more pronounced in larger vessels. Quantitative data are presented in Table 3. Lumen sizes were larger by OCT than by 3D QCA: SD 2.70 ± 0.65 mm vs 2.57 ± 0.61 mm ($p < 0.001$); LD 3.11 ± 0.72 mm vs 2.80 ± 0.62 mm ($p < 0.001$); Area 7.01 ± 3.28 mm^2 vs 5.93 ± 2.66 mm^2 ($p < 0.001$) in frame-based analysis. The difference was 0.14 mm (5.3%) in SD, 0.30 mm (10.2%) in LD, and 1.07 mm2 (16.5%) in area. Vessel-based analysis showed similar discrepancies: SD 2.71 ± 0.46 mm vs 2.57 ± 0.43 mm ($p < 0.001$); LD 3.11 ± 0.52 mm vs 2.81 ± 0.45 mm ($p < 0.001$); Area 7.02 ± 2.34 mm^2 vs 5.94 ± 1.91 mm^2 ($p < 0.001$).

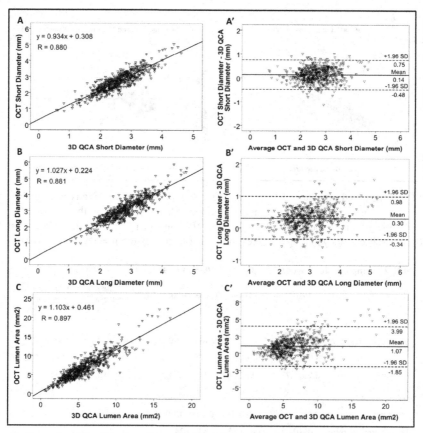

Figure 7. Frame-based comparison between 3D QCA and OCT. Correlations in assessing short diameter (A), long diameter (B), and area (C). Bland-Altman plots show the differences of the measurements in short diameter (A'), long diameter (B'), and area (C'). There is an increasing bias towards larger discrepancy in long diameter and area at larger vessels. n = 541 in 40 vessels.

Table 3. Comparison between 3D QCA and OCT in Assessing Lumen Size

	OCT	3D QCA	Difference (95% CI)	Intra-observer variability*	Inter-observer variability*
Positions, n = 541					
Short diameter (mm)	2.70±0.65	2.57±0.61	0.14 (0.11-0.16) [†]	0.000±0.013	0.003±0.029
Long diameter (mm)	3.11±0.72	2.80±0.62	0.30 (0.27-0.33) [†]	0.003±0.024	0.006±0.035
Lumen area (mm²)	7.01±3.28	5.93±2.66	1.07 (0.95-1.20) [†]	0.002±0.039	0.021±0.059
Vessels, n = 40					
Short diameter (mm)	2.71±0.46	2.57±0.43	0.14 (0.09-0.19) [†]	-	-
Long diameter (mm)	3.11±0.52	2.81±0.45	0.30 (0.24-0.37) [†]	-	-
Lumen area (mm²)	7.02±2.34	5.94±1.91	1.08 (0.80-1.37) [†]	-	-

*Observer variability was calculated from 165 positions from the first 10 vessels. CI = confidence interval; [†]$p < 0.001$.

5. Discussions

In this work a new system for the integration of coronary X-ray angiography and intracoronary imaging devices in 3D was presented, enabling the fusion of 3D QCA and IVUS/OCT in a single application. The feasibility of the system in supporting coronary interventions was demonstrated in a number of clinical cases and the accuracy of the co-registration was validated in both phantom and in-vivo data [17, 26].

Co-registration of X-ray angiography and IVUS/OCT

Over the past years, the continuous development in coronary quantitative analysis has been motivated by the increasing need to assess the true dimensions of vascular structures more accurately and by the on-line support of coronary interventions in the catheterization laboratories. It has been shown that suboptimal stent selection and deployment techniques are associated with significant risks of restenosis and stent thrombosis [1]. The choice of the correct stent size is therefore important for the outcome of stenting procedures [8]. In modern catheterization laboratories, multiple imaging modalities including X-ray angiography and intracoronary imaging such as IVUS or OCT are widely available. The role of IVUS/OCT in assessing plaque extent and distribution to optimize the treatment strategy has been well acknowledged. However, to implement the course of planning has been limited by the difficulty in corresponding IVUS/OCT anatomically with the X-ray images.

The current workflow by mentally mapping the landing zones from IVUS/OCT to the X-ray images can be quite challenging when no clear landmark is present near or at the lesion. In other cases when the diseased vessel has multiple sidebranches, e.g., the LAD with many septal and diagonal branches, the mental mapping could be confused or even become completely mismatched due to the fact that not all sidebranches are well presented in the same IVUS/OCT L-View. In such cases, the co-registration of X-ray angiography and IVUS/OCT can establish a point-to-point correspondence between these two complementary imaging modalities. As a result, the interpretation of the vessel morphology is greatly simplified and the sizing and positioning of the stent could be improved.

Lumen sizing assessed by different imaging modalities

For meticulous tailoring of individual PCI treatment, the diameter of the stent and the balloon is also of great importance, especially for some bioresorbable vascular scaffolds which are prone to fracture if overdilated during revascularization procedures. In current practice, when X-ray angiography is performed in conjunction with IVUS or OCT, lumen dimensions often show discrepancies in these imaging modalities. De Scheerder [27] reported smaller lumen size as assessed by IVUS in both normal and diseased coronary arteries, while Tsuchida [28] showed that IVUS measured larger lumen size in stented vessel, as compared to QCA. The difference can be attributed to some extent to the limitations in conventional QCA. In order to measure absolute lumen dimensions, a calibration procedure is required in conventional QCA, which can increase the measurement variability and introduce the out-of-plane magnification error [16, 29]. When the vessel of interest is not aligned in the same plane as the calibration object, the lumen size can be overestimated or underestimated depending on the assessed position. Another important limitation in the assumption of circular cross-sections might lead to inaccurate assessments of noncircular lesions.

To address the limitations in conventional QCA, 3D QCA was proposed and developed. By restoring vascular structures in their nature shape, 3D QCA was able to resolve some of these limitations, e.g., the vessel foreshortening and out-of-plane magnification errors, and reveal more details in the arterial cross-sections. In a bench study, it was shown that 3D QCA was able to measure the lumen dimensions with high accuracy and low variability on a wide range of acquisition angles [14]. When applied in patients with coronary artery disease, 3D QCA results agreed very well with vessel segment length as compared to IVUS using motorized pullback at constant pullback speed [16] and with true balloon length [30]. In addition, 3D QCA can be integrated with IVUS or OCT to optimize the stent sizing and positioning during the interventional procedures [23, 26]. While IVUS or OCT provides a wealth of information of the vessel wall, 3D QCA provides unique and complementary information including vessel tortuosity, curvature, and optimal viewing angles [5, 6]. Such combined systems have high potential to be widely applied in routine clinical practice if a seamless workflow is implemented. It is thus desirable to understand the systematic discrepancy in order to interpret and combine different imaging modalities, especially for diffusely diseased vessels when coupled with imaging artifacts.

At present, however, limited evidence is available on the comparison between 3D QCA and IVUS or OCT. Bruining [31] evaluated 16 patients receiving a biodegradable stent and found that lumen diameter and area were smaller by IVUS than by 3D QCA. However, only vessel-based comparison was performed resulting in a small sample size (11 vessels were evaluated by 3D QCA) and limited evidence. Schuurbiers [32] compared 3D QCA with IVUS on 1157 cross-sections in 10 coronary arteries using an offline co-registration tool to establish the correspondence between X-ray and IVUS images. The authors reported that 3D QCA systematically underestimated lumen area, as compared to quantitative IVUS. However, the evidence was limited by the fact that injection of diluted contrast agent during angiographic image acquisitions was required, which reduced the quality of the angiographic images. To our knowledge, there is no direct comparison between 3D QCA and OCT in co-registered datasets. Therefore, we developed and used a novel, real-time co-registration approach to compare 3D QCA with IVUS and OCT. Our data demonstrated that both IVUS and OCT correlated well with 3D QCA in assessing the lumen size at corresponding positions [17]. The lumen size was larger by both IVUS and OCT, however, the agreement with 3D QCA tended to be slightly better by OCT than by IVUS: The differences between OCT and 3D QCA in short diameter, long diameter, and area were 0.14 mm (5.3%), 0.30 mm (10.2%), and 1.07 mm^2 (16.5%), respectively, while the differences between IVUS and 3D QCA were 0.16 mm (6.6%), 0.39 mm (13.8%), and 1.21 mm2 (21.3%), respectively. These results are in line with a recent study by Okamura [33], who evaluated the optical frequency domain imaging (OFDI) in comparison to IVUS and QCA in 19 patients undergoing stent implantation. The lumen area was found the largest by IVUS, followed by OFDI, and was the smallest by QCA. New in our study is that non-stented vessel segments were evaluated and 3D QCA was applied. Besides that, a real-time co-registration approach was used to establish the point-to-point correspondence between different imaging modalities. Our results are also in agreement with previous studies by Gonzalo [34] and Suzuki [35], which showed that compared to histology, both IVUS and OCT measured larger lumen size and the discrepancy was more pronounced by IVUS. Nevertheless, it should be borne in mind that our study does not allow a direct comparison between IVUS and OCT, since IVUS and OCT imaging were not performed in the same vessels. In addition, our study compared 3D QCA at the end-diastolic phase with OCT images which could correspond to any moment in the cardiac cycle, while 3D QCA was compared to IVUS images which were both selected at the end-diastolic phase. Finally, although the correspondence between different imaging modalities was established by the co-registration approach, the relatively slow pullback speed in IVUS imaging could increase local errors in the registration when coupled with patient respirations, resulting in a suboptimal match for the comparison between 3D QCA and IVUS.

Similar to the findings by Schuurbiers [32] in the comparison between 3D QCA and IVUS, our data showed that the lumen area was larger by IVUS than by 3D QCA. However, the difference that we found by Bland-Altman plots indicated that the discrepancy was more pronounced in larger vessels, while Schuurbiers reported that the trend (lumen area was larger in IVUS) tended to reverse in larger vessels (difference lumen area = 0.013 - 0.058 × average lumen area, $p < 0.05$). The difference could be explained by the fact that suboptimal angiographic image quality using diluted contrast agent was used by Schuurbiers, while we used angiographic images with vessels well filled with pure contrast agent. In addition, different 3D QCA software packages were applied. Finally, there was no official guideline in the image acquisition dedicated for 3D QCA in a broad clinical setting, making the interpretation of different studies difficult.

Of note, we showed that vessel-based discrepancy between 3D QCA and IVUS or OCT tended to increase with the vessel curvature, especially in assessing the long diameter [17]. Tortuous vessels with high vessel curvature could lead to oblique imaging, i.e., the imaging catheter was positioned obliquely inside the lumen, and hence the circular lumen appeared elliptical in shape, resulting in overestimation of the long diameter by IVUS or by OCT. This could partly explain our finding that the discrepancy between 3D QCA and IVUS or OCT was more pronounced in the long diameter than in the short diameter. Actually, the discrepancy in the long diameter, as demonstrated in this study, was about two times larger than in the short diameter, indicating that attention should be given when sizing the stent based on the long diameter from IVUS or OCT. An optimal stent selection should be applied from multiple assessments when combined with individual characteristics of the target vessel.

6. Conclusions

We have presented in this book chapter a novel, user-friendly system for the fusion of X-ray angiography and IVUS/OCT for coronary interventions. The system uses 3D angiographic reconstruction as a roadmap to integrate the IVUS and OCT images, allowing detailed lesion morphology assessment and careful tailoring of the procedural strategy before the intervention. Despite the fact that the accumulated evidence has been limited so far to retrospective studies and case reports, it is expected that the present paradigm of angiographic guided PCI will develop into a more meticulously tailored approach. The integration of X-ray angiography with intracoronary imaging devices will likely evolve in a rapid pace in the coming years, with the potential of improving outcomes and reducing costs in the treatment of obstructive coronary artery disease.

Acknowledgements

We thank Gerhard Koning, Pieter Kitslaar, Andrei Rareş, Joan Tuinenburg, Evelyn Regar, Jurgen Lighthart, Karen Witberg, Stylianos A. Pyxaras, William Wijns, Zheng Huang, Liang Xu, and Bo Xu for their contributions in the development and validation of the system.

References

1. Costa MA, Angiolillo DJ, Tannenbaum M, et al. Impact of stent deployment procedural factors on long-term effectiveness and safety of sirolimus-eluting stents (final results of the multicenter prospective STLLR trial). Am J Cardiol 2008; 101:1704–1711.
2. Reiber JHC, Tuinenburg JC, Koning G, et al. Quantitative coronary arteriography. In: Coronary Radiology 2nd Revised Edition, Oudkerk M, Reiser MF (Eds.), Series: Medical Radiology, Sub series: Diagnostic Imaging, Baert AL, Knauth M, Sartor K (Eds.). Springer-Verlag, Berlin-Heidelberg, 2009:41–65.
3. Reiber JHC, Serruys PW, Kooijman CJ, et al. Assessment of short-, medium-, and long-term variations in arterial dimensions from computer-assisted quantitation of coronary cineangiograms. Circulation 1985; 71:280–288.
4. Lansky A, Tuinenburg J, Costa M, et al., on behalf of the European Bifurcation Angiographic Sub-Committee. Quantitative Angiographic methods for bifurcation lesions: A consensus statement from the European Bifurcation Group. Cath Cardiovasc Interventions 2009; 73:258–266.
5. Tu S, Hao P, Koning G, et al. In-vivo assessment of optimal viewing angles from X-ray coronary angiograms. EuroIntervention 2011; 7:112–120.
6. Tu S, Jing J, Holm NR, et al. In-vivo Assessments of Bifurcation Optimal Viewing Angles and Bifurcation Angles by Three-dimensional (3D) Quantitative Coronary Angiography. Int J Cardiovasc Imaging 2012; 28:1617–1625.
7. Green NE, Chen SJ, Hansgen AR, et al. Angiographic Views Used for Percutaneous Coronary Interventions: A Three Dimensional Analysis of Physician-Determined vs. Computer-Generated Views. Catheterization and Cardiovascular Interventions 2005; 64:451–459.
8. Gollapudi RR, Valencia R, Lee SS, et al. Utility of three-dimensional reconstruction of coronary angiography to guide percutaneous coronary intervention. Catheter Cardiovasc Interv 2007; 69:479–482.
9. Glagov S, Weisenberg E, Zarins CK, et al. Compensatory enlargement of human atherosclerotic coronary arteries. N Engl J Med 1987; 316:1371–1375.
10. Virmani R, Kolodgie FD, Burke AP, et al. Atherosclerotic plaque progression and vulnerability to rupture: angiogenesis as a source of intraplaque hemorrhage. Arterioscler Thromb Vasc Biol 2005; 25:2054–2061.

11. Dumay ACM. Image Reconstruction from Biplane Angiographic Projections. Dissertation 1992, Delft University of Technology.
12. Wahle A, Wellnhofer E, Mugaragu I, et al. Assessment of Diffuse Coronary Artery Disease by Quantitative Analysis of Coronary Morphology Based upon 3-D Reconstruction from Biplane Angiograms. IEEE Trans Med Imaging 1995; 14:230–241.
13. Chen SJ, Carroll JD, Messenger JC. Quantitative Analysis of Reconstructed 3-D Coronary Arterial Tree and Intracoronary Devices. IEEE Trans Med Imaging 2002; 21:724–740.
14. Tu S, Holm NR, Koning G. The impact of acquisition angle difference on three-dimensional quantitative coronary angiography. Catheter Cardiovasc Interv 2011; 78:214–222.
15. Tu S, Koning G, Jukema W, et al. Assessment of obstruction length and optimal viewing angle from biplane X-ray angiograms. Int J Cardiovasc Imaging 2010; 26:5–17.
16. Tu S, Huang Z, Koning G, et al. A novel three-dimensional quantitative coronary angiography system: in vivo comparison with intravascular ultrasound for assessing arterial segment length. Catheter Cardiovasc Interv 2010; 76:291–298.
17. Tu S, Xu L, Ligthart J, Xu B, et al. In-vivo Comparison of Arterial Lumen Dimensions Assessed by Co-registered Three-dimensional (3D) Quantitative Coronary Angiography, Intravascular Ultrasound and Optical Coherence Tomography. Int J Cardiovasc Imaging 2012; 8:1315–1327.
18. Tuinenburg JC, Koning G, Rares A, et al. Dedicated bifurcation analysis: basic principles. Int J Cardiovasc Imaging 2010; 26:169–174.
19. Janssen JP, Rares A, Tuinenburg JC, et al. New approaches for the assessment of vessel sizes in quantitative (cardio-)vascular X-ray analysis. Int J Cardiovasc Imaging 2010; 26:259–271.
20. Slager CJ, Wentzel JJ, Schuurbiers JCH, et al. True 3-Dimensional Reconstruction of Coronary Arteries in Patients by Fusion of Angiography and IVUS (ANGUS) and Its Quantitative Validation. Circulation 2000; 102:511–516.
21. Wahle A, Lopez JJ, Olszewski ME, et al. Plaque development, vessel curvature, and wall shear stress in coronary arteries assessed by X-ray angiography and intravascular ultrasound. Medical Image Analysis 2006; 10:615–631.
22. Rotger D, Radeva P, Canero C, et al. Corresponding IVUS and Angiogram Image Data. Proceedings of Computers in Cardiology 2001; 28:273–276.
23. Tu S, Holm NR, Christiansen EH, et al. First Presentation of 3-Dimensional Reconstruction and Centerline-guided Assessment of Coronary Bifurcation by Fusion of X-ray Angiography and Optical Coherence Tomography. JACC Cardiovascular Interventions 2012, 5:884–885.
24. Koning G, Dijkstra J, Birgelen C von, et al. Advanced contour detection for three-dimensional intracoronary ultrasound: a validation – in vitro and in vivo. Int J Cardiovasc Imaging 2002; 18:235–248.
25. Tu S, Koning G, Tuinenburg JC, et al. Coronary angiography enhancement for visualization. Int J Cardiovasc imaging 2009; 25:657–667.
26. Tu S, Holm NR, Koning G, Huang Z, et al. Fusion of 3D QCA and IVUS/OCT. Int J Cardiovasc imaging 2011; 27:197–207.
27. De Scheerder I, De Man F, Herregods MC, et al. Intravascular ultrasound versus angiography for measurement of luminal diameters in normal and diseased coronary arteries. Am Heart J 1994; 127:243–251.
28. Tsuchida K, Serruys PW, Bruining N, et al. Two-year serial coronary angiographic and intravascular ultrasound analysis of in-stent angiographic late lumen loss and ultrasonic neointimal volume from the TAXUS II trial. Am J Cardiol 2007; 99:607–615.
29. Koning G, Hekking E, Kemppainen JS, et al. Suitability of the Cordis StabilizerTM marker guide wire for quantitative coronary angiography calibration: An in vitro and in vivo study. Catheterization and Cardiovascular Interventions 2001; 52:334–341.

30. Rittger H, Schertel B, Schmidt M, et al. Three-dimensional reconstruction allows accurate quantification and length measurements of coronary artery stenoses. EuroIntervention 2009; 5:127–132.
31. Bruining N, Tanimoto S, Otsuka M, et al. Quantitative multi-modality imaging analysis of a bioabsorbable poly-L-lactid acid stent design in the acute phase: a comparison between 2 and 3D-QCA, QCU and QMSCT-CA. EuroIntervention 2008; 4:285–291.
32. Schuurbiers JC, Lopez NG, Ligthart J, et al. In vivo validation of CAAS QCA-3D coronary reconstruction using fusion of angiography and intravascular ultrasound (ANGUS). Catheter Cardiovasc Interv 2009; 73:620–626.
33. Okamura T, Onuma Y, Garcia-Garcia HM, et al. First-in-man evaluation of intravascular optical frequency domain imaging (OFDI) of Terumo: a comparison with intravascular ultrasound and quantitative coronary angiography. EuroIntervention 2011; 6:1037–1045.
34. Gonzalo N, Serruys PW, García-García HM, et al. Quantitative ex vivo and in vivo comparison of lumen dimensions measured by optical coherence tomography and intravascular ultrasound in human coronary arteries. Rev Esp Cardiol 2009; 62:615–624.
35. Suzuki Y, Ikeno F, Koizumi T, et al. In vivo comparison between optical coherence tomography and intravascular ultrasound for detecting small degrees of in-stent neointima after stent implantation. JACC Cardiovasc Interv 2008; 1:168–173.

CHAPTER 10

THREE-DIMENSIONAL RECONSTRUCTION METHODS IN NEAR-FIELD CODED APERTURE FOR SPECT IMAGING SYSTEM

Stephen Baoming Hong

12 Sorrel Rd, Concord, MA 01742, USA
E-mail: baoming.hong@yale.edu

Coded aperture imaging was originally developed in X-ray astronomy. It has been investigated extensively in two-dimensional (2D) planar objects in the past, whereas little success has been achieved in three-dimensional (3D) object imaging using this technique. In this chapter, we introduce a near-field coded aperture imaging technique and 3D image reconstruction methods for high sensitivity and high resolution single photon emission computerized tomography (SPECT). Multiangular coded aperture projections are acquired and a stack of 2D images is first decoded separately from each of the projections. The projections are then corrected by viable magnification of near-field coded aperture imaging. The ordered subset expectation maximization (OSEM) method is finally employed to reconstruct the cross-sectional image slices from the decoded images. Experiments were conducted using a customized capillary tube phantom and a micro hot rod phantom. The experimental results have demonstrated the feasibility of the 3D reconstruction algorithm in coded aperture imaging for high sensitivity and high resolution SPECT systems.

1. Introduction

SPECT is a nuclear emission tomographic imaging technique which measures the emission of single photons of a given energy from radioactive tracers to construct images of the distribution of the tracers in the patient. SPECT scan is capable of providing information about blood flow to tissue and visualizing functional information about a patient's specific organ or body system. The radioactive isotope/tracer (e.g., Tc-99m, I-123) decays, resulting in the emission of gamma rays. These gamma rays collected from the detectors of SPECT systems give us a picture of what's happening inside the patient's body.

SPECT imaging is performed by using a gamma camera to acquire multiple 2D projection images from multiple angles. A tomographic reconstruction algorithm is then applied on the collected multiple projections to generate 3D object data. Visualization of thin slices representing the radionuclide distribution can be performed along cross-sections of the patient's body by manipulating the reconstructed 3D data. However, SPECT imaging typically suffers from low count sensitivity and low image resolution (10~15 mm) due to collimation. The image resolution can be improved using pinhole collimators [1-3], whereas the count sensitivity using the pinholes is considerably poor [3,4].

Multipinhole collimation has recently gained a lot of attention in the effort to develop high sensitivity and high resolution SPECT imaging systems [4,5,6,7]. In comparison to conventional pinhole imaging, SPECT imaging with multipinhole collimators offers substantially higher count sensitivity while maintaining high image resolution. A trade-off exists, however, since multipinhole collimators provide a smaller field of view for the same detector size than conventional pinhole imaging. To improve the count sensitivity with a larger field of view for imaging, near-field coded aperture imaging technique has been recently applied to conventional SPECT imaging systems. Near-field coded aperture imaging is known to have superior image resolution and count sensitivity over conventional parallel-hole collimated nuclear imaging. There have been comprehensive investigations in 2D planar imaging using coded aperture imaging technologies [8,9,10,11]. Nevertheless, little success has been achieved in imaging 3D objects using this technique.

In this chapter, we introduce a 3D object image reconstruction approach driven by iterative computation. This approach directly uses maximal likelihood-based expectation maximization (MLEM) [12,13,14,15], assuming the projection has Poisson distribution, for image decoding and incorporated with the depth-dependent correction factor in the MLEM algorithm for 3D near-field coded aperture images. This method can improve deconvolution performance of a specific slice of the 3D object by removing artifact influence from other slices to the specific slice and hence accomplish 3D reconstruction by ordered subset expectation maximization approach [16,17].

2. Theory & Method

2.1. *Coded aperture imaging and decoding*

Coded aperture imaging is a technique originally proposed for astronomical imaging [8], where the incident rays from a very distant point source are parallel to each other. The coded aperture mask is a thin shield with numerous apertures drilled in a certain pattern. The mask is placed parallel to the detector surface. Each star projects onto the detector a shadow of the coded aperture mask weighted by the intensity of the star, and the location of the shadow depends on the direction of the incident rays from the star. As a result, the image of the stars is a summation of the shadows projected from all the stars within the field-of-view (FOV) of the imaging system.

Mathematically, the coded aperture imaging system can be modeled by convolution [18,19] as

$$p = f * h + n ,\tag{1}$$

where p is the coded image, f is the original source distribution; h is the mask pattern (as shown in Figure 1), n is the random noise associated with the imaging process, and $*$ denotes convolution operator.

The source image, f can be estimated by decoding, i.e., correlating the acquired coded aperture image, p with a decoding mask pattern, g. This decoding procedure can be represented as an inverse restoration for Eq. (1),

$$\hat{f} = p \otimes g = f * (h \otimes g) + n \otimes g ,\tag{2}$$

where $\otimes$ represents the correlation operator, $\hat{f}$ denotes an estimate of the original image and g is the decoding pattern which is usually an inverse filter of h, satisfying that

$$h \otimes g \approx \delta ,\tag{3}$$

Eq. (2) becomes

$$\hat{f} = f + n \otimes g,\tag{4}$$

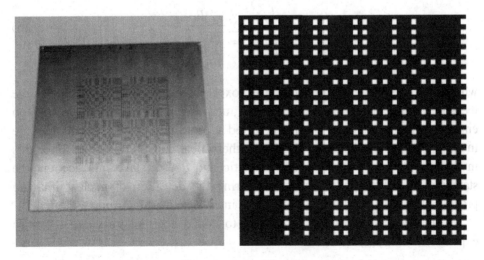

Fig. 1. Near-field coded aperture mask
(left: a real code aperture mask; right: a diagram of digitized basic pattern of the coded aperture mask).

The noise, n, can be assumed to have zero-mean and be uncorrelated with g such that the expectation (mean value) of $n \otimes g$ in Eq. (4) is zero. However, the statistics of n does not always hold since g is normally of finite size, which inevitably causes image artifacts, such as negative pixel values in the decoded image.

In conventional coded aperture imaging, the mask is usually a mosaic of four identical basic aperture patterns [18,19,20]. Only the projection of the central area of the mosaic pattern is used as p which defines the FOV. The use of the mosaic pattern is to ensure that p is truly a circular convolution of the image within the FOV and the basic mask pattern as expressed in Eq. (1).

2.2. Iterative reconstruction of 2D coded aperture SPECT imaging

The maximum likelihood estimation-based expectation maximization approach is an iterative image reconstruction method for SPECT. Since MLEM allows more accurate modeling of the imaging system by including statistical Poisson model for photo emission, the iterative reconstruction procedure can control noise suppression and is hence superior to the filtered back-projection method in the reconstruction of emission tomography [21]. This kind of method yields superior results in noise suppression and artifact removal and is particularly suitable for the deconvolution of coded aperture images [17]. Since the probabilistic nature of radioactive decay during the SPECT imaging process is described by the Poisson distribution, the MLEM algorithm can be written as [12,13]

$$f_j^{(k+1)} = \frac{f_j^{(k)}}{\sum\limits_{i=1}^{n} C_{ij}} \sum_{i=1}^{n} \frac{p_i C_{ij}}{\sum\limits_{j=1}^{m} C_{ij} f_j^{(k)}}, \tag{5}$$

where $f_j^{(k)}$ is the value of the image voxel j for the kth iteration, p_i is the measured value of the projection pixel i, and C_{ij} is the probability of photon emitted from image voxel j being detected at projection pixel i. Coded aperture imaging process can be described by mathematical convolution [19]. Since this inverse restoration method is deterministic and doesn't take into account the statistical model of photon emission during the detection of nuclear imaging process, it might not achieve a good result in noise and artifact suppression.

When the EM algorithm is applied to coded aperture imaging, it can be expressed by [20,22]:

$$f^{(k+1)}(x,y) = f^{(k)}(x,y)[\frac{p_c(x,y)}{f^{(k)}(x,y) * h(x,y)} \otimes h(x,y)] \tag{6}$$

where $f^{(k)}$ is current estimate of the original signal f, p_c is the projection measurement which has been corrected by angular and collimation effect [20]. h is a known coding mask pattern. $*$ and $\otimes$ are the convolution and correlation operators, respectively. Eq. (6) is particularly suitable for image reconstruction of a 2D planar object. As seen, this algorithm includes two major procedures: forward-projection and back-projection. The convolution represents the forward-projection step using current estimate of $f^{(k)}$, and the correlation with the correction ratio resulted from the division step of p_c represents the back-projection step.

2.3. *Iterative reconstruction of 3D coded aperture SPECT imaging*

A 3D object can be represented by a stack of 2D slices along the z direction. Each of these slices located at a specific depth z_0 can be viewed as a 2D planar object

$$p(x,y) = \sum_z f(x,y,z) * h_z(x,y), \tag{7}$$

where h_z denotes the mask shadow produced by source at distance z. When the EM method is applied to a specific slice of coded aperture imaging, the slice can be reconstructed according to Eq. (6),

$$f_{z_0}^{(k+1)}(x,y) = f_{z_0}^{(k)}(x,y)[\frac{p_c(x,y)}{f_{z_0}^{(k)}(x,y) * h_{z_0}(x,y)} \otimes h_{z_0}(x,y)], \tag{8}$$

where f_{z_0} represents a reconstructed image at slice ($z = z_0$). However, image reconstruction using this approach for 3D coded aperture images will inevitably cause a blurring effect along the z direction since the sources from the out-of-focus planes ($z \neq z_0$) also contribute to the reconstruction of the in-focus plane ($z = z_0$). To remove this depth-dependent blur, we introduced an out-of-focus correction factor into Eq. (8). The modified iterative EM algorithm for slice reconstruction from a 3D object can be rewritten as [17]

$$f_{z_0}^{(k+1)}(x,y) = \frac{f_{z_0}^{(k)}(x,y)}{\sum_z h_z(x,y)} \left\{ \frac{p_c(x,y) - \sum_{z \neq z_0} f_z^{(k)}(x,y) * h_z(x,y)}{f_{z_0}^{(k)}(x,y) * h_{z_0}(x,y)} \otimes h_{z_0}(x,y) \right\},$$

$$\tag{9}$$

where z denotes the object-to-detector distance, $f_z(x,y)$ is the reconstruction of the object slice at z, and $h_z(x,y)$ is the mask shadow pattern at z. thus, a 3D object consisting of a stack of slices at different depth z_0 along the z direction can be reconstructed using Eq. (9). By doing so, each slice reconstruction no longer contains other slices' information due to the removal of the out-of-focus information from the other slices. Nevertheless, the image resolution in the z direction is expected to be still limited since the images are reconstructed from projections acquired in the same axial z direction.

2.4. *OSEM reconstruction in coded aperture SPECT images*

For a full 3D image reconstruction, the object is placed on a rotation stage and usually carried on using a rotational camera or detector as shown in Figure 2. It is necessary to acquire multiple angles of projections and reconstruct each set of the projections. Since the magnification factor varies as the object-mask distance changes, the pixel size at different slice is different due to changes of the geometry structure. These facts present a serious challenge to the conventional EM algorithm (e.g., Eq. (8)) where pixel sizes have to fixed so that the relationship between projections and object is tractable. However, this problem can be solved by using ordered subset expectation maximization (OSEM) method [16].

The reconstructed slices for each angle are subsequently summed to generate a "clean" in-focus projection for each angle. This summation process is similar to the tomography projection process. If slice thickness is set as less than size of the finest detail of the object image, the resolution of the reconstruction should meet reconstruction condition of the finest image details from theoretically. Ultimately, the OSEM method is used to reconstruct the 3D object from the deconvoluted projections of the different acquisition angles. In SPECT imaging, two sets of projection data (one from coded aperture and the other one from parallel-hole collimator) are simultaneously acquired. Subset selection of OSEM may naturally correspond to groups of projections. The projection data in the OSEM method are grouped in a series of subsets arranged in certain order and each subset contains multiple projections. The OSEM algorithm is designed as follows,

- Iterates until converge
- Repeat n_1 iterations from 1 to N_1
- Repeat n_2 iterations from 1 to N_2
  - Reconstruct f using projection $p(n_1, n_2)$
  - Rotate and interpolate f to fit the coordinate system of next projection.

where N_1 denotes the partitioned group number of subsets and N_2 denotes projection number contained in each subset. For example, we can partition a total of 60 projections into 15 subjects and each subset contains 4 projections. Generally, partition of the subsets among the projections is benefit in a balance way so that pixel activity contributes equally to any subset and it directly associated with the convergence speed. A good subset partition of projections has typically two pairs of opposite projections that are orthogonal to each other. Because the consecutive projections are orthogonal to each other, this arrangement provides the most different view and least redundant information and the OSEM algorithm is expected to converge fast.

3. Coded Aperture SPECT Imaging Systems and Phantom Experimental Results

3.1. *Coded aperture SPECT imaging systems*

A dual-head SPECT imaging system (Varicam, GE Medical Systems, Waukesha, WI) with an intrinsic resolution of 3.9 mm was used in our image acquisitions [22]. The dual-head SPECT camera was equipped with a coded aperture module on one head and a pinhole collimator on the other head. For the pinhole collimator, the diameter of the pinhole was 1 mm and the pinhole-to-detector distance was 12 cm. For the coded aperture module, the mask was placed in parallel to the detector and at 32.2 cm from the detector. The basic pattern of the coded aperture mask was a 46×46 NTHT [10] MURA [18,23]. The aperture diameter was 1.1 mm and the mask thickness was 2.0 mm. A diagram of the basic pattern of the coded aperture mask digitized is shown in Figure 1. The size of the basic mask pattern was 5.06×5.06 cm^2 and the full mask consisted of a mosaic of four basic patterns. The radiation sensitive area on the detector heads was 39×51 cm^2. An image matrix of 512×512 with a pixel size of 1.105×1.105 mm^2 was used in image acquisitions.

Multiangular projections were acquired by rotating the object instead of the camera heads because the coded aperture mask was too close to the camera rotating axis. More specifically, the maximal camera arm extension was 68 cm and the mask-to-detector distance was 32.2 cm, leaving only a cylindrical shape space with a diameter less than 4 cm for the object. Although rotating the object in one direction is conceptually equivalent to rotating the camera heads in the opposite direction, in reality it is not a trivial task to establish this equivalence because the object rotating axis needs to be coincided with that of the camera heads. Some image degradation is expected in the reconstructed images due to the potential axis misalignment. Figure 2 depicts the imaging systems used in our phantom experiments. The object was secured by a metal bar attached to a stepping motor, and the stepping motor was placed on an L-shaped frame clamped on the imaging table. Before image acquisitions, the object's rotating axis was first checked using a level to ensure that the axis was parallel to the detector surface, and the axis was then visually aligned with the rows of the pinhole image seen on the image acquisition monitor.

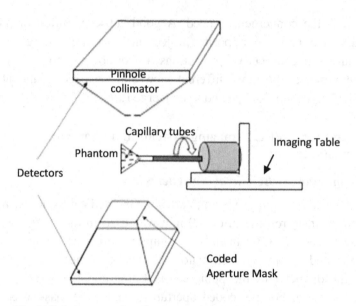

Fig. 2. Coded aperture imaging setup using dual-head SPECT system.

3.2. Experimental setup

3.2(a) Reconstruct a simple 3D pyramid shaped phantom

The phantom was made of four capillary tubes in this experiment. Each had a length of 6.5 cm, an inner diameter of 1 mm, and a wall thickness of 0.2 mm. The capillary tubes were each filled with 75 Ci of ^{99m}Tc solution and attached radially along the slope to the inner wall of a small funnel, as demonstrated in Figure 2. The metal bar attached to the rotating motor was screwed into the cylindrical opening of the funnel to secure the phantom. Because the conic part of the funnel had an opening angle of approximately 60°, the cross section of this object should include four ellipse-shaped point sources with different separations. This phantom was placed in such a way that its central axis rotating axis was 5.5 cm away from the pinhole and 18.5 cm away from the coded aperture mask. Pinhole and coded aperture projections were acquired simultaneously over a full 360° phantom rotation using a step-and-shoot imaging protocol 2 min/step. A total of 48 projections (24 from pinhole plus 24 from coded aperture) were acquired. As compared to pin- hole collimated imaging, coded aperture imaging resulted in a 50-fold increase in count sensitivity in this phantom experiment (1.1×10^6 counts/projection vs 2.2×10^4 counts/projection), despite the much larger object-to-mask distance for the coded aperture module.

For each coded aperture projection, a 3D image stack was reconstructed using Eq. (9). A total of nine images in each image stack were reconstructed using 200 iterations of the MLEM algorithm. The large number of iterations is needed because the image stack was reconstructed from a single projection, and the algorithm was expected to converge at a lower speed than the OSEM using multi-angular projections. Each of the reconstructed images in the stack corresponds to an object depth 5 mm slice thickness ranging from 165 to 205 mm away from the mask. The slice thickness of 5 mm is selected empirically as a result of a trade-off between computational efficiency and the effectiveness of removing the out-of-focus blur. Figure 3 shows one of these reconstructed image stacks. Cross-sectional images of the capillary tube phantom were reconstructed using the OSEM with four subsets and five iterations. Figure 4 shows six representative slices from the reconstructed 3D images. As expected, the slice images show clearly four objects with decreasing separations. In the reconstructed images, the voxel size was 0.57 mm based on the in-plane pixel size in the nearest slice to the mask 165 mm [22]. As seen in Figure 4, the reconstructed images are of excellent image resolution, exhibiting much reduced background noise between the objects.

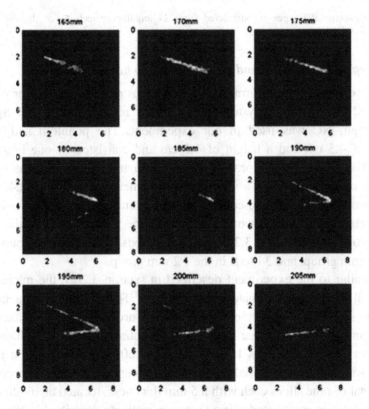

Fig. 3. Reconstructed image slices at object-to-mask distances from 165 to 205 mm.

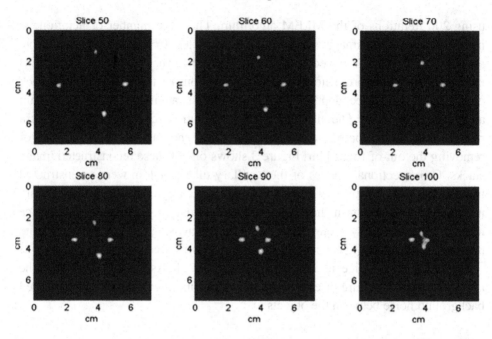

Fig. 4. Cross-sectional images reconstructed from 24 angular projections of the capillary tube phantom using the OSEM.

3.2(b) *Experimental setup and results for micro hot rod phantom*

To further evaluate the performance of 3D reconstruction method for the coded aperture SPECT imaging system, a micro hot rod phantom Data Spectrum, Hillsborough, NC was used in our experiment. The phantom had an inner diameter of 4.5 cm and a height of 6.3 cm and consisted of one large central rod and six groups of microrods arranged in a triangular shape as shown in Figure 5(a). The rods in the six groups had diameters of 1.2, 1.6, 2.4, 3.2, 4.0, and 4.8 mm, and the center-to-center spacing within each group were twice of the rod diameter in the corresponding group. There were 3 rods in the 4.0 and 4.8 mm groups, 6 rods in the 3.2 mm group, 10 rods in the 2.4 mm group, 19 rods in the 1.6 mm group, and 34 rods in the 1.2 mm group.

As similar to the experiment described in section 3.2(a), the micro hot rod phantom filled with approximately 900 Ci of ^{99m}Tc solution was attached to the metal bar so that the object could be rotated around its central axis by the stepping motor. The distance between the central axis of the phantom and the coded aperture mask was 18 cm. A total of 60 projections over a full 360° phantom rotation were acquired using a step-and-shoot imaging protocol 2 min/step. A total of nine slices each with a 5 mm thickness, located at 16–20 cm from the mask, were reconstructed using the same methods described in the previous section with the deviations described below. Because the hot rods were composed of small cylindrical shaped rods, the cross sections of the phantom were identical. Figure 5(b) shows the reconstructed image using the OSEM method with ten subsets and ten iterations. As seen, the six groups of rods in triangular shape can be identified visually from the reconstructed image. In addition, the hot rods in four of the groups, with rod diameters ranging from 2.4 to 4.8 mm, can be visually resolved. This result is particularly encouraging given the suboptimal imaging conditions including the small magnification due to the large object-to-mask distance and the possible errors introduced by the imperfect rotating mechanism [22].

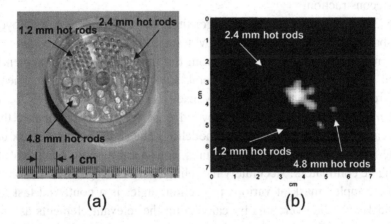

Fig. 5. Experimental results of micro hot rod phantom (adopted from [22]).

4. Discussions

We have demonstrated with experimental results the feasibilities of our near-field coded aperture imaging technique and novel image reconstruction methods for 3D SPECT. While the reconstructed image quality obtained from the preliminary phantom results is quite promising, a number of limitations in our experimental systems have undermined our efforts to improve the image reconstruction. Among them, the most prominent limitation was the large mask-to-detector distance of the coded aperture module, which forced us to rotate the object instead of the cameras during image acquisitions. Detailed system calibrations including precise rotation axis alignment were not performed in this study. As a result, the geometry of cross-sectional slices of the object varied from one projection to another and the imperfect imaging geometry inevitably corrupted the quality of image reconstruction, particularly for a complex object such as the micro hot rod phantom used in this study.

In our phantom experiments, the objects had to be placed quite far from the detector to avoid image truncation [20] due to the large size of the mask used, resulting in a small magnification. Additional sources of error were the imperfect object placement and rotating mechanism as mentioned above, which in turn introduced degradation in the image reconstruction. As such, given the early stage of the research and the imperfection of the experimental system, it would be premature to perform quantitative analysis on image reconstruction quality or comparison with other existing imaging modalities, such as pinhole or multipinhole collimated 3D SPECT imaging. However, we feel that the results presented herein are quite encouraging, particularly in the situations of the existing system limitations and the small number of projections used in our 3D SPECT reconstruction.

The 3D image reconstruction algorithm introduced herein employed the MLEM-based OSEM algorithm that provides a fast path to full 3D coded aperture SPECT image reconstruction. Aside from the implementation convenience, the proposed two-step approach has several advantages compared to the direct MLEM reconstruction method widely used for multipinhole SPECT. Direct MLEM method requires detailed knowledge of the transition matrix through either measurements or mathematical modeling. The coded aperture mask used in our experiments has hundreds of apertures, considerably more complicated than multipinhole collimators. Accurately modeling or measuring the transition matrix of such a complex mask at various projection angles is a nontrivial task. While this obstacle may be overcome by calculating the relevant elements as they are needed in the OSEM reconstruction, this approach would be inefficient and impractical for coded aperture because the masks are substantially more complex than multipinhole collimators and it would require longer time to calculate those elements on the fly. In contrast, the proposed approach decouples the 3D reconstruction problem into two steps, resulting in significant data reduction as well as computing efficiency. The partial 3D reconstruction in Eq. (9) uses only the mask shadow, which is derived from the mask matrix and the magnification factor. This step is identical for all projections in which the same mask shadows are used, providing the desired flexibility. The next step, i.e., the OSEM step, is well established and the implementation is straightforward. Above all, the proposed method does not require measurement or storage of a terabyte sized transition matrix.

5. Conclusion

A novel 3D image reconstruction approach has been proposed to near-field coded aperture SPECT imaging and we evaluated this method using a customized capillary tube phantom and a complex micro hot rod phantom. The experimental results have demonstrated that our approaches to near-field coded aperture SPECT imaging and the MLEM image reconstruction may have the potential for high sensitivity and high resolution SPECT. Future studies on the optimization of coded aperture mask design, algorithms for the 3D reconstruction of coded aperture SPECT imaging with a small number of projections, and the correction for photon attenuation are warranted for the systems to be readily used in clinical applications.

Acknowledgements

The chapter is written based on our previous publications. The author would like to thank Prof. Y. Liu and Dr. Z. Mu's contributions in the near-field coded aperture imaging and reconstruction for SPECT.

References

[1] R. J. Jaszczak, J. Li, H. Wang, Z. M.R., and R. E. Coleman, "Pinhole collimation for ultrahigh resolution, small-field-of-view SPECT," *Phys Med Biol*, vol. 39, pp. 425-437, 1994.

[2] K. Ogawa, T. Kawade, K. Nakamura, A. Kubo, and T. Ichihara, "Ultra high resolution pinhole SPECT for small animal study," *IEEE Trans Med Imag*, vol. 45, pp. 3122-3126, 1998.

[3] T. Zeniya, H. *et al.*, "A new reconstruction strategy for image improvement in pinhole SPECT," *Eur J Nucl Med Mod Imaging*, vol. 31, pp. 1166-1172, 2004.

[4] S. Meikle, P. Kench, M. Kassiou, and R. Banati, "Small animal SPECT and its place in the matrix of molecular imaging technologies," Phys. Med. Biol. 50 (22), pp. 45-61, 2005.

[5] Y.-H. Liu, G. P. Fernando, and A. J. Sinusas, "A new method for hot-spot quantification of hybrid SPECT/CT cardiac images: methodology and preliminary phantom validation," IEEE Trans. Nucl. Sci. 53, 2814-2821, 2006.

[6] T. Funk *et al.*, "A multipinhole small animal SPECT system with submillimete spatial resolution," Med. Phys. 33(5), pp. 1259-1268, 2006.

[7] N. Schramm *et al.*, "High-resolution SPECT using multipinhole collimation," IEEE Trans. Nucl. Sci. 50(3), 315-320, 2003.

[8] E. Caroli, J. Stephen, G. D. Cocco, L. Natalucci, and A. Spizzichino, "Coded aperture imaging in x- and gamma-ray astronomy," *Space Sci Rev*, vol. 45, pp. 349-403, 1987.

[9] E. E. Fenimore and T. M. Cannon, "Coded aperture imaging with uniformly redundant arrays," *Appl Opt*, vol. 17, pp. 337-347, 1978.

[10] R. Accorsi and R. Lanza, "Near-field artifact reduction in planar coded aperture imaging," *Appl Opt*, vol. 40, pp. 4697-4705, 2001.

[11] S. R. Meikle *et al.*, "A prototype coded aperture detector for small animal SPECT," *IEEE Trans Nucl Sci*, vol. 49, pp. 2167-2171, 2002.

[12] L. A. Shepp, and Y. Vardi, "Maximum likelihood reconstruction for emission tomography," IEEE Trans. Med. Imag., vol. MI-1, pp.113-122, 1982.

[13] Y. Vardi, L. A. Shepp, L. Kaufman, "A statistical model for positron emission tomography," J. American Statistical Association, vol. 80, pp. 8-20, 1985.

[14] K. Lange and R. Carson, "EM reconstruction algorithms for emission and transmission tomography," J. Computer Assited Tomography, vol. 8, pp. 306-316, 1984.

[15] Y. H. Liu *et al.*, "A novel geometry for SPECT imaging associated with the EM-type blind deconvolution method," IEEE TNS, vol. 45, pp. 2095-2101, 1998.

[16] H, M. Hudson and R. S. Larkin, "Accelerated image reconstruction using ordered subsets of projection data," IEEE Trans Med. Imag., vol. 13, 1994.

[17] B. Hong, Z. Mu, and Y. Liu, "A new approach of 3D SPECT reconstruction for near-field coded aperture imaging," Proc. SPIE 6142, 2006.

[18] E. E. Fenimore and T. M. Cannon, "Uniformly redundant arrays: digital reconstruction methods," *Appl Opt*, vol. 20, pp. 1858-1864, 1981.

[19] E. E. Fenimore and T. M. Cannon, "Coded aperture imaging: predicted performance of uniformly redundant arrays," *Appl Opt*, vol. 17, pp. 3562-3570, 1978.

[20] Z. Mu and Y. Liu, "Aperture collimation correction and maximum- likelihood image reconstruction for near-field coded aperture imaging of single photon emission computerized tomography," IEEE Trans. Med. Imaging, vol. 25 no. 6, 701-711, 2006.

[21] E. J. Soares, C. L. Byrne, S. J. Glick, "Noise characterization of block-iterative reconstruction algorithms: I. theory," IEEE Trans Med. Imag., vol. 19, pp. 261-270, 2000.

[22] Z. Mu, B. Hong S. Li and Y. Liu, "A novel three-dimensional image reconstruction for near-field coded aperture single photon emission computerized tomography," Medical Physics, vol. 36, no. 5, 1533-1542, 2009.

[23] S. Gottesman and E. E. Fenimore, "New family of binary arrays for coded aperture imaging," *Appl Opt*, vol. 28, pp. 4344-4352, 1989.

CHAPTER 11

ULTRASOUND VOLUME RECONSTRUCTION BASED ON DIRECT FRAME INTERPOLATION

Sergei Koptenko[1,*], Rachel Remlinger[2,†], Martin Lachaine[3,‡],
Tony Falco[4,§], and Ulrich Scheipers[5,¶]

[1,2]*URS-US Medical Technologies Inc., Toronto, Canada*
[3,4]*Elekta Ltd, Montreal, Canada*
[5]*Prognortis Technologies GmbH,München, Germany*
E-mail: sergei.koptenko@urs-us.com
†*E-mail: rachel.remlinger@urs-us.com*
‡*E-mail: martin.lachaine@elekta.com*
§*E-mail: tony.falco@elekta.com*
¶*E-mail: ulrich.scheipers@prognortis.com*

An alternative approach for 3-D ultrasound volume reconstruction is discussed. The proposed direct frame interpolation (DFI) method creates additional intermediate image frames by directly interpolating between two or more adjacent image frames of the series of high resolution ultrasound B-mode image frames (an image series). The target volume is filled using the original frames in combination with the additionally constructed frames. The DFI method is based on a forward approach making use of *a priori* information about the position and shape of the B-mode image frames (*e.g.*, masking information) to optimize the reconstruction procedure and to reduce computation times and memory requirements. The DFI method can be considered as a valuable alternative to conventional 3-D ultrasound reconstruction methods based on pixel or a voxel nearest neighbor approaches, offering better quality and competitive reconstruction time.

1. Introduction

The clinical application of three or four dimensional (3-D or 4-D) ultrasound is gaining importance in medical diagnostics as well as in other areas, such as planning and verification of various therapies [1-10, 36-40]. In comparison to computed tomography (CT), and especially in comparison to magnetic resonance imaging (MRI), the application of ultrasound is economically priced, fast and straightforward. Soft-tissue contrast is high compared with CT and no ionizing radiation is applied during ultrasound imaging [4]. Ultrasound scanners are generally small and light and thus, can easily be integrated into existing

189

diagnostic or therapeutic environments. Although 3-D and 4-D ultrasound was formerly available exclusively on premium systems, the current generation of mid-range and portable systems already provides 3-D and 4-D imaging solutions at competitive prices.

Presently, even with the advent of true 3-D ultrasound volume acquisition methods and systems [40, 41], the most typical way to obtain a 3-D ultrasound data set is to reconstruct it from a series of 2-D images produced by either a mechanically steered transducer or by freehand scanning. The freehand tracked 3-D ultrasound imaging system consist of two components: an ultrasound imaging device that acquires a series of non-uniformly spaced and arbitrary aligned 2-D image frames by manually scanning over the organ or region of interest, and a motion tracking system that marks the position and spatial orientation of the ultrasound probe at the time of frame acquisition [36]. The choice of the tracking method is dependent on the particulars of the task.

The typical tracking system employs electromagnetic or optical position sensors that are complimentary to one another in terms of their capabilities. The electromagnetic tracking does not require direct line of sight to the tracked object (sensor), while optical tracking systems generally have larger range, better accuracy, and are oblivious to the presence of metallic objects [11-12]. An electronically or mechanically steered 3-D ultrasound transducer has the inherent advantage of precise positioning of frames within the scanned volume; however, it still may require an external tracking system when it being used as a part of a treatment modality, as will be discussed below.

There are also a number of sensorless freehand 3-D ultrasound imaging techniques that are based on various image registration and motion tracking techniques such as speckle decorrelation. Even though we did not test the DFI algorithm with such data sets, one might expect to get similar improvements in the volume reconstruction results as with ones produced by the tracked freehand DFI volume reconstructions.

The choice of the coordinate system of the reconstructed volume depends on the application. In cases when ultrasound data are acquired only to visualize the volume, *e.g.*, for diagnostic reasons, with no further interaction with other imaging or treatment modalities, there is generally no need for a common coordinate system. In cases when using imaging volumes for tracking, monitoring, or targeting for treatments such as radiotherapy, navigated surgery, or biopsy procedures, or to do a volumetric fusion with modalities like CT, MRI, single photon emission computed tomography (SPECT), or positron emission tomography (PET), a common coordinate system is necessary. In many cases, the coordinate system of the reconstructed 3-D space resembles the coordinate system within the diagnostic or therapy room, although different orientations have been proposed in the literature [13-14].

Freehand ultrasound data acquisition is typically performed on a non-uniformly spaced grid; however, typical tasks such as visualization of the acquired data and subsequent analysis, registration and segmentation of image volumes are based on regularly spaced grids as a rule. Hence, the interpolation or approximation of the acquired ultrasound image data must be performed by the 3-D ultrasound system during conversion of the data from the original positions of the ultrasound B-mode image frames to the new positions within the target volume. Conversion from original pixel data to voxel data is not a trivial step and many different methods have been proposed in the literature [15-17, 37, 42-43].

2. Overview of volume reconstruction methods

The majority of volume reconstruction methods can be categorized into two different classes, namely forward and reverse reconstruction approaches [16-18]. In the forward approach, we start with the pixel of a 2-D image frame, find a voxel within the reconstructed volume with coordinates being the closest match to the pixel's coordinates, and assign the brightness value of that pixel to the voxel. In methods based on reverse approach, we do the opposite. First we define the voxels grid, then for every voxel we try to find the closest pixel within the given set of B-mode image frames and assign its value to the voxel. Although both classes have several minor advantages and disadvantages, which will be discussed later, the forward approach has the important advantage of allowing the inclusion of a priori information about the position (*i.e.*, probe position and scanning direction) and shape or geometry (*e.g.*, masking information) of the underlying B-mode image frames into solving the reconstruction problem [19]. This knowledge of the scanning direction, shape and/or geometry of the B-mode images can be used to significantly decrease the computational load and memory requirements of the reconstruction algorithm. For instance, applying masking information during the voxel-filling step can considerably reduce the computational burden when working on scan-converted B-mode images originating from curved or phased arrays that typically contain numerous empty, *i.e.*, black, pixels surrounding the actual image data.

Voxel Nearest Neighbor

The VNN method assigns to each voxel of the target volume the value of the nearest pixel(s) of the image frame series and thus belongs to the class of reverse reconstruction methods. The most straightforward and computationally acceptable implementation of this method is to assign the value of a nearest single pixel to the corresponding voxel. However, in cases where the slices of the volume are not parallel to the original B-mode image frames, which is typically the case in freehand ultrasound, the contribution of different input image frames to one slice of the reconstructed volume can result in artifacts, *e.g.*, steps or jumps and other visually unsatisfying effects in the reconstructed volume, especially if the calibration lacks accuracy [20-22]. To handle these artifact-producing situations, instead of the single nearest pixel, a certain number of neighboring pixels are typically averaged to estimate the value of the voxel. Thus, VNN methods using $n > 1$ nearest neighbors actually perform spatial compounding to prevent artifacts [23]. This averaging technique has the trade-off between potentially blurring image details and a general loss of resolution within the volume.

Using VNN methods, two parameters must be defined: n - the number of pixels to average for each voxel, and d_{max} - the maximum distance within which to look for neighboring pixels. Both parameters must be adjusted precisely according to the specific scanning setup. If n is chosen too small, reconstruction artifacts may deteriorate the volume, whereas if it is chosen too large, the volume may be blurred. If d_{max} is chosen too small, undesired gaps can occur within the volume, whereas an overly large d_{max} can lead to exaggerated unnatural fillings of large gaps between the acquired B-mode image frames that lead to 'stripes' within the target volume.

This method can be computationally fast if a single transformation that defines the position of all image frames within the volume can be found. Another important advantage of the VNN method is the straightforward portability of the problem to multithreading environments. Although all threads require access to the original B-mode image frames and their positions within the 3-D space, the target volume can easily be divided into several sub-volumes with every thread running on one of the sub-volumes and parallel reading of the same B-mode image frames. When two abovementioned conditions are fulfilled, the VNN method is probably the fastest method.

Pixel Nearest Neighbor

The PNN method, which belongs to the forward reconstruction class of methods, has been extensively discussed in the literature [3, 5, 9, 15, 16, 19, 24-29].

PNN methods generally incorporate two steps. During the first step, all acquired ultrasound B-mode image frames are taken and the volume is filled starting from the first pixel of the first ultrasound B-mode image and ending with the last pixel of the last acquired frame. After the first step is completed, a reconstruction volume with uneven data density is obtained. In some areas there will be an excessive amount of information, with more than one pixel being assigned to one voxel; other areas will be filled with empty voxels without any pixels assigned. If these empty voxels lie within the reconstructed area, they must be filled during the second step of the PNN method.

In cases when more than one pixel position overlaps within a single voxel, these overlapping pixels are typically averaged to estimate a value that is used to fill the voxel. In addition to averaging the pixels, taking the maximum value or taking defined ratios between the maximum value and the average value have been proposed. In most cases, however, the average value is used because of its smoothing or speckle-reducing nature. Volumes reconstructed using average values appear to be less noisy than volumes reconstructed using maximum values which can be explained by the spatial compounding effect [5, 23]. Using average values also has a useful property of preserving the gray-value histogram of the underlying data, which may be practical for additional post processing steps performed on the ultrasound volume. Using maximum values instead of mean values does not preserve the general characteristics of the gray-level histogram because of the nonlinearity of the max operator. In other situations, where very high contrast is required, *e.g.*, certain muscular skeletal examinations, choosing the maximum value may lead to better visual representations of boundaries.

The first step of the PNN method can be performed relatively quickly if there is no pixel averaging. If we introduce averaging of pixels assigned to the same voxel position, the computational costs and the memory requirements rise. Considering that typical image series encountered in 3-D ultrasound consist of several million pixels, averaging gray value information at numerous positions can easily pose a computationally demanding problem; however, such averaging is highly recommended to achieve smooth volume reconstructions.

After the first step is completed, the second step is to fill the empty voxels. Several different methods of filling empty voxels have been suggested in the literature. In each case, nearby voxels are interpolated to find the missing entries. Most methods consist of simply averaging values in each empty voxel's neighborhood, only taking previously filled voxels into account, although Gaussian or other radial basis functions have been proposed for weighting the distance of neighboring voxels [13, 14 19, 30]. The number and the position of the surrounding voxels to be included differ from method to method. Generally, all methods begin by searching for entries within the direct (connected) neighbors of an empty voxel. If all direct neighbors of an empty voxel are empty as well, the search volume is linearly expanded. This step is iteratively repeated for a specified maximum number of iterations or for a maximum distance d_{max} from the original voxel. If the maximum number of iterations is reached, the gap is considered to be too large to be filled and the voxel is left empty. Three such methods of filling empty voxels that we selected as our benchmark are discussed in detail below in the next section.

It is worth stressing that empty voxels are filled using previously reconstructed data, which is derived from the original high-resolution image frames and thus has a lower resolution than the original images. This property can be disadvantageous compared with methods that directly derive the data for all voxels from the high-resolution original data.

Artifacts within the reconstructed volume may occur with this method when part of a volume slice is reconstructed during the first processing step by using original B-mode image data and another part of a volume slice is reconstructed during the second step by interpolating or averaging the original data. In these cases, blurred regions resulting from averaging of neighboring voxels are visually evident in comparison to the sharp reconstructions originating from the first step. Low-accuracy calibrations increase the severity of these artifacts because pixels with different gray values actually originating from different positions can become aligned and thus are averaged during the second step of the procedure producing grayscale values which are unnatural for the actual position.

Description of Pixel Nearest Neighbor Methods Selected as a Test Benchmark

In this study we compare three different PNN methods with the proposed DFI method [43]. The PNN method was selected for this comparison instead of the VNN scheme due to the previously described advantages of forward methods for freehand acquisition, along with its general popularity. All three PNN algorithms are identical, with the exception of the neighborhoods used to fill empty voxels. In a first method, the 26 nearest not-empty neighboring voxels (*i.e.*, 3^3-1) in the volume were used to fill each empty voxel. If no entries could be found within the 26 direct neighbors, the search volume was linearly expanded to the 98 next neighboring voxels (*i.e.*, 5^3-3^3), then to 218 neighboring voxels (*i.e.*, 7^3-5^3), and to 386 neighboring voxels (*i.e.*, 9^3-7^3). The PNN method is typically adjusted and tweaked for a specific setup and is not sufficiently flexible to be applied to highly varying scanning conditions. In the setup used for experiments in this work, most of the empty voxels were filled after a maximum of only two iterations. Because this method of filling empty voxels is computationally extensive, different alternative methods have been proposed.

In a second scheme, which has a lower computational demand compared with the first method, only the six closest non-empty neighbors of an empty voxel were averaged to estimate its value. The evaluated area of this method can iteratively be expanded by linearly extending the distances between the original empty voxel and its six neighboring voxels. Thus, regardless of the number of times the search area has to be expanded, only six values need to be averaged at a time to find the value for a missing entry in the volume. Although this method lacks the mathematical accuracy of the 26-neighbor method, it has the advantage of being fast, allowing a compact form of coding and resulting in volumes that exhibit a good visual quality. Instead of generating blurred areas in interpolation zones that can easily be distinguished from sharp areas in zones filled with original pixel data, zones that have been reconstructed by interpolation using the six-neighbor method are qualitatively noisier rather than blurred. Interesting enough, the noisy character of such reconstructed volumes is more satisfying to the eye than the blurring effects caused by the first PNN method probably because its noisy character more closely resembles the typical character or visual cues of medical ultrasound.

A third method, which on average has a lowest computational demand of all three methods, uses only two neighboring voxels to find the value for a missing entry. For this method, the average trajectory of the probe movement was estimated from the position data. The two neighboring voxels were chosen to lie approximately on the trajectory of the probe movement. In iterative steps, the probe trajectory was followed and extended in search of neighboring non-empty voxels. This method ensures that interpolations are performed between the data of independent image frames, as opposed to data originating from the same image frame. In addition, this method is considered to be the fastest way of filling empty voxels using the PNN method, because a maximum of only two voxels needs to be averaged in each iteration. However, in cases were wide gaps between image frames must be filled, this method may become slower than the six-neighbor method because of the numerous iterations which can be required to reach non-empty voxels.

Other Methods

The VNN and PNN methods are the two conventional and most widely used approaches for volume reconstruction. In addition to it, there is a host of less popular volume reconstruction methods being described in the literature. The forward reconstruction method based on a distance weighting (DW) approach described by Barry *et al.* [23] and Rohling *et al.* [17] presented a third popular option after the PNN and VNN methods. In DW method, the voxel's value is determined by a weighted average of all pixels found within a predefined volume around the voxel. Weights assigned to the pixels are inversely proportional to the distance between the pixel and the voxel. The DW interpolation approach can be useful when reduction of shadowing and speckle noise is desired. However, DW averaging can introduce a significant blurring of image details. To reduce image blurring associated with pixel averaging in DW, various distance weighted interpolation methods such as squared-distance-weighted interpolation were advanced [37, 42]. Coupe *et al.* [31] and Reis *et al.* [37] additionally take the underlying probe trajectory into consideration.

Rohling *et al.* [16-17] have developed a forward method based on radial basis function interpolation of pixel data which has been extensively applied to numerous applications, e.g., surface rendering of ultrasound data [32]. Prager *et al.* [20-22, 33] and Ji *et al.* [41] omit the task of reconstructing volumes altogether and directly visualize arbitrary slices through the originally acquired B-mode image data by using fast real-time interpolation methods. Each of these methods has certain advantages and disadvantages compared with the methods described within this chapter. The interested reader is encouraged to consult the references cited for detailed descriptions of the methods.

3. Description of the direct frame interpolation method

Volume reconstruction using the DFI method is performed in three major steps. A detailed block diagram of all of processing steps that will be thoroughly discussed subsequently is shown in Fig. 1.

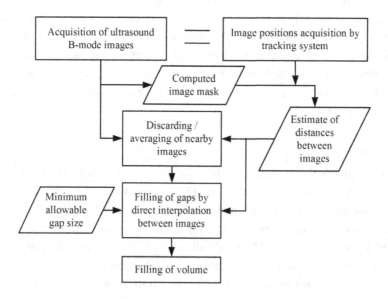

Figure 1. Block diagram of direct frame interpolation method (DFI). The method consists of three main steps: averaging and discarding of close B-mode image frames, interpolation and insertion of new intermediate B-mode image frames, conversion of image frames to volume.

During the first step of the DFI, the largest distance between any two adjacent images is estimated. The largest distance is found by calculating the distance between the extremes of the two adjacent frame planes. If the distance is smaller than the size of the voxels, both of the pixels of the neighboring image frames as well as the frame positions are averaged, creating a new frame with a new position and this newly created image frame is integrated into the series of B-mode image frames. This step is repeated for the all image frames in the series. This first step has minimal computation expense because averaging the adjacent image frames is a fast operation and vector operations implemented in modern CPUs can be used. The speed of this step can be further improved if we consider that in medical ultrasound, the elevational resolution is relatively low in comparison to the lateral or axial resolution. Thus, adjacent images at very close positions can be considered to be highly correlated and the process of creating a new averaged frame could be replaced by simply copying the content of one of the adjacent image frames, averaging the positions of the two adjacent image frames, and assigning the result to the new frame. However, during this study, image frames were averaged to maintain the highest possible accuracy of the reconstruction procedure.

On the second step of the DFI method, gaps between adjacent image frames are again evaluated. If the size of a gap, *i.e.*, the maximum distance between two adjacent image frames, is larger than the size of the voxels, new intermediate image frames are created by interpolating between the adjacent images [34]. In most cases, linear interpolation between two adjacent image frames works sufficiently well, considering the results discussed in the next paragraph. However, polynomial interpolation between four adjacent image frames as an intermediate solution, and between six adjacent image frames as the most complex approach, were evaluated in this study together with the fastest solution, nearest neighbor interpolation.

The only parameter which must be defined before applying the DFI method is the maximum distance d_{max} between image frames to be interpolated. In practice, a maximum distance between image frames to be interpolated of around 40 voxels was found to lead to satisfying results for the chosen setup of the system. The d_{max} of 40 voxels was manually selected for the underlying data after reviewing many reconstructed volumes of the study. For a voxel size of $0.2 \times 0.2 \times 0.2$ mm on a cubic grid and d_{max} equal to 40 voxels, we will obtain a maximum interpolation distance of 8 mm. Such a maximum interpolation distance can be considered a good starting point. However, when applying the proposed DFI algorithm, the user must experimentally determine the optimum maximum interpolation distance according to their setup, *i.e.*, image resolution, voxel size, typical scanning pattern and application. If the user observes artifacts, *e.g.*, gray stripes or smearing effects, a reduction in maximum interpolation distance will reduce or completely overcome the artifacts. However, if the maximum interpolation distance is reduced too drastically, the method could create gaps within the reconstructed volume. We have not found the trade-off between excessive interpolation and gaps to be an issue in our clinical setup as long as a reasonable interpolation distance is chosen. An example of image series consisting of 165 frames acquired under laboratory conditions is shown in Fig. 2 as a typical example of the positions and orientation of frames.

Figure 3 illustrates the difference in voxel treatment between DFI and PNN methods. In the figure the voxels are schematically shown as a rectangular 2-D grid, where voxel a_{22}, for example, is the voxel that needs to be filled with values of pixels p from neighboring frames F_j and F_{j+1} represented in the figure by their scan lines Lo_j and Lo_{J+1} correspondingly. Using the direct frame interpolation method, the intermediate frame Fint is created (shown in the figure is the scan line $Lint_K$ that belongs to this image frame and that passes close to voxel a_{22}). Then, voxel a_{22} receives the value of the pixel closest to it, in this case the pixel $p_{nn} = (p_{n1} + p_{n2})/2$. Using the PNN method the voxel a_{22} is filled by averaging the neighborhoods' non-empty voxels, or in this particular case: $a_{22} = (a_{11} + a_{12} + a_{13} + a_{21} + a_{23} + a_{31} + a_{32} + a_{33})/8 = (p_{11} + p_{12} + p_{13} + p_{21} + p_{23} + p_{31} + p_{32} + p_{33})/8$ which would produce more smoothing than the proposed DFI method.

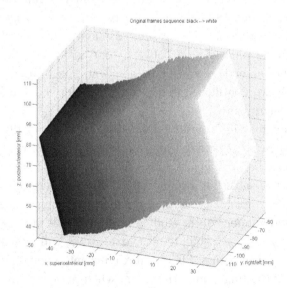

Figure 2. Example of frames spatial positions and orientation within the series of 165 frames taken from the clinical image series. Relatively slow and constant scanning speeds were used for the laboratory data sets while faster and irregular scans were typically found in the clinical data sets.

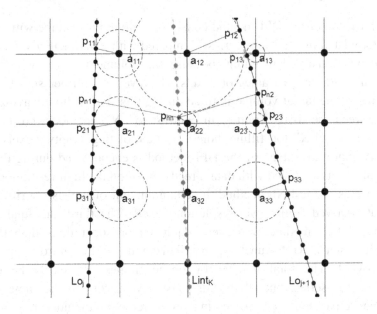

Figure 3. Schematic example of voxel treatment in DFI method.

In this study, spherical linear interpolation (SLERP) of quaternions was used to determine the position of new image frames instead of interpolating position matrices directly [35]. The SLERP algorithm calculates a unit quaternion q' which lies between two known unit quaternions, q_1 and q_2 that represent positions of two adjacent image frames to be interpolated. The angle Ω between these two image frames is calculated by estimating the dot product between q_1 and q_2; and u can take values between 0 and 1 and stands for the distance of the new image frame from the first original image frame:

$$q' = \frac{q_1 \, sin\big((1-u)\Omega\big) + q_2 \, sin(u\Omega)}{sin\Omega}$$

where $\Omega = \arccos(q_1 \cdot q_2)$.

The SLERP method follows the shortest great arc on a unit sphere, hence, the shortest possible spherical interpolation path between two image frames. Consequently, this interpolation has a constant angular velocity, and represents the optimal interpolation curve between two rotations.

The second step of the DFI method is more computationally demanding than the first step. Therefore, using multiple threads may be desirable to speed up the processing of a large image series. Dividing the total number of image frames into several sub-series and interpolating between image frames of only one sub-series per thread can again be used for running the algorithm in multiple threads.

The third step of the DFI method consists of filling the volume with the data of the interpolated image frame series. Compared with PNN methods, this step is more computationally demanding, because the volume is filled with a much larger number of image frames or pixels. However, no further step is needed because the whole target volume is filled during this step without leaving empty voxels between the image frames. In contrast to PNN methods, no additional procedure is required for filling holes or interpolating empty voxels in the volume. A major advantage of the DFI method is encountered during this step, because all voxels are filled with data directly based on the high-resolution image series, whereas in the PNN method, a certain amount of voxels are filled using image data derived from lower-resolution voxels. The third and final step of the proposed DFI method, however, requires more operations than the first and second steps. Unfortunately, parallelization of the third step is not straightforward. The total number of image frames can easily be divided into several sub-series, but all threads must have access to the same volume during the conversion step. Accepting an increase in memory requirements, multithreading is possible if multiple volumes are created. Then, after completion of the conversion from pixel data to voxel data, the multiple volumes would have to be merged in an additional step. This proposed procedure could reduce the overall processing time, however, the additional computational overhead needed for merging the multiple volumes must also be taken into account when estimating the overall computational burden.

4. Methods

In total, our experimental data set consists of 81 image series of the head and neck region that were acquired using the Clarity ultrasound-based radiotherapy guidance system (Resonant Medical, Montreal, Quebec, now Elekta Ltd). Each image series consisted of several 2-D ultrasound B-mode image frames sequentially acquired in the course of one ultrasound scan. All image series were acquired during a period of two months and from different patients. Eight image series were acquired under optimum conditions in a laboratory environment, paying close attention to accurate and precise calibrations in combination with a slow and uniform scanning speed with average size of the set $507 \times 551 \times 503$ voxels; 73 image series were acquired under clinical conditions with average size of the set $422 \times 379 \times 402$ voxels.

All examinations were performed with a conventional L12-5 linear probe (Ultrasonix Corp., Richmond, BC, Canada) running at a transmit center frequency of 10 MHz. Imaging depth was varied between 3 cm and 6 cm. The frame rate was dependent on the overall system settings (*e.g.*, imaging depth, number of foci, image filtering) and varied between 15 and 25 frames per second. A custom-made optical position sensor based on four active elements (infrared light emitting diodes) was attached to the probe as part of the Clarity system's optical tracking setup based on the NDI Polaris optical tracking unit (Northern Digital Inc., Waterloo, ON, Canada). The voxel size chosen for all experiments was $0.2 \times 0.2 \times 0.2$ mm on a cubic grid as a good compromise between image quality, memory consumption, and speed.

5. Results

Seven different configurations of the DFI and PNN methods were evaluated. An overview is given in Table I. For comparison of the accuracy of the different volume reconstruction methods, the gray level errors or gray value differences between different setups of the same volume reconstruction method have been estimated [16, 17]. The DFI method directly interpolates high-resolution B-mode image data to estimate the voxel values. Although the results of this method could therefore be considered more precise than the results of any other method interpolating lower resolution voxel data only, the different methods are too diverse to allow a direct numerical comparison. The whole 3-D ultrasound reconstruction problem can be regarded as an interpolation task. The better the interpolation, the better the method is able to make up for missing data.

Table I. Overview of reconstruction methods.

Reconstruction method	Interp. order	Comment
Direct frame interpolation	1	Nearest-neighbor interpolation between image frames. The pixel is filled with the same gray value as the nearest pixel.
	2	SLERP based linear interpolation between two image frames
	4	SLERP based four-point interpolation between four image frames
	6	SLERP based six-point interpolation between six image frames
PNN interpolation	2	Linear interpolation between the two nearest voxels encountered on the scanning path of the transducer.
	6	Linear interpolation between the six nearest voxels
	26	Linear interpolation between the 26 nearest voxels

The ideal way to calculate a realistic error estimate for the reconstruction algorithms would be to define a gold standard. Choosing a particular method as a gold standard would be arbitrary, however, and thus comparisons can only be performed between the different methods themselves. As a compromise, every method was compared with the best possible volume reconstruction based on the same method. To accomplish this, volumes were reconstructed using the two methods primarily discussed in this paper, the DFI and PNN methods, while reducing the number of original image frames that went into the reconstruction. More precisely, at first, volumes were reconstructed using the full number of image frames available, and then, volumes were reconstructed using only 50% of the original images frames by discarding every second image frame of the original image frame series. The volumes that originated from the reduced set of image frames were compared voxel by voxel to the volumes that originated from the full set of image frames. A reconstruction method is considered of good quality if the result of the reconstruction using a reduced set of image frames is similar to the volume based on the full set of image frames.

Gray level error

The results of the comparison within the different volume reconstruction methods are shown in Fig. 4, and are additionally given in Table II. The differences between the volumes are estimated using the average gray level error defined in the following equation [16, 17],

$$V = \frac{1}{N} \sum_{n=1}^{N} |v_n - v'_n|$$

where N is the total number of voxels within the reconstructed volume, and v and v' are the gray value of voxel n of the first or second volume, respectively.

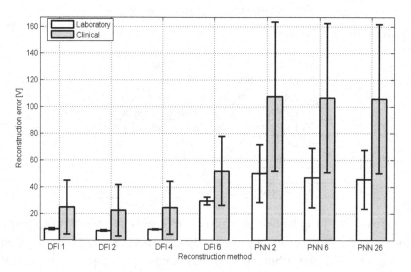

Figure 4. Laboratory (white bars) and clinical (gray bars) data sets of mean errors or gray value differences together with their standard deviations (error bars) over data sets between volume reconstructions based on original B-mode image series and on reduced image series containing only 50% of the original B-mode image frames. DFI stands for direct frame interpolation method while PNN stands for PNN method.

Table II. Overview of reconstruction errors and reconstruction times.

Error & Time	Environment	Measure	Reconstruction method						
			Direct frame interpolation				PNN		
			1	2	4	6	2	6	26
Error / V	Laboratory	Mean value	9	7	8	30	50	47	46
		Standard dev.	1	1	1	3	22	22	22
	Clinic	Mean value	25	23	25	52	108	107	106
		Standard dev.	20	19	20	26	56	56	56
Time / s	Laboratory	Mean value	129	142	161	169	73	77	107
		Standard dev.	18	15	18	19	12	13	18
	Clinic	Mean value	85	92	107	117	21	21	26
		Standard dev.	34	37	42	46	9	10	13

In Fig. 4, and Table II, the differences between the reconstructed volumes are given as the mean value and as the standard deviation over the image series. Regarding the results of the laboratory data set shown as white bars in Fig. 4, a decrease in error was observed between the nearest-neighbor interpolation and the linear interpolation of the DFI method. Interestingly, the error increased again slightly between the linear interpolation and the four-point interpolation while the largest error was observed using the most complex interpolation, the six point interpolation. The decrease in error between the nearest neighbor interpolation and the linear interpolation is not surprising. However, the increase in error for higher orders of interpolation requires explanation. Every second image frame of the original series has been discarded for the reconstruction test. Therefore, using higher interpolation orders combines image data originating from image frame positions which are more distant from the position to be filled than from using lower interpolation orders. Linear interpolation only combines image data of the adjacent image frames, and is therefore not overly sensitive to wider gaps in the image frame series which can lead to an increase in error with the higher interpolation orders.

In comparison to the DFI method, the error of the PNN method does not increase for larger neighborhoods. This can be attributed to differences in the way the interpolation is performed in two methods. Filling wide gaps in the original image frame series, the DFI method always combines the specific number of pixels that are required by the selected interpolation order whereas the PNN method only searches for neighboring pixels until non-empty voxels are found. However, the errors estimated for the PNN method are approximately five times larger than the errors found for the DFI method.

The results of the volume reconstructions are shown as gray bars in Fig. 4. Taking the results of the DFI method into account, a decrease in error is again observed between the nearest neighbor and the linear interpolation and errors increase for four-point and six-point interpolation schemes. Interestingly, the results of the PNN method are approximately the same for all three neighborhoods and only a very slight decrease in error can be observed for larger neighborhoods. As with the laboratory data set, the error of the PNN method is about five times larger than the error of the DFI method. When comparing the results of the laboratory and clinical data sets, it can be observed that the mean errors of all interpolation methods have approximately increased by a factor of between two and three. The standard deviations of all interpolation methods have increased disproportionably, which can be explained by the high variation of imaging parameters and within the general setup found in the clinical data sets (*i.e.*, number of foci, imaging depth, imaging filters, extended field of view, *etc.*).

Computation Times

In Fig. 5 and in Table II, a comparison of the computation times required by the methods is shown. It should be remembered that the computation times can only give a rough estimation of the computational costs of the methods. All experiments were run under the same environment. All methods were coded in Matlab (the MathWorks, Natick, MA) but the code was highly optimized. Using production C++ code and optimization techniques, the computational load can conceivably be decreased at least several times. However, the relationship between the different methods observed in Fig. 5 can be used to evaluate the expected general complexity of the algorithms. Finding a closed form expression for the complexity of the discussed methods is not a straightforward task, because the complexity depends not only on the number of pixels and the size of the volume to be reconstructed, but also on the position of the pixels within the volume.

Differences in reconstruction accuracy and computational efficiency were expected *a priori* between results originating from data series acquired under optimum laboratory environments and those acquired under clinical conditions. Therefore, it was decided to run each method on two different data sets, one ideal data set consisting of image frame series acquired in a laboratory environment only and the other data set recorded in a clinical environment. Although the proposed reconstruction method performs best if image series are acquired using linear sweeps or fan shaped series, good results are also achieved with irregular scanning paths. A steady increase in computation time can be observed as the complexity of the different interpolation methods increased, the highest being the six-point DFI method and to the lowest being the two-neighbor PNN method.

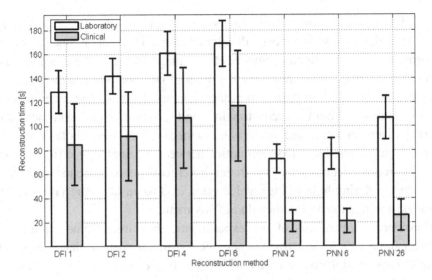

Figure 5. Laboratory (white bars) and clinical (gray bars) data set of mean execution times of volume reconstruction for different reconstruction methods together with their standard deviations (error bars). DFI stands for direct frame interpolation method while PNN stands for PNN method.

For the clinical data set, the difference between the two reconstruction methods is larger. Although the overall computation times for the clinical data set are smaller than the laboratory data set, which can be explained by the shorter image frame series recorded in the clinic, an approximately linear increase over the complexity of the DFI methods can still be observed. For the laboratory data set, the DFI methods took approximately twice as long as the PNN methods, whereas for the clinical data sets they took approximately four times as long.

6. Conclusion

The direct frame interpolation method can be seen as a valuable addition to the suite of volume reconstruction methods. While the pixel near neighbor method may offer faster reconstruction times, the DFI algorithm presents a trade off of computational speed for much higher accuracy of the reconstructed volume.

In most cases, solving a volume reconstruction problem with the DFI can be achieved by using the linear interpolation between adjacent image frames that provides acceptable computational time and low reconstruction errors. In an environment with higher tolerance to calibration error, scanning speed and scanning uniformity, it must be decided whether or not additional computational costs can be balanced by a gain in accuracy.

An additional advantage of the described method is that the original gray value histogram is preserved and no overshoots in the gray values are produced during the voxels creation. This allows direct application of CAD or image processing algorithms previously developed for 2-D B-mode images on the reconstructed volume. Another important advantage of the DFI method is that it is only dependent on two parameters: the order of interpolation and the maximum interpolation distance between two adjacent image frames. The latter property leads to uniform volume reconstruction and poses a significant advantage in comparison to other reconstruction methods since the whole volume is reconstructed in one step. Discontinuities between qualitatively different zones (such as zones reconstructed by direct pixel-to-voxel conversion and zones reconstructed during hole filling) which often lead to unsatisfying visual results, do not exist in this method as they do in PNN methods.

Considering the results of the experiments, the direct frame interpolation method can be seen as an attractive new reconstruction method that is especially advantageous in high tolerance environments, like clinical settings, where fast and irregular scanning patterns are encountered.

Acknowledgements

We would like to thank the research and development team at Elekta (Resonant Medical), Montreal, Canada, for their help with the image data.

References

[1] A. Fenster and D. B. Downey, "Three-dimensional ultrasound imaging," *Annu. Rev. Biomed. Eng.*, vol. 20, no. 2, pp. 457–475, 2000.

[2] A. Fenster, D. B. Downey, and H. N. Cardinal, "Three-dimensional ultrasound imaging," *Phys. Med. Biol.*, vol. 46, no. 5, pp. 67–99, 2001.

[3] T. R. Nelson and D. H. Pretorius, "Three-dimensional ultrasound imaging," *Ultrasound Med. Biol.*, vol. 24, no. 9, pp. 1243–1270, 1998.

[4] A. H. Gee, R. W. Prager, G. M. Treece, and L. H. Berman, "Engineering a freehand 3-D ultrasound system," *Pattern Recognit. Lett.*, vol. 24, no. 4–5, pp. 757–777, 2003.

[5] D. F. Leotta and R. W. Martin, "Three-dimensional ultrasound imaging of the rotator cuff: Spatial compounding and tendon thickness measurement," *Ultras. Med. Biol.*, v.26(4), pp. 509–525, 2000.

[6] A. Salustri and J. R. T. C. Roelandt, "Ultrasonic three-dimensional reconstruction of the heart," *Ultrasound Med. Biol.*, vol. 21, no. 3, pp. 281–293, 1995.

[7] R. N. Rankin, A. Fenster, D. B. Downey, P. L. Munk, M. F. Levin, and A. D. Vellet, "Three-dimensional sonographic reconstruction: Techniques and diagnostic applications," *AJR Am. J. Roentgenol.*, vol. 161, no. 4, pp. 695–702, 1993.

[8] F. Hottier and A. C. Billon, "3-D Echography, status and perspective," in *3-D Imaging in Medicine: Algorithms, Systems, Applications*, Berlin, Germany: Springer, Verlag, 1990, pp. 21–41.

[9] T. R. Nelson and D. H. Pretorius, "Interactive acquisition, analysis and visualization of sonographic volume data," *Int. J. Imaging Syst. Technol.*, vol. 8, pp. 26–37, 1997.

[10] A. Fenster and D. B. Downey, "3-D ultrasound imaging: A review," *IEEE Eng. Med. Biol. Mag.*, vol. 15, no. 6, pp. 41–51, 1996.

[11] P. R. Detmer, G. Bashein, T. Hodges, K. W. Beach, E. P. Filer, D. H. Burns, and D. E. Strandness, "3-D ultrasonic image feature location based on magnetic scan head tracking: In vitro calibration and validation," *Ultrasound Med. Biol.*, vol. 20, no. 9, pp. 923–936, 1994.

[12] S. W. Hughes, T. J. D'Arcy, D. J. Maxwell, W. Chiu, A. Milner, J. E. Saunders, and R. J. Sheppard, "Volume estimation from multiplanar 2D ultrasound images using a remote electromagnetic position and orientation sensor," *Ultras. Med. Biol.*, v.22(5), pp. 561–572, 1996.

[13] R. San Jose-Estepar, M. Martin-Fernandez, P. P. Caballero-Martinez, C. Alberola-Lopez, and J. Ruiz-Alzola, "A theoretical framework to three-dimensional ultrasound reconstruction from irregularly sampled data," *Ultrasound Med. Biol.*, vol. 29, no. 2, pp. 255–269, 2003.

[14] R. San Jose-Estepar, M. Martin-Fernandez, C. Alberola-Lopez, J. Ellsmere, R. Kikinis, and C. F. Westin, "Freehand ultrasound reconstruction based on RO I prior modeling and normalized convolution," in *MICCAI 2003, Lecture Notes in Computer Science*, vol. 2879, pp. 382–390.

[15] R. N. Rohling, A. H. Gee, and L. Berman, "3-D spatial compounding of ultrasound images," *Med. Image Anal.*, vol. 1, no. 3, pp. 177–193, 1997.

[16] R. N. Rohling, A. H. Gee, and L. Berman, "Radial basis function interpolation for 3-D ultrasound," *Cambridge Univ. Dept. Engineering, Tech. report CUED/F-INFENG/TR 327*, 1998.

[17] R. N. Rohling, A. H. Gee, and L. Berman, "A comparison of freehand three-dimensional ultrasound reconstruction techniques," *Med. Image Anal.*, vol. 3, no. 4, pp. 339–359, 1999.

[18] O. V. Solberg, F. Lindseth, H. Torp, R. E. Blake, and T. A. Hernes, "Freehand 3-D ultrasound reconstruction algorithms- A review," *Ultrasound Med. Biol.*, v.33(7), pp. 991–1009, 2007.

[19] R. Ohbuchi, D. Chen, and H. Fuchs, "Incremental volume reconstruction and rendering for 3-D ultrasound imaging," *Proc. SPIE*, vol. 1808, pp. 312–323, 1992.

[20] R. W. Prager, A. H. Gee, and L. Berman, "StradX: Real-time acquisition and visualization of freehand 3-D ultrasound," *Cambridge Univ. Technical report CUED/F-INFENG/TR 319*, 1998.

[21] R. W. Prager, R. Rohling, A. H. Gee, and L. Berman, "Rapid calibration for 3-D freehand ultrasound," *Ultrasound Med. Biol.*, vol. 24, no. 6, pp. 855–869, 1998.

[22] R. W. Prager, A. H. Gee, and L. Berman, "3-D ultrasound without voxels," in *Proc. Medical Image Understanding and Analysis*, Leeds, UK, 1998, pp. 93–96.

[23] C. D. Barry, C. P. Allott, N. W. John, P. M. Mellor, P. A. Arundel, D. S. Thomson, and J. C. Waterton, "Three-dimensional freehand ultrasound, image reconstruction and volume analysis," *Ultrasound Med. Biol.*, vol. 23, no. 8, pp. 1209–1224, 1997.

[24] D. Fine, S. Perring, J. Herbetko, C. N. Hacking, J. S. Fleming, and K. C. Dewbury, "Three-dimensional (3-D) ultrasound imaging of the gallbladder and dilated biliary tree: Reconstruction from real-time B-scans," *Br. J. Radiol.*, vol. 64, pp. 1056–1057, 1991.

[25] H. A. McCann, J. C. Sharp, T. M. Kinter, C. N. McEwan, C. Barillot, and J. F. Greenleaf, "Multidimensional ultrasonic imaging for cardiology," *Proc. IEEE*, v.76(9), pp. 1063–1072, 1988.

[26] J. W. Trobaugh, D. J. Trobaugh, and W. D. Richard, "Three-dimensional imaging with stereotactic ultrasonography," *Comput. Med. Imaging Graph.*, vol. 18, no. 5, pp. 315–323, 1994.

[27] S. Berg, H. Torp, D. Martens, E. Steen, S. Samstad, I. Høivik, and B. Olstad, "Dynamic three-dimensional freehand echocardiography using raw digital ultrasound data," *Ultrasound Med. Biol.*, vol. 25, no. 5, pp. 745–753, 1999.

[28] J. N. Welch, J. A. Johnson, M. R. Bax, R. Badr, and R. A. Shahidi, "Real-time freehand 3-D ultrasound system for image-guided surgery," *IEEE Ultrasonics Symp.*, v.2, pp. 1601–1604, 2000.

[29] M. Belohlavek, D. A. Foley, J. B. Seward, and J. F. Greenleaf, "3-D echocardiography: Reconstruction algorithm and diagnostic performance of resulting images," *Proc. SPIE*, v.2359, pp.680–692, 1994.

[30] S. Meairs, J. Beyer, and M. Hennerici, "Reconstruction and visualization of irregularly sampled three- and four-dimensional ultrasound data for cerebrovascular applications," *Ultrasound Med. Biol.*, vol. 26, no. 2, pp. 263–272, 2000.

[31] P. Coupe, P. Hellier, N. Azzabou, and C. Barillot, "3-D freehand ultrasound reconstruction based on probe trajectory," *MICCAI 2005, Lecture Notes in Computer Science*, v.3749, pp. 597–564.

[32] W. Y. Zhang, R. N. Rohling, and D. K. Pai, "Surface extraction with a three-dimensional freehand ultrasound system," *Ultrasound Med. Biol.*, vol. 30, no. 11, pp. 1461–1473, 2004.

[33] R. W. Prager, A. H. Gee, G. Treece, and L. Berman, "Freehand 3-D ultrasound without voxels: volume measurement and visualization using the Stradx system," *Ultrasonics*, v.40, pp. 109–115, 2002.

[34] R. C. Lalouche, D. Bickmore, F. Tessler, N. J. Mankovich, H. K. Huang, and H. Kangarloo, "Three-dimensional reconstruction of ultrasound images," *Proc. SPIE*, v.1092, pp. 450–457, 1989.

[35] K. Shoemake, "Animating rotation with quaternion curves," in *Proc. 12th Annu. Conf. Computer Graphics and Interactive Techniques*, pp. 245–254, 1985.

[36] G. M. Treece, A. H. Gee, R. W. Prager, C. J. C. Cash, and L. H. Berman, "High resolution freehand 3D ultrasound," *Technical Report CUED/F-INFENG/TR 438*. Cambridge U., (2002).

[37] G. Reis, M. Bertram, R. H. van Lengen, and H. Hagen "Adaptive Volume Construction from Ultrasound Images of a Human Heart," *Joint EUROGRAPHICS - IEEE TCVG Symposium on Visualization*, pp. 321–330 (2003).

[38] D. Miller, C. Lippert, V. Vollmar, O. Bozinov, L. Benes, D. M. Schulte, and U. Sure, "Comparison of different reconstruction algorithms for threedimensional ultrasound imaging in a neurosurgical setting," *Int. Journal of Medical Robotics and Computer Assisted Surgery*, 8(3) pp. 348–359, 2012.

[39] O. V. Solberg, F. Lindseth, L. E. Bø, S. Muller, J. B. Bakeng, G. Tangen, and T. Hernes, "3D ultrasound reconstruction algorithms from analog and digital data," *Ultrasonics* 51 pp. 405–419, 2011.

[40] J. Hung, R. Lang, F. Flachskampf, S. K. Shernan, M. L. McCulloch, D. B. Adams, J. Thomas, M. Vannan, and T. Ryan, "3D Echocardiography: A Review of the Current Status and Future Directions," *J. Am. Soc. Echocardiography* 20(3), pp. 213–33, 2007.

[41] S. Ji, D. W. Roberts, A. Hartov, and K. D. Paulsen, "Real-time interpolation for true 3-dimensional ultrasound image volumes," *J Ultrasound Med.* 30(2), pp. 243–52, 2011.

[42] Q. H. Huang and Y. P. Zheng, "An adaptive squared-distance-weighted interpolation for volume reconstruction in 3D freehand ultrasound," *Ultrasonics*, 44 Suppl, pp. e73-77, 2006.

[43] U. Scheipers, S. Koptenko, R. Remlinger, T. Falco, and M. Lachaine, "3-D Ultrasound Volume Reconstruction Using the Direct Frame Interpolation Method", *IEEE Trans. on Ultrasonics, Ferroelectrics, and Frequency Control*, vol. 57, No. 11, pp. 2460–2470, 2010.

CHAPTER 12

DECONVOLUTION TECHNIQUE FOR ENHANCING AND CLASSIFYING THE RETINAL IMAGES

Uvais A. Qidwai[1,*] and Umair A. Qidwai[2]

[1]*Department of Computer Science & Engineering Qatar University*
P.O.Box 2713, Doha, Qatar
[2]*Department of Ophthalmology, Isra Postgraduate Institute of Ophthalmology*
Karachi, Pakistan
[*]E-mail: uqidwai@qu.edu.qa

In this chapter, a new technique is presented to enhance the blurred images obtained from retinal imaging; Fundus Photographs, and Fluorescein Angiograms. While most of the cases in clinical practice, the retinal images produced are quite clean and easily used by the ophthalmologists, there are many cases in which these images come out to be very blurred due to ocular opacities such as cataract, vitritis etc. In such cases, having an enhanced image can enable the ophthalmologists to come to the diagnosis and start the appropriate treatment for the underlying disease. The proposed research utilizes the algorithmic techniques from Digital Image Processing field. Especially, Blind Deconvolution of the blurred images using Maximum Likelihood Estimation approach with an initial Gaussian kernel. Further post-processing steps have been proposed as well to extract specific regions from the deconvolved images automatically to assist ophthalmologists in visualizing these regions related to very specific diseases. These steps include Image color space conversions, thresholding, Region Growing, and Edge detection. The mathematical formulation was implemented in MATLAB™ software Version 7.7.0.471 (R2008b) and its Image Processing Toolbox Version 6.2 (R2008b). The proposed deconvolution approach has shown promising results and will be further explored and converted into a clinical tool that will be very useful in examining the eye in a better way and correctly diagnosing the problem without risking un-necessary medical and surgical procedures. The post processing steps enable the usage of the system on another level where specific areas of the eye can by automatically identified and further enhanced.

This chapter is based upon the paper from same authors in Journal of Medical Imaging and Health Informatics, Vol. 1, 2011, pp. 1-10.

1. Introduction

Eye is the organ of the human body that provides vision sense to the brain and it works like a camera. Human Eye is made up of many layers e.g., outer, inner and middle. The inner layer of the human eye is called Retina. It is the most essential part of the human eye like a camera roll in photographic cameras. The examination of the inner layer (retina) of human eye with instruments such as slit lamp biomicroscope, direct ophthalmoscope and indirect ophthalmoscope is called Fundoscopy. Fundoscopy is the most important part of detailed ophthalmologic examination because so many disease effects retina most frequently. Diabetes Mellitus is the most rapidly growing disease globally, its effects of human eye results in "Diabetic Retinopathy". Diabetic retinopathy is one of the leading causes of blindness in the present world. The global prevalence for diabetic retinopathy is 34.6%, [1]there are multiple findings on the retina to look for during Fundoscopy in order to detect diabetic retinopathy in any patient. These includes, retinal hemorrhages and certain vascular abnormalities. Early diagnosis gives the patient best chance of preventing decrease in vision by undergoing treatment. Similarly delay in diagnosis will result in serious visual consequences, like diabetic retinopathy, there are many more commoner diseases as well that affect the retina, these includes, "Age related macular degeneration" which affects the most important part of the retina that is macula, "central retinal vein occlusion", affecting the whole retinal and results in multiple retinal hemorrhages in patients with high blood pressure. Therefore, Fundoscopy is not only essential in diagnosing these diseases but to perform treatments as well in the form of laser photocoagulation, preventing visual deterioration.

In order to perform Fundoscopy light must pass thru the outer clear parts of the human eye and these parts include, from the order of anterior to posterior, Cornea, aqueous humour, lens and vitreous. Thus, light has to pass thru all these parts in order to reach retina and then reflects back from retina and again pass thru these parts in order to be visualized by the examiner. Any hindrance in the passage of light will prevent clear Fundoscopy. Hindrance can be due to either opacities in cornea (corneal opacities, trauma, corneal edema, corneal degenerations and corneal dystrophies), aqueous humour (blood in aqueous, Hyphema, inflammatory cells in aqueous), lens (cataract, implanted intraocular lens with opacities on its surface and posterior capsule opacification) or vitreous (vitreous hemorrhage, inflammation of vitreous).

In order to elaborate this lets take an examples of a patient who visits an ophthalmologists, had a history of diabetes for more than 10 years and comes with the complaint of gradual decrease in vision for last 5 months. When ophthalmologist examines this patient he observes significant cataract in his one eye leading to inability in detailed Fundoscopy. The question that bothers the ophthalmologist is that is there any macular edema a finding of diabetic retinopathy in this patient or not. Because if there is than there is significant risk that when this patient will undergo cataract surgery this edema can increase and further decrease the patients' vision. Thus the ideal treatment would be to treat the macular edema first before undergoing cataract surgery by either treating it with laser photocoagulation or giving an off-labeled treatment with very high success such as intravitreal injection of Bevacizumab drug before performing cataract surgery, thus preventing the progression of diabetic retinopathy related to cataract surgery. On the other hand if ophthalmologist is unable to diagnose macular edema in this patient's eye he will be only left with one option of letting the patient undergo cataract surgery first and then reevaluate for macular edema. By that time the factors that lead to progression of macular edema after cataract surgery might have been released inside the eye, thus resulting in progression of macular edema and more difficulty in treatment of this macular edema. Figure 1 shows a comparative view of a blurred and a clean retinal image. One can appreciate the level of difficulty even from the visual inspection. However, the structural complications are far more difficult when designing a machine vision system.

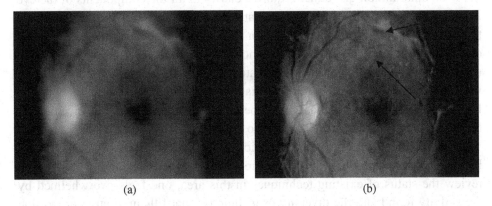

(a)   (b)

Figure 1. Comparative view of Retinal Images, (a) Blurred, and (b) clean. The arrows in (b) indicate possible indications of diabetic edema which is completely invisible in the blurred image.

2. Background

While the clinical technology related to ophthalmology is very advanced and easy to use, there are many areas that are still open for further enhancement. One of the key examination procedures is called fundus photography in which a specific type of fundus image is obtained. Figure1 shows one such image with areas of interest.

In two most commonly used retinal imaging techniques; Fundoscopy and Fluorescein Angiography (FA), as the attempt is made to see the inner portions of the eye light needs to pass through different parts of the eye. In most of the clinical tests, these images are quite clear. However, a large number of cases are also found where the obtained images are not very clear. Any abnormality in cornea such as corneal edema can lead to hazy view of the inner parts of the eye. If even cornea is clear but there are opacities in the aqueous humour such as inflammatory cells in case of uveitis, than again the view of inner parts of the eye will be difficult due to haziness. Cataract is the post common cause of hazy view of the fundus and optic disc. Other possibilities such as vitritis, vitreous hemorrhage, and asteroid hyalosis can again lead to hazy view of fundus and optic disc [1].

Diabetic retinopathy is a very highly prevalent condition all over the world and it can only be diagnosed when fundus is thoroughly viewed. Similarly many other retinal vascular disorders such as retinal vein obstruction, hypertensive retinopathies etc. are all diagnosed by looking into the fundus of the patients eyes. Also, glaucoma is a sight threatening condition and in order to diagnose it and to see its progression or efficacy of treatment again we need to look at the optic disc. In order to diagnose above mentioned diseases of the eye and many more, an ophthalmologist either require a clarity in all the components of the eye from where light passes through or treatment of the cause of the haziness first than to look for the other diseases, for example if a patient has cataract and diabetic retinopathy, but his fundus cannot be seen due to cataract so his diabetic retinopathy cannot be diagnosed nor treated. It can only be treated and diagnosed when cataract is removed surgically than reexamined for diabetic retinopathy. Every day delay in the diagnosis of diabetic retinopathy leads to advancement of the disease until it reaches the point of no return of lost vision.

There has been an extensive application of various techniques from the Image Processing domain on this application area. In fact, when visiting the literature to review the status of existing techniques in this area, one feels overwhelmed by the activity found and the diversity of techniques that fills up a large proportion of the known scientific knowledge. Researchers have applied almost every known technique during the past five years to improve and automate the ophthalmologic inspection procedures. Some of these techniques are summarized in the following.

It has been observed that the information found in different layers of the RGB image has specific information contents that can be used for isolating subject-specific information [2]. Adaptive Equalization of the gray-scale has been used extensively as well for improving the image of vessels and optical disc [2, 3].

Several classical computational approaches are also used such as the Principal Component Analysis [3], Wavelet decomposition [4], Otsu's Maximum Entropy method [5] and sharpening filters [6, 7]. In addition to these methods, all possible morphological operations from the Image processing domain have been used for post-processing the images. These include Erosion, Dilation, opening, and closing operators [3, 5], as well as adaptive thresholding for appropriate conversion to binary masks [5], and selective subtraction [8]. A very comprehensive survey of the techniques used in enhancing the retinal images has been given in [9, 10].

With respect to Fluorescence Angiography, one of the latest works is related to the application of Fuzzy C-mean clustering algorithm to isolate the vessels from the background images as well as the disease-related spots (exudates) [11]. The results are quite good in terms of automatic classification but works well with already very clean images. Adaptive Equalization of the gray-scale has been used extensively as well for improving the image of vessels and optical disc [12]. In addition to these methods, all possible morphological operations from the Image processing domain have been used for post-processing the images. These include Erosion, Dilation, opening, and closing operators [13]. A more classical approach is also found using Bayesian classification principles in FA images [14]. A very comprehensive survey of the techniques used in enhancing the FA images has been given in [15].

However, irrespective of the merits and performance of these reported techniques, one remarkable commonality is the use of very clean images in the processing as the starting point. Most of the reported techniques are focused on automatic detection of the various areas of interest in the retinal images and hence they assume that the image is quite clean and nothing is occluded. The proposed solution attempts to utilize the basic examination data from retinopathy's standard clinical procedures and improves the quality of the same to an extent that the doctors can make a better informed decision without having to resort to more expensive and invasive techniques. Above reported techniques can be used further on these resulting images for automated classification of various components in the image.

3. The Deconvolutional Model

As a general notation, the retinal images are considered as the matrix representation in x and y coordinates and usually are colored in the RGB (the Red-Green-Blue fundamental color triad used in digital images) color space hence producing an $N \times M \times 3$ image; referring to a height of M pixels and width of N pixels. Ignoring the notation for the third layer (RGB related) the actual concepts can be elaborated in considering the images as strictly 2D entities. As the light from the source enters into the eye, (Figure 2), it ultimately gets reflected from the retina extracting its true image, $f(m, n)$. However, in its path, it sees several distorting factors (as mentioned above) which can be represented cumulatively as $h(m, n)$. The effect of this distortion is scattering of the light from its ideal path which creates further internal reflections that get mixed-up in a fashion that it appears as a hazy, blurred image which is actually measured/stored by the camera. This observed image, $g(m, n)$, is mathematically explained to have gone through a process called Convolution which is defined as sums of products of translated segments of one function over the other [16]. Further noise, $v(m, n)$, can get added into this blurred image through electronic or optical channels.

Figure 3 is a block-diagram representation of the convolution process and the overall imaging process.

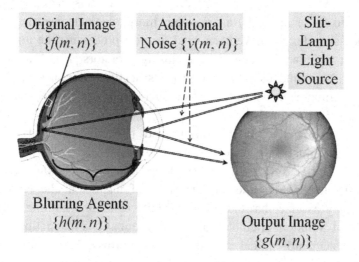

Figure 2. Basic ray diagram to represent the image model.

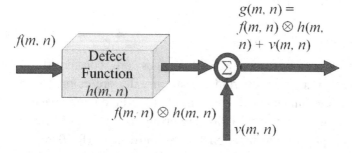

Figure 3. Block diagram for the image deconvolution model.

Hence, the observed image *g(m, n)* is given by:

$$g(m,n) = f(m,n) \otimes h(m,n) + v(m,n) \tag{1}$$

where $h(m,n)$ represents the degradation model and $\otimes$ represents the 2-D convolution operation which can be further defined as:

$$f(m,n) \otimes h(m,n) = \sum_{x=-\frac{M}{2}}^{\frac{M}{2}} \sum_{y=-\frac{N}{2}}^{\frac{N}{2}} h(x,y) f(m-x,n-y) \tag{2}$$

4. Restoration of Images

The principal technique in any image restoration scheme is finding out an inverse procedure to cancel out the effect of the blurring function. This is also called deconvolution or inverse filtering. Given the image model of (1) without noise (an assumption that is either backed-up by pre-filtering the image for removing the noise or is tackled directly by the deconvolution algorithm), and further assuming for simplification $F = f(m, n)$, $G = g(m, n)$, and $H = h(m, n)$, then

$$G = H \otimes F \quad \Leftrightarrow \quad \tilde{G} = \tilde{H}\tilde{F} \tag{3}$$

where $\tilde{G}$, $\tilde{H}$, and $\tilde{F}$ are the Fourier Transforms for *G*, *H*, and *F* respectively [16]. Therefore by inverse filtering or deconvolution operation, the original image can be retrieved as follows:

$$\tilde{F} = \tilde{H}^{-1}\tilde{G} \quad \Leftrightarrow \quad F = \left(\Im^{-1}\tilde{H}^{-1}\right) \otimes G \tag{4}$$

where $\Im^{-1}$ represents the inverse Fourier Transform. This seemingly simple problem is not so simple in reality. In many practical cases, it is useless or even impossible to apply it as given by (2) and (3). This is mostly due to the reason that the blurring function is usually unknown and is often zero in wide ranges. Hence H^{-1} will be infinite in this case. When the blurring function $h(m, n)$ is not accurately known, then $h(m, n)$ must be estimated prior to inverse filtering. Since the attempt is to deconvolve the degraded image $g(m, n)$ without any prior knowledge of the cause that is producing the degradation, such a procedure is called Blind Deconvolution, as it is blind to the source of the degradation.

5. Problem Formulation

Given a degraded image *g(m, n)* (Figure 3), with the characteristics of both *h(m, n)* and *v(m, n)* being unknown, the problem is to recover *f(m, n)* by deconvolving the degraded image *g(m, n)*.

Maximum likelihood deconvolution (MLD) is an improved subset of Iterative Constrained optimization algorithms [17]. The iteration is designed based upon a probability model. Among all known approaches, the Maximum Likelihood approach has proved to provide the best quality images [18, 19]. Usually, in MLD, it is known that the function H belongs to a certain family of distributions so that deconvolution problem reduces to estimating the parameters that define such a class. Hence, for the parametric set, θ_0 (referred to as the "true value" of the parameters), it is desirable to find some $\hat{\theta}$ (the estimated parameters) which would be as close to the true value θ_0 as possible.

5.1. *The Retinal images*

The images used in this work were obtained as part of the Fundoscopy as well as Fluorescence Angiography in which the image of the retina and its surrounding is obtained either using a standard Fundus photographic camera alone, or after injecting the Fluorescence dye. The images used belong to patients having diabetes mellitus and Cataract. Figure 4 shows sample images used in this work.

In contrast to most of the presented work, the presented case is extremely difficult to be tackled by using the previously reported techniques such as contrast stretching, histogram equalization, filtering, and Region of Interest (ROI) techniques [2-15]. Also, most of the available databanks (e.g., [20]) containing these images also have the cleaner images.

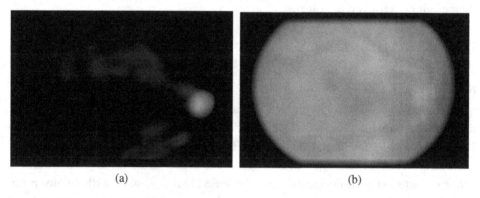

(a)   (b)

Figure 4. The actual blurred image used in this work, (a) RGB image from standard Fundoscopy, and (b) FA image.

6. Proposed Algorithm

For a black-box problem, as the one in hand, the inverse approach to getting the actual image from its blurred measurement is called blind deconvolution. In order to use the method of maximum likelihood deconvolution, one first starts with a 'guess' for the blurring function. Looking at the obtained images in detail, they appear to be similar to out-of-focus blurred images. Such images are modeled with a Gaussian function so that the size of the Gaussian hump becomes the main defining class of the blurring functions, which in turn, is defined by the mean, variance, and the base size of the function. Specifies the joint density function for all observations. The measured image is deconvolved using this estimated function and the error between the resulting and the input images is calculated. The size of the Gaussian function as well as the mean have been kept fixed in this work and the variance is changed based on the error norm values. The resulting image then becomes the input for the next iteration and is deconvolved using the new blurring function. The iterative process continues in this manner until the error norm does not change significantly. At this stage, the resulting image becomes the final deconvolved image which is the main objective of the technique. The general algorithm proposed in this work is shown in Figure 5.

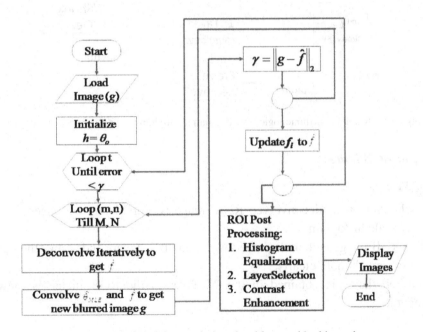

Figure 5. The blind deconvolution algorithm used in this work.

Once the deconvolution loop (Loop *t*) finishes, the resulting image, $\hat{f}$ which is the estimated deconvolved image after iteration *t*, is quite improved in terms of its visual appearance. For manual inspection purposes this image is sufficiently improved for most of the ophthalmologic parameters. However, post processing steps are also proposed here to identify the two most important components in a retinal image that corresponds to the diagnosis of diabetic retinopathy; Major Vessels, and Macula. The post-processing steps are related to the Region of Interest (ROI) processing and are outlined in the following as well as displayed as block diagram as shown in Figure 6.

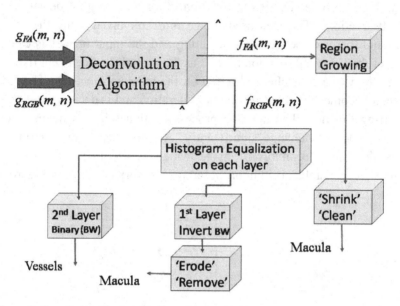

Figure 6. Overall algorithmic logic flow diagram highlighting the post-processing steps.

6.1. *For RGB Images*

Major Vessels

1. Each layer of the deconvolved RGB image is individually equalized for the gray-scale histogram.
2. The RGB image is then displayed with equalized layers and shows the major vessels much more clearly.
3. Further clarity is obtained in the 2nd layer in the RGB image is viewed separately.

Macula

1. Isolate the 1st layer of the deconvolved and equalized RGB image and convert it to binary at 90% thresholding.
2. Further removal of artifacts is done using Morphological operators "Erode" and "Remove" successively [16, 21]
3. The ROI (macula) is then isolated and further contrast enhancement is done to enhance the RGB image area corresponding to the isolated binary mask.

6.2. For Fluorescence Angiographic Images

Macula detection

1. Locate the center of the deconvolved image say at (m_0, n_0).
2. Start expanding outwards by selecting $m_0 \pm \Delta$ rows and $n_0 \pm \Delta$ columns. Δ can be selected in an ad hoc manner to cover enough areas where making a gray vs. light-gray distinction can be done. In this work, this was selected to be approximately 5% of the row and column lengths averaged.
3. This selected area is then converted to binary by thresholding at 30% grayscale. The 30% level is suitable for low contrast areas, such as the one between the actual Macula in the image and the background.
4. Further removal of artifacts is done using Morphological operators "Shrink" and "Clean" successively [16, 21]
5. The ROI (macula) is then marked and further contrast enhancement is done to enhance the RGB image area corresponding to the isolated binary mask.

6.3. Region Growing for FA

Since the region growing is an iterative procedure, a mathematical measure is developed to automatically stop the algorithm at the appropriate point where the Macula can be detected. The measure was selected to be the entropy of the binary thresholded image. Entropy is defined as the degree of uncertainty in the image [16, 21]. It is given by

$$E = -\sum_{i=1}^{K} p_i \log p_i \qquad (5)$$

where p_i represents the probability of the ith bin out of K bins from the histogram mapping of the image. A 2D histogram is first calculated which gives K bins to be used by Equation (5). The entropy first increases until a complete macula is in sight and then decreases until additional artifacts are in sight. The first turning point is not very reliable since initial increase could be a result of the initial approximations only, while the continuous decreasing in entropy after that results in a better view of the macula in the region under consideration. This corresponds to the reduction of uncertainties of artifacts in the region of view. However, after a certain stage, the entropy starts to increase again due to the boundary effects in image reconstruction as well as due to appearance of other artifacts as the region grows. This gives a 2nd knee-point that has been used as a terminal point to stop the iterations. Figure 7 shows one such trend.

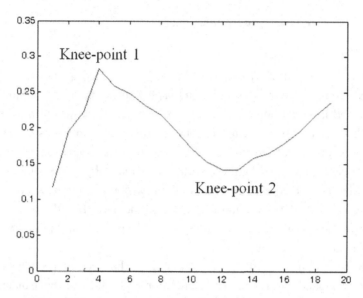

Figure 7. The entropy trend observed in the region-growing step.

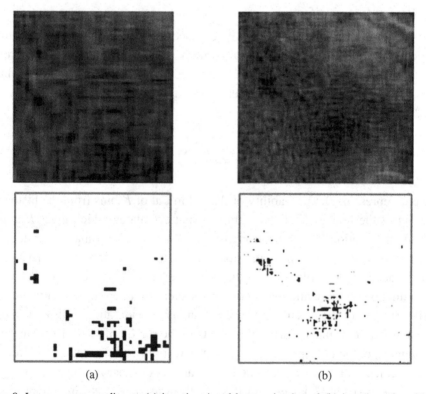

(a)   (b)

Figure 8. Images corresponding to (a) iteration 4 and knee point 1, and (b) iteration 12 and knee point 2.

The x-axis in Figure 7 represents the iteration number while y-axis represents the entropy value. Images corresponding to the two knee points are shown in Figure 8. The top gray-scales images in this figure represent the actual gray-scale area from the deconvolved image under study. The binary images below these gray-scale images correspond to their 30% thresholded binary versions respectively. As can be seen, initially there isn't much information available but that grows further with the iterative procedures. Further enhancement of the binary region is done using the morphological operators that convert the binary patches into a connected closed area which is then superimposed on the deconvolved image to locate the Macula more prominently. Related results are shown in the next section.

7. Results and Discussion

The algorithm is implemented in MATLAB using the Image Processing toolbox [21]. While the results were found to be quite consistent with various patients, only one such result is presented here.

The process of deconvolution was initiated with a general purpose Gaussian kernel as the estimated blurring function. Figure 9 shows the initial and the final blurring kernel resulted as a result of the deconvolution process.

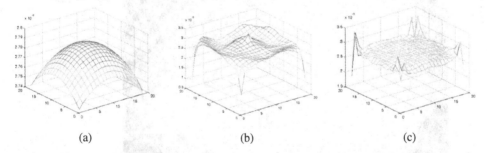

(a)   (b)   (c)

Figure 9. Blurring functions, (a) initial estimate of a standard Gaussian function, (b) final estimate at which the deconvolution iterations were stopped for the RGB images, and (c) final estimate at which the deconvolution iterations were stopped for the FA image.

7.1. *Image Enhancement for RGB Images*

Using the blurred image from Figure 4, the first step was to resize the image to 25% in order to speed up the processing. Figure 10 shows the resulting image after the application of the blind deconvolution.

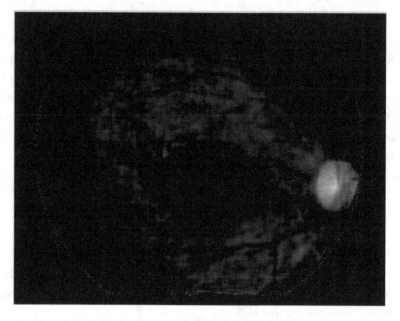

Figure 10. The deconvolved RGB image.

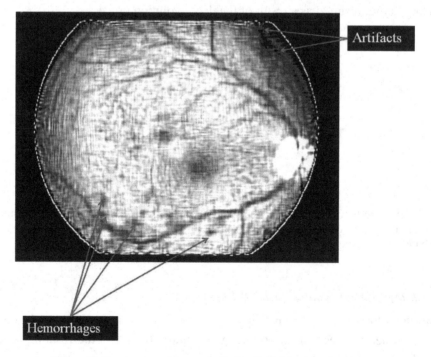

Figure 11. Post processed image to display the hemorrhaged regions.

While the deconvolved image is already a lot enhanced in terms of visual quality, further clarity is achieved through post-processing steps. First of all, only second slice of the RGB image was displayed and was found to be much more clearing terms of its details related to identifying the vessels and the related hemorrhages. This is shown as labeled image in Figure 11.

In addition to the correct spotting of the hemorrhages, the clear detection of Macula is done as shown in Figure 12. Some artifacts are also pointed out but these are ruled out as artifacts due to their location. These artifacts are a result of imaging errors and are usually negligible. Once located, the area under the binary mask with some percentage extension, can be further enhanced by using the contrast enhancement and histogram equalization.

 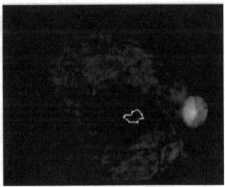

Figure 12. Detecting the location of the macula, (a) binary mask, and (b) mask superimposed on the actual deconvolved image.

For the FA images, the images were recorded for the two eyes for almost 9 minutes after injecting the Fluorescein. Initially more frequent images were obtained and then the frequency was reduced. In a normal eye, the images correspond to several phases of the dye actions as outlined below:

- "Choroidal phase" is within 8-12 seconds after the dye has been injected. It shows the choroid due to leakage of dye through the leaky choroidal vessels.
- "Arterial phase" shows arterial filling in retina.
- "Arteriovenous phase" shows complete filling of the arteries and capillaries with early lamellar flow in the veins.
- "Venous Phase" is further divided into early, mid and late venous phases. Early venous phase shows marked lamellar flow in veins while mid venous

phase displays complete filling of retinal veins. Late venous phase shows the reduction of dye in arteries.

- "Elimination phase" shoes effects of elimination of dye.

The obtained images are in gray-scale format and the dye injection effect is shown at various time instances. Since the degradation source remains the same as the images are obtained in the same session for the same patient. However, the deconvolution is carried out independently with the same flat initial estimate. Hence different points are localized at different stage in the whole FA procedure and each phase has information related to certain parts of the eye that ophthalmologists are looking for. Figure 13 shows the resulting image after the application of the blind deconvolution.

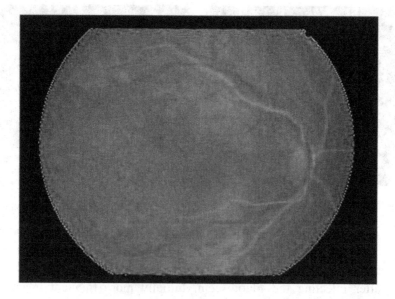

Figure 13. The deconvolved FA image.

While the deconvolved image is already a lot enhanced in terms of visual quality, further clarity is achieved through post-processing steps. By locating the possible location of Macula, the image becomes more informative for the ophthalmologists. Figures 14 through 16 show the results of the application of the algorithm to the images corresponding to the images taken at 15th, 28th, and 52nd second. Each result is comprised of three images, the original blurred image, the deconvolved image, and the marked image for the macula. As the time a progress, the effect of the injected dye becomes prominent first and then slowly starts to diminish.

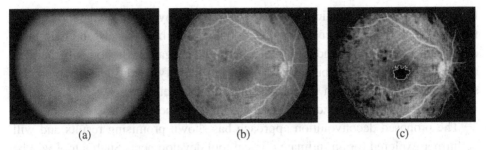

Figure 14. Results of image enhancement for FA image at 15th second (a) original blurred image, (b) deconvolved image, and (c) Post processed image to locate Macula.

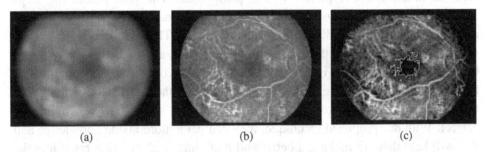

Figure 15. Results of image enhancement for FA image at 28th second (a) original blurred image, (b) deconvolved image, and (c) Post processed image to locate Macula.

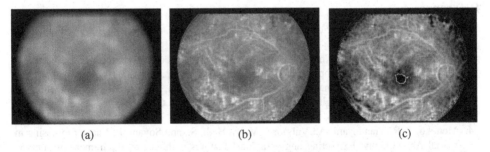

Figure 16. Results of image enhancement for FA image at 52nd second (a) original blurred image, (b) deconvolved image, and (c) Post processed image to locate Macula.

8. Conclusion

The image processing technique used in this paper will help ophthalmologists in enhancing the blurred fundus photographs either by corneal opacities, corneal edema, uvietis, cataract or vitritis, especially in conditions when the patient is also a diabetic, in order to diagnose and treat the diabetic retinopathy. In this way an early diagnosis and hence early treatment will be possible which will prevent life threatening complications of diabetic retinopathy. This image processing technique not only enhances the fundus photographs but will also be helpful in enhancing the blurred fundus angiograms, which again will not only help in confirming the diagnosis but will also help in identifying the leaks in vascular system that can be seen in patients having diabetic retinopathy, so that need of intensive treatment can be identified on the earliest if needed.

The proposed deconvolution approach has shown promising results and will be further explored for an ultimate clinical tool development. Such a tool will be very useful for the ophthalmological experts in examining the eye in a better way and without risking un-necessary medical and surgical procedures on the eye in order to obtain a better picture of the pathologies. The post processing steps enable the usage of the system on another level where specific areas of the eye can by automatically identified and further enhanced. The main importance of the work is the extraction of these important areas from a very bad quality image. Getting such an image is usually not very common, but when it is obtained, it leaves the doctors guessing what to do next. Usually they will start some type of treatment based on their understanding of the disease which may or may not be correct. With our proposed technique, they can get a more inside knowledge and that will help them in making a better and more informed decision regarding the illness. Further work is underway to make the proposed algorithm more reliable and more robust to other naturally occurring factors.

References

1. Jack, J. K., Retinal vascular disease, Clinical Ophthalmology, 6th Edition, Elsevier Publishing Company, 2007. pp. 569.
2. Xu, Z., Guo, X., Hu, X., Cheng, X., and Wang, Z., The blood vessel recognition of ocular fundus, 7th Argentinean Symposium on Artificial Intelligence. 2005:183-190.
3. Sagar, A. V., Balasubramanian, S., and Chandrasekaran, V., Automatic Detection of anatomical structures in digital fundus retinal images, IAPR Conference on Machine Vision Applications. 2007:483-486.
4. Mengko, T. R., Handayani, A., Valindria, V. V., Hadi, S., and Sovani, I., Image processing in retinal Abgiography: Extracting angiographical features without the requirement of contrast agents, IAPR Conference on Machine Vision Applications. 2007:451-454.
5. Youssif, A., Ghalwash, A., and Ghoneim, A., Comparative study of contrast enhancement and illumination equalization methods for retinal vasculature segmentation, Cairo International Biomedical Engineering Conference. 2006:1-5.
6. Walter, T., Klein, J., Massin, P., and Erginay, A., A contribution of image processing to the diagnosis of diabetic retinopathy – detection of exudates in color fundus images of human retina, IEEE Transactions on Medical Imaging. 2002; 21(10):1236-1243.
7. Li, H., and Chutatape, O., Fundus image feature extraction, IEEE 22nd Annual EMBS International Conference. 2000:3071-73.
8. Hani, A., Izhar, L., and Nugroho, H., Analysis of Foveal A vascular zone in color fundus image for grading of diabetic retinopathy, International Journal of Recent Trends in Engineering. 2009; 2(6):101-4.

9. Iqbal, M., Aibinu, A., Gubbal, N., and Khan, A., Automatic diagnosis of diabetic retinopathy using fundus images, Master thesis, Belkinge Institute of Technology, Sweden, 2006.

10. Youssif, A., Ghalwash, A., and Ghoneim, A., Comparative study of contrast enhancement and illumination equalization methods for retinal vasculature segmentation, Cairo International Biomedical Engineering Conference, 2006, pp. 1-5.

11. G. B. Kande, T. S. Savithri, and P. V. Subbaiah, Segmentation of Vessels in Fundus Images using Spatially Weighted Fuzzy c-Means Clustering Algorithm, International Journal of Computer Science and Network Security. 2007; 7(12):102.

12. V. Dimitroula, FUNAGES: Fundus AnGiography Expert System, M.Sc. thesis, Department of Medical Informatics, Aristotle University, Thessaloniki, Greece, 2001.

13. J. Gutierrez, I. Epifanio, E. De Ves, and F. J. Ferri, An Active Contour Model for the Automatic Detection of the Fovea in Fluorescein Angiographies, Proc. Int. Conf. on Pattern Recognition, Barcelona, Spain, IEEE Computer Society Press, 2000.

14. M. Ibanez, and A. Simo, Bayesian detection of the fovea in eye fundus angiographies, Pattern Recognition Letters, Vol. 20, pp. 229-240, 1999.

15. S. Dimitrakos, Thirty years of fundus Fluorescein angiography, Ophthalmology. 1992; 4:86-98.

16. Qidwai, U., and Chen, C. H., Digital Image Processing: An Algorithmic approach with MATLAB, CRC Press, November 2009, p. 104, 160, 161, 175-186.

17. Holmes, T. J., Background of Deconvolution, Media Cybernetics Application Note, August 2006. http://www.mediacy.com/pdfs/Applications/BackgroundofDeconvolution.pdf

18. Verveer, P., Computational and Optical Methods for Improving Resolution and Signal Quality in Fluorescence Microscopy, PhD Thesis, Tecnische Universiteit Delft, 1998.

19. Holmes, T., Bhattacharyya, et al., Light Microscopic Images Reconstructed by Maximum Likelihood Deconvolution, Ch. 24, Handbook of Biological Confocal Microscopy, J. Pawley, Plenum, 1995.

20. The Stare database: http://www.ces.clemson.edu/~ahoover/stare/

21. Manual of Image processing Toolbox (version 6.2, August 2008) in MATLAB (version 7.7, R2008b), Specific Function Reference: BWMORPH.

22. Jack, J. K., Imaging Techniques, 6th Edition, Elsevier Publishing Company, 2007. pp. 35-42.

CHAPTER 13

MEDICAL ULTRASOUND DIGITAL SIGNAL PROCESSING IN THE GPU COMPUTING ERA

Marcin Lewandowski

Institute of Fundamental Technological Research
Pawiński ego 5B str., 02-106 Warsaw, Poland
E-mail: mlew@ippt.pan.pl

Medical ultrasound systems require computation of complex algorithms for real-time digital signal processing. The rapid development of electronics and computational systems is followed by the constant development and implementation of new advanced processing and visualisation algorithms. In the recent years, graphics processing units (GPU) have become a new tool for computing, offering the processing power of yesterday's supercomputers. This section covers methods and systems for implementation of digital signal processing in ultrasonography. Standard signal processing chains in the ultrasound system, the hardware and internal communication architecture are discussed. Uses of GPUs in medical ultrasound imaging, based on literature and own research are presented. The issues and problems with practical implementation of GPU computing systems based on ultrasound imaging with synthetic aperture are indicated.

1. Foreword

Multichannel medical ultrasound digital signal processing always required the use of very efficient solutions. The classification into front-end and a back-end processing is related to device division into hardware section for multichannel processing and software section capable of imaging data processing. Since a single ultrasound data acquisition channel generates data stream of approx. 120 MB/s, a total stream of 15.4 GB/s is generated for a mid-range 128 channel device. Real time transmission and computing of such amounts of data, even by today's standards, is a serious engineering challenge.

Over the last few years, a visible trend to migrate hardware signal processing to software was noticeable. It is possible due to the dynamic development of parallel processing technology, especially multi-core processors (CPU) and graphics processing units (GPU). The development of tools and programming methods to facilitate implementation of new and existing algorithm codes is also significant.

The rapid development of parallel processing systems over the last few years was caused by GPUs and their use. At the beginning of the 2000s, the rapidly growing processing capabilities of GPUs led to the concept of using them for GPGPU (General-Purpose Computing on Graphics Processing Units). The Nvidia GeForce 8800 graphics card with unified internal architecture introduced in 2006 determined the course of further development of the technology. The uniform architecture of general-purpose processors with relatively high programming capabilities enabled the implementation of not only 3D graphics, but also all other signal processing algorithms. The next stage of the development of the technology was the introduction in 2007 of the CUDA (Compute Unified Device Architecture) and the software by Nvidia for programming parallel algorithms for GPUs with the direct use of the C programming language. As of today, GPUs are used in a wide range of applications from computing clusters, desktop and laptop computers to mobile systems and mobile phones. The currently available GPU graphics cards reach the efficiency measured in TFLOPS (1e12 floating-point operations per seconds) with total power input below 300 W. GPUs are the new signal processing tool, providing new capabilities for complex algorithm computing without specialized hardware solutions. Also, their general availability and low cost contributed to the extreme popularity of GPUs in processing and acceleration both using specialized scientific software and application software, hence the term "GPU computing era"[1].

This section covers methods and systems for implementation of digital system processing in ultrasonography. The methods include image reconstruction by beamforming, Doppler processing and other visualisation and computing algorithms. Ultrasound image processing and reconstruction architecture, as well as computational requirements and data throughput are discussed. Properties, comparison and applicability of various processing systems are presented with examples of the solutions used. The scope of GPU applications in ultrasound systems based on existing literature and own research data is presented. The SAFT imaging technique (Synthetic Aperture Focusing Technique) and its implementation on GPUs are presented. The issues and problems involved in the practical use of GPU based ultrasound systems are also indicated.

2. Signal architecture and processing in ultrasonography

Ultrasonography involves the use of an entire spectrum of methods and algorithms for digital signal processing, both one and multidimensional[2] (Fig. 1).

Various imaging and processing modes may require specific send/receive patterns, i.e. methods of ultrasonic beam scanning. The basic imaging modes include M-mode (Motion) for visualisation of a single line in time and B-Mode (Brightness), i.e. standard grey-scale 2D image. The Doppler methods for the assessment and visualisation of blood flow are also a standard feature in today's devices. Advanced ultrasonic methods: parametric imaging (e.g. elastography - strain images of soft tissue), harmonic imaging and complex post-processing methods are limited to high-end devices.

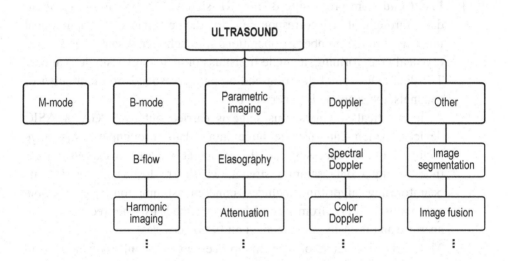

Fig. 1. Ultrasonic methods and algorithms.

Currently available ultrasound systems are complex electronic systems with multi-channel A/D conversion and parallel digital signal processing. The transmission beam scanning process and scanline generation based on the echo received by each transducer element is digital, usually carried out by FPGA devices (Field Programmable Gate Array). Each image scanline in B-mode is generated in the beamforming process based on RF ultrasonic echoes from the receiver unit aperture. The number of parallel received and processed echo signals depends on device class and varies from 16 channels for low-end systems through 128-256 channels for mid-range systems to 512 or more channels for high-end systems.

The standard frequency range of transmitted ultrasonic waves in medical applications is 2 to 20 MHz, whereas the top limit of receiving signal band may reach 40 MHz in harmonic imaging (transmitting frequency second harmonic). Special integrated multi-channel amplifiers and A/D converters with 40–80 MSPS sampling rate and 10–14 bit resolutions are used for A/D conversion. A single channel from A/D converter generates 80 to 160 MB/s data stream. Assuming an average data stream of 120 MB/s, multiplied by the number of parallel channels, the total data throughput is from 1.9 GB/s (16 channels), 15.4 GB/s (128 channels) up to 61.4 GB/s (512 channels). It is a continuous data stream, which requires real-time processing and visualisation.

The signal processing chain in ultrasonography usually includes three stages (Fig. 2):

1. **Front-end** - pre-processing of raw RF signals and beamforming. Input data throughput is corresponding to the estimates. Computational intensity, i.e. the number of operations for each signal sample is low. In classical beamforming, a single transmission generates a single scanline. The data reduction at the front-end output corresponds to the number of channels, the scanline is generated by.

   In practical solutions, this stage is carried out by FPGA or ASIC devices, which can manage huge input data throughput. This stage includes stream processing, i.e. the computations are carried out in real-time on input data samples stream, which are lost (not stored). The beamforming algorithm includes coherent summation with variable contribution delay from channels determined by the receiving unit aperture and is easily implemented on FPGA devices.

2. **Mid-end** - demodulation and post-processing of scanlines generated in the beamforming process. The order of beamforming and demodulation is reversed in some solutions[3]. The demodulation process consists in the removal of ultrasonic carrier frequency from the signal to obtain an envelope signal (so called: video signal). The envelope signal's band is narrow, and may be decimated, allowing for the further reduction of data stream. The demodulation and decimation algorithms can also be used in hardware implementations. At this stage, the output data stream does not exceed 10 MB/s.

3. **Back-end** - Mid-end image lines (i.e. scanlines) are combined into an image, which is further processed (filtration, interpolation, format change etc.). Doppler methods also use scanlines, although generated by different send/receive patterns. The amount of data for processing is reduced from initial GB/s to MB/s, but the complexity of algorithms is higher. Back-end functions are usually implemented on signal processors or directly on embedded PCs, which also carry out control, UI and display functions.

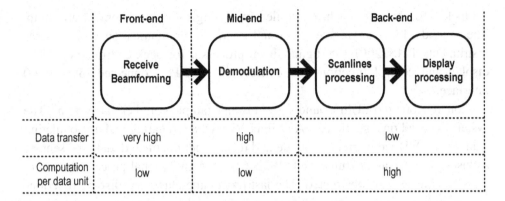

Fig. 2. Signal processing chain in ultrasonography.

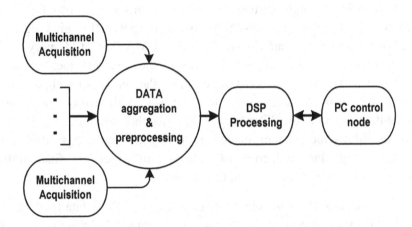

Fig. 3. Standard communication and processing architecture in ultrasound systems.

3. Hardware architecture

Fig. 3 shows a standard block diagram of ultrasound system communication. Data acquisition process in small systems (16–64 channels) may be implemented on a single FPGA device. The acquisition channels in larger systems are grouped physically (as modules) or logically, 8–32 channels in each group. Each module provides A/D conversion, pre-processing and the first beamformer stage. The second FPGA device provides data aggregation from each block and the second beamformer stage. Mid-end processing functions are also hardware implemented. Imaging data is sent for software processing.

The example system using this architecture is the ULAoP ultrasound research system.[4] The system features 64 parallel data acquisition channels divided into

4 blocks, 16 channels each, controlled by a single FPGA Altera Stratix chip. The second FPGA aggregates data and controls communication with a Texas Instruments TMS320C6455 digital signal processor for back-end functions. The display and control functions are carried out by a PC connected to USB 2.0 interface.

Zonare z.one ultra Ultrasound system is an example commercial system.[5] The system is based on a single FPGA (Xilinx Virtex), aggregating and demodulating data from A/D converters. The demodulated and decimated data is sent to a cluster of 3 Texas Instruments TMS320C6455 digital signal processors, where the USG image is reconstructed. The last processing stage and display functions are carried out by a PowerPC microprocessor. The system uses zone image reconstruction using synthetic aperture instead of classical beamforming.

The new architecture of internal structure and signal processing was used in the Verasonic research system (http://www.verasonics.com). The system supports 64–128 receive and 128–256 transmit channels. RF digital signals are streamed directly to a high-end PC via PCIe. The DMA (Direct Memory Access) transfer method from data acquisition cards to the memory does not require active CPU use. The image reconstruction and other processing algorithms are implemented in software. The system does not use a GPU for computation, but the availability of data in the PC memory allows for this solution.

Standard ultrasonic system design is based on multistage digital data processing and gradual reduction of data stream to enable final software processing. This approach has several limitations:

- No access to RF echo signals for each channel. Raw data from channels is processed in real time and not stored. Selected platforms (especially research) allow for limited RF data access, usually in post-processing mode.

- Some processing methods, which require access to RF echo signals, must be implemented directly on the FPGA device, which is a complex issue, especially for more complex algorithms.

- The implementation of new processing methods requires complex partitioning of processes between hardware and software and time consuming implementation on the FPGA.

- Problems with channel number scalability - a single system, limited data which may be effectively aggregated and transmitted for further processing. It requires more complex and expensive FPGA devices, capable of providing a required number of signals, throughput and processing power.

4. GPUs

Use of GPUs in ultrasonic signal computing creates new opportunities in real-time implementation of complex algorithms. Hardware to software migration of signal processing solutions has been a lasting trend. Creating and running algorithms is easier in software solutions, which are also less expensive than FPGA based hardware systems. On the other hand, the variety of solutions and the complexity of parallel programming methods makes it difficult to create an optimum solution.

4.1. *GPU Software & Hardware*

The development of GPU use in computing started in 1999 with the first programmable GPU - Nvidia GeForce 256. In its initial phase, GPUs were configured for standard graphical 3D pipeline with shader processing on specific stages. Shader programming was implemented in the DirectX and OpenGL libraries. Despite the significant limitations in shader data access (resulting from the intended use for 3D pipeline processing), they were used for the implementation of non-graphic processing functions.[6,7] In 2004 Buck *et al.*[8] developed the Brook programming language for the implementation of general purpose computing on GPUs. Brook introduced a new method to describe parallelism within the code, using streams and compute kernels, setting the direction for further development of GPU programming tools. In 2006 Nvidia introduced GeForce 8800 with unified internal architecture and the CUDA (Compute Unified Device Architecture) programming language for the implementation of computing on GPUs.[9] The availability of more and more powerful GPUs and easy to use development tools significantly improved GPGPU (General-Purpose computing on GPU) techniques. Nowadays, GPU acceleration is not only used for computation and engineering applications, but also for application software (http://www.nvidia.com/object/gpu-applications.html).

The next step was the development of OpenCL (Open Computing Language) specification by Apple in 2008 – it is a framework for writing programs that execute across heterogeneous platforms consisting of various processing units.[10] OpenCL, currently developed by Khronos Group, is supported by all main GPU (Nvidia, AMD) and CPU (Intel, AMD, ARM, Samsung) manufacturers. The framework consists of C99 based programming language for writing, executing and controlling compute kernels and APIs (Application Programming Interfaces). The important advantages of OpenCL are open access, portability, support for heterogeneous systems, and the rapidly growing base of compatible products (http://www.khronos.org/conformance/adopters/conformant-products). Its high potential is attested by its implementation on FPGA devices.[11] The solution may be an interesting alternative to the currently used HSL (High Level Synthesis) environments and lead to further unification of software and hardware solutions.

The most powerful GPU solutions are available for PCs in the form of PCIe graphics cards. Due to their significant power input (150–600 W), efficient power supply and cooling systems are required. Fig. 4 shows a typical GPU architecture in a standard PC. In previous solutions (to 2009), GPUs were connected via a North Bridge, also used as a memory controller. Currently, both the memory controller and the PCIe interface for graphics cards are CPU-integrated. PCIe x16 interfaces normally used for graphics cards have the following theoretical throughput in both directions: 8 GB/s for PCIe Gen 2 and 16 GB/s for Gen 3. Practical throughput is lower[12] and reaches in CPU→GPU direction approx. 4 GB/s for PCIe Gen 2 and approx. 5.7 GB/s for PCIe Gen 3. Bandwidth GPU to GPU memory is significantly higher, up to 150 GB/s for the most powerful solutions.

Data transfer from CPU memory to GPU may require additional transfer within the CPU memory. Depending on the controller and GPU support, the controller may require data transfer to special allocated buffers within the CPU memory. In the latest solutions, memory transfer is limited, and hardware DMA of the GPU is used for asynchronous memory transfer without additional CPU load.

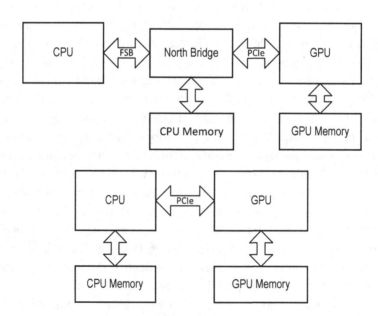

Fig. 4. CPU↔GPU connection architecture in a standard PC: with North Bridge (top), CPU-integrated memory controller and PCIe (bottom).

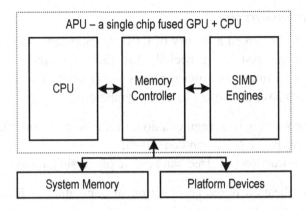

Fig. 5. AMD-Fusion architecture.

The next step for CPU and GPU integration is the hybrid AMD-Fusion architecture (Fig. 5). APU (Accelerated Processing Unit) integrates: CPU, GPU and memory controller. Lee *et al.*[13] compared the data transfer rates of APU AMD Llano between the CPU and integrated GPU or external GPU (AMD HD5870). The buffer reading speed in system memory via the integrated GPU was 11 times higher, and writing speed was 3.9 times higher compared to the external GPU connected via PCIe. Although the performance of the integrated GPU is lower compared to discrete solutions, the higher local memory access may determine the overall performance in some applications.

Another, equally important component of high GPU based processing power is the optimization of the algorithm and effective use of memory and computational resources. The purpose of parallel code is to provide computations for the highest possible number of processing units. The total GPU performance is in most cases many times higher than the total GPU memory throughput. Balanced use of resources requires high arithmetic intensity, i.e. number of computational operations per single memory access.[14] Lack of balance may cause the algorithm efficiency to be memory-bound or computational-bound. The other issue is the complex GPU memory hierarchy, including global, shared, and local memory as well as registers. The modification of data system in the GPU memory may significantly improve performance; Baghsorkhi *et al.*[15] obtained a 2.4 to 14.8 acceleration for operations on sparse arrays.

In ultrasonic imaging, where the transferred data system is forced by the data acquisition system, algorithm optimization will include maximising locality in memory accessing. A change in the direction of computation: along the columns vs. along the rows may significantly affect memory access patterns, and thus performance.

4.2. *Use in ultrasonography*

Pratxa and Xing[14] presented a history of GPU development, optimization issues and use in medical systems, especially for PET, CT image reconstruction, radiation therapy planning and image processing (recording and segmentation). Many applications have their roots in 2D/3D graphics:

- image processing (e.g. segmentation, filtration, recognition),
- geometry change (e.g. scan-converter),
- 3D reconstruction (e.g. free hand image processing, tomography).

The other application is the acceleration of computations for simulation of ultrasonic field and other issues of wave and medium interaction. Selected reports on GPU application in ultrasound imaging and Doppler methods are presented below.

Color-Doppler processing on GPUs was described by Chang *et al.*[16] The authors implemented a complete Doppler processing chain: filtration (clutter filter), flow estimation, velocity signal post-processing and colour image generation and filtration. For input data consisting of 500 scanlines extending to a depth of 128 gates with an ensemble length of 8, image processing rate of up to 174 fps on Nvidia GeForce 8800GT GPU was achieved. The result for implementation on Intel Core2 Duo E4500 CPU was 70 times lower (2.5 fps). The method was however in favour of GPU implementation, since generic code was used for the CPU, without the use of MMX/SSE/SSE2 instruction sets.

Grønvold in his master thesis[17] implemented a classical beamforming method. Input data from 128 channels at 40 MHz and 12 bit resolution was transferred to Nvidia Tesla C870 graphics card memory. Since the required input data throughput (9.5 GB/s) exceeded PCIe capabilities, the tests were carried out in the GPU memory. The author achieved real-time processing for a simple algorithm only (without interpolation), resulting in low imaging quality. An algorithm with interpolation required 4 GPUs working in parallel.

While in beamforming a single scanline is reconstructed from a single transmission, synthetic aperture allows for the synthesis of the entire image (LRI low-resolution image). The DAS (Delay and Sum) process is similar to beamforming. LRIs are the subjected to coherent summing in order to generate a high-resolution image (HRI). For 128 channel data, the number of scanlines reconstructed for each data transfer in SAFT method is 128, and in standard beamforming it is 1. The amount of data for processing is thus identical for both methods, whereas the number of computations in SAFT method is significantly higher. Such an algorithm was implemented by Yiu *et al.*[18,19] For 32 channel echoes acquired at the depth of 15 cm with 40 MHz sampling and for an output image resolution of 512x255 pixels, the authors obtained 3000 fps for HRI reconstruction process. The result required the use of a GPU cluster including: 2x Nvidia GTX-480 and 1x Nvidia GTX-470.

The SAFT implementation was analysed on different software platforms by So *et al.*[20] The authors compared the reconstruction rate and energy efficiency of high-performance GPUs (Nvidia GTX-480), energy efficient GPUs (Nvidia 9600M and ION) and various CPUs. For 128 channel input data with 40 MHz sampling and reconstructed 512x256 pixels image, the rate was 1000 fps for Nvidia GTX-480, approx. 100 fps for energy efficient GPUs and approx. 10 fps for CPUs. The highest energy efficiency (quotient of power and efficiency) was achieved for the high performance GPUs GTX-480, and it was 10–100 times lower for the tested CPUs.

Thus, GPU capabilities are sufficient even to the most demanding USG reconstruction algorithms, e.g. SAFT, although the bottleneck of data transfer is noticeable. The CPU↔GPU interface throughput is still an issue for many applications, and it becomes critical in real-time processing, e.g. ultrasonography.

4.3. *GPU implementation issues*

In all studies on implementation of ultrasound image algorithms with GPUs, an issue of data transfer to GPU is always mentioned. As far as the author is aware, the literature presents only simulation tests of algorithm efficiency, sometimes considering data transfer from CPU to GPU memory. The design of a complete ultrasound system requires efficient data transfer from the data acquisition module to PC memory, and from PC memory to GPU. The number of available PCIe ports in a standard PC and their total throughput limits the possibility of integration of a large number of data acquisition modules and GPU cards. The other issue is thermal power and electromagnetic interferences generated by high current power supplies and their effects on sensitive receiving units. The issue of GPU algorithm optimisation must also be addressed. High GPU processing performance requires optimum use of memory and computational resources. Complex structure of memory hierarchy and CPU means that the algorithm optimisation process is time-consuming and laborious. The availability of universal developer tools allows for achieving quick results but does not guarantee optimum processor use.

This whole range of design issues is considered in the projects (http://us4us.eu), whose aim is to develop a concept and prototypes of ultrasound platforms with signal processing implemented on GPUs. The research platform is to provide a scalable number of data acquisition channels (64–192). The developed data acquisition card RX64 (Fig. 6) allows receiving and processing data from 64 analog channels and data streaming via PCIe Gen 2 x8 to the CPU memory[21]. FPGA Altera Stratix 4 used on RX64 implements data acquisition and pre-processing functions (e.g. demodulation). The use of external enclosures with PCIe backplane will allow 1–4 RX64 cards and 1–3 GPU cards (Fig. 6). The solution will ensure scalability of the number of channels and computing resources. Migration to PCI Gen 3 will be possible in the future in order to improve throughput.

The second developed system is a mobile platform, enabling parallel processing of 32 ultrasound channels with energy efficient GPUs.[22] Model implementation of SAFT reconstruction on a PC with AMD APU T56N (15 W total power input) showed that real-time imaging was possible with reduced image resolution.

In both systems, hardware processing is limited to pre-processing of RF digital signals and optional demodulation. Effective DMA hardware data streaming to CPU and GPU guarantees the optimum use of available PCIe throughput. The costs and complexity of demodulation implementation on FPGA are relatively low. Also, the demodulated data may be decimated, further reducing the amount of data. The majority of ultrasound processing methods use baseband signal (post demodulation).

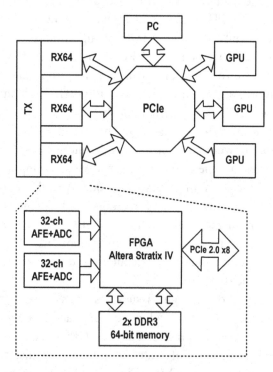

Fig. 6. Ultrasound platform (top) and RX64 (bottom) architecture.

Asynchronous data transfer between RX64 and RAM CPU was 3 GB/s (theoretically 3.8 GB/s for PCIe Gen 2 x8). Single SAFT acquisition frame transfer rate with 128 channels, 65 MPSP sampling and imaging depth of 19 cm (4MB = 128ch x 16kS x 2B) is approx. 1.3 ms, allowing for an acquisition frame rate to CPU memory of 769 Hz. Data transfer from CPU memory to GPU memory was 5.2 GB/s. Actual data transfer rate from CPU to GPU for 256x256 pixels LRI using a single GPU GTX-580 was 450 Hz.[23]

4.3.1. *Optimisation of SAFT implementation on GPU*

Synthetic aperture focusing is an extended version of delay-and-sum used in a classical beamforming method. A single transducer element is emitting a signal, which is interpreted as a spherical wave. For a medium with constant speed of sound one can assume that geometrical rays can be used to calculate time-of-flight between the transmit element, the scattering point and the receiving element. Coherently delaying and summing the contributions for each and every transmit-receive pair one can obtain a focused signal in each pixel of the resulting image.

The delay-and-sum algorithm for SAFT was implemented on GPU and a number of improvements were developed in order to shorten the time needed to reconstruct a single HRI. Most of the used acceleration techniques were applied in order to minimize the cost of data readings and writings that the algorithm has to perform.

- For the classical synthetic aperture imaging every pair of transducers participates in the data acquisition twice, exchanging roles of transmitter and receiver. The data obtained in these acquisitions are processed with use of the same time delay values. Thus, instead of reconstructing the image twice for each transducer pair, the I/Q signals can be summed in pairs before the reconstruction. This, in turn, reduces the input data nearly by half. Each transmitter-receiver pair is represented by a single element of the scheme. The I/Q data related to the elements placed symmetrically with respect to the scheme diagonal, are summed together.
- The spatial locality is optimized by issuing readings that are close to one another on the same GPU SM (Streaming Multiprocessor), which allows to increase the L1 and L2 cache utilization. This is done by batch processing of few adjacent horizontal image lines.
- The writing operations can be substantially eliminated by saving the processing results in per-chip registers and accessing them only at the

very end of the processing. This, in turn, eliminates the issue of reading/writing race conditions.

- Multiple low-level optimizations were made. These operations include setting proper compiler flags (e.g. -use_fast_math), using specialized functions (e.g. sincosf) and minimizing the number of registers needed to improve overall occupancy.
- Computation of the indexes for the reading operations is accelerated by a memory trade-off by preprocessing the distances and saving them in shared memory or computing inner frames in the right order.

The above optimizations were applied to the naïve implementation of the reconstruction algorithm. The best performance was achieved with a modified algorithm, in which transmitter-pixel-receiver sets were grouped into geometrically identical pattern. The delays for each pattern are computed only once. The best optimized implementation was almost twice as fast as the first naïve implementation.

The results show that with innovative optimization strategies we can greatly increase the device utilization and implementation performance. However, new generation GPUs may give different results and require different optimization strategies.

5. Summary and outlook

GPUs have a large potential for implementation of complex digital signal processing algorithms in many applications, particularly in ultrasonography. The constant development of GPUs, parallel programming tools and methods sets the direction for continuous performance improvements. The trend to switch from hardware signal processing to software solutions will probably continue. Excellent GPU's floating point performance means that many advanced algorithms that were unpractical for real-time processing before, are now considered for practical use. One of the algorithms is USG imaging using synthetic aperture method. The review of literature and own research results shows, that today's GPUs provide sufficient performance for the practical implementation of those methods.

The developed general-purpose GPU computation oriented ultrasound research platform will allow for the testing and implementation of various types of ultrasound methods. We believe that the developed system will become a new tool for researchers and programmers, contributing to the further development of ultrasound applications.

Acknowledgments

Project POIG.01.03.01-14-012/08-00 co-financed by the European Regional Development Fund under the Innovative Economy Operational Programme.

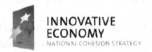 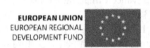

I would like to thank my colleagues from the Ultrasound Department, who work hard with me to implement real-time GPU based ultrasound scanner.

References

1. J. Nickolls, W. J. Dally, The GPU Computing Era, IEEE Micro, vol.30, no.2, pp.56–69 (2010).
2. R. S. C. Cobbold, *Foundations of Biomedical Ultrasound* (Oxford University Press, 2006).
3. F. K. Schneider, Fully-Programmable Computing Architecture for Medical Ultrasound Machines. Ph.D. Dissertation. University of Washington, Seattle, WA, USA (2006).
4. P. Tortoli, L. Bassi, E. Boni, A. Dallai, F. Guidi, S. Ricci, ULA-OP: an Advanced Open Platform for ULtrasound Research, IEEE Trans. Ultrason., Ferroelect., Freq. Contr, 56:10, pp.2207-2216 (2009).
5. G. McLaughlin, DSPs and Zone Sonography Enable Portable Ultrasound, RTC Magazine, http://www.rtcmagazine.com/articles/view/100693 (July 2006).
6. R. Fernando (ed.), *GPU Gems: Programming Techniques, Tips and Tricks for Real-Time Graphics* (Addison-Wesley, 2004).
7. M. Pharr, R. Fernando (eds), *GPU Gems 2: Programming Techniques for High-performance Graphics and General-purpose Computation* (Addison-Wesley Professional, 2005).
8. I. Buck, T. Foley, D. Horn, J. Sugerman, K. Fatahalian, M. Houston, P. Hanrahan, Brook for GPUs: Stream Computing on Graphics Hardware, ACM TRANSACTIONS ON GRAPHICS, vol.23, pp.777–786 (2004).
9. S. Cook, *CUDA Programming: A Developer's Guide to Parallel Computing with GPUs* (Morgan Kaufmann, 2012).
10. B. Gaster, *Heterogeneous Computing with OpenCL* (Morgan Kaufmann, 2011).
11. Altera Corporation, Implementing FPGA Design with the OpenCL Standard, white paper WP-01173-2.0 (2012).
12. G. Louel, PCI Express 3.0: impact on performance – BeHardware, URL: http://www.behardware.com/art/lire/850 (January 20, 2012).
13. K. Lee, H. Lin, W. Ch. Feng, Performance characterization of data-intensive kernels on AMD Fusion architectures, Comput Sci Res Dev, DOI 10.1007/s00450-012-0209-1 (2012).
14. G. Pratxa, L. Xing, GPU computing in medical physics: A review, Med. Phys. 38, pp.2685–2697 (2011).
15. S. S. Baghsorkhi, I. Gelado, M. Delahaye, W. W. Hwu, Efficient performance evaluation of memory hierarchy for highly multithreaded graphics processors, in Proceedings of the 17th ACM SIGPLAN symposium on Principles and Practice of Parallel Programming, pp.23–34, ACM (February 2012).
16. L. W. Chang, K. H. Hsu, P. Ch. Li, Graphics processing unit-based high-frame-rate color doppler ultrasound processing, IEEE TUFFC, vol.56, no.9, pp.1856–1860 (2009).

17. L. Grønvold, Implementing Ultrasound Beamforming on the GPU using CUDA, Master Thesis, Norwegian University of Science and Technology, Department of Engineering Cybernetics (2008).
18. B. Y. S. Yiu, I. K. H. Tsang, A. C. H. Yu, Real-time GPU-based software beamformer designed for advanced imaging methods research, Ultrasonics Symposium (IUS), 2010 IEEE, pp.1920–1923 (11–14 Oct. 2010).
19. B. Y. S. Yiu, I. K. H. Tsang; A. C. H. Yu, GPU-based beamformer: Fast realization of plane wave compounding and synthetic aperture imaging, Ultrasonics, Ferroelectrics and Frequency Control, IEEE Transactions on, vol.58, no.8, pp.1698–1705 (August 2011).
20. H. K. H. So, J. Chen, B. Y. S. Yiu, A. C. H. Yu, Medical Ultrasound Imaging: To GPU or Not to GPU?, IEEE Micro, vol.31, no.5, pp.54–65 (2011).
21. M. Lewandowski, M. Walczak, B. Witek, P. Kulesza, K. Sielewicz, Modular & Scalable Ultrasound Platform with GPU Processing, IEEE International Ultrasonics Symposium, Dresden, Germany (October 7–10, 2012).
22. M. Lewandowski, K. Sielewicz, M. Walczak, A Low-cost 32-channel Module with High-speed Digital Interfaces for Portable Ultrasound Systems, IEEE International Ultrasonics Symposium, Dresden, Germany (October 7–10, 2012).
23. M. Lewandowski, P. Karwat, J. Kudelka, T. Kleczek, GPU Implementation of the STA Algorithm on I/Q Data, IEEE International Ultrasonics Symposium, Dresden, Germany (October 7–10, 2012).

CHAPTER 14

DEVELOPING MEDICAL IMAGE PROCESSING ALGORITHMS FOR GPU ASSISTED PARALLEL COMPUTATION

Mathias Broxvall[*,1,2] and Marios Daoutis[†,1,2]

[1]*Centre for Biomedical Image Processing, Örebro University Hospital*
[2]*School of Science and Technology, Örebro University*
Örebro, Sweden
[*]E-mail: mathias.broxvall@oru.se
[†]E-mail: marios.daoutis@oru.se

GPU's have recently emerged as a significantly more powerful computing platform, capable of several orders of magnitude faster computations compared to CPU based approaches. However, they require significant changes in the algorithmic designing compared to traditional programming paradigms. In this chapter we specifically introduce the reader to an overview of GPGPU development tools and the potential algorithmic pitfalls and bottlenecks when developing medical imaging algorithms for the GPU. We present a few general methodologies and building blocks for implementing fast image processing on GPUs. More specifically they include: methods for performing fast image convolutions and filtering; line detection, and bandwidth and memory considerations when processing volumetric datasets. Finally we conclude with a discourse on numerical precision as well as on mixing single floating-point versus double floating-point code.

1. Introduction

Recent developments of medical imaging technologies routinely deliver high resolution 3-D or 4-D images and volume scans of superior image quality, greater accuracy and higher resolution. This poses an increasing computational challenge when processing these datasets, at least one dimension more compute-intensive than standard two-dimensional (2-D) image processing applications. The higher computational cost of medical image analysis together with the time constraints imposed by the medical procedures, are the main reasons that limit the deployment of advanced medical imaging technologies and algorithms in clinical settings.

However typical medical imaging datasets are largely constituted by similar elements, such as voxels in tomographic imaging volumes. Hence medical image processing algorithms can benefit from parallel processing, since the processing of such datasets can often be accelerated by distributing the computation over many parallel processing elements, and therefore they show very good data level parallelism (i.e., can be parallelized on the data level instead of the task/algorithmic level). Although not all algorithms can be parallelized, many applications can benefit from the massive parallel processing capacity of graphics processors (GPUs) which emerged as a versatile platform for running massively parallel computation and thus dramatically reducing the processing times of parallelizable problems.

GPUs are becoming popular in medical imaging as well as many other disciplines, partly because of the data-parallel nature of many computational problems, but also due to the increasing capabilities of modern GPU hardware (i.e., high memory bandwidth and shared-memory model, high computation throughput, support for floating-point double-precision arithmetic, built-in mathematical functions and compute-oriented programming interfaces). For example modern GPUs have significantly more computational performance on floating point operations compared to the current mainstream multi-core Central Processing Units (CPUs). Furthermore, GPU cores have become increasingly sophisticated with rich instruction sets capable of delivering raw computational performance often one or two orders of magnitude (10-100) times faster than modern CPUs, and operating with a memory bandwidth as high as 593 GB/s (NVidia Tesla S2050 1U GPU Computing System). The use of GPUs for general-purpose computing has become popularly known as General Purpose GPU (GPGPU) with a growing research community[1] around it.

Even though the ability to perform general-purpose computation on the GPU was first demonstrated in 1994 [3], only recently GPUS became a mainstream research topic. Not surprisingly, the multitude of applications which utilize GPUs to to substantially decrease the processing time, span across different medical imaging modalities such as CT and ultrasound. GPU computations can be applicable in many medical imaging pipeline processing steps such as image de-noising [12, 20], real-time tracking [18] as well as image registration [7] and segmentation [17]. However programming these specialized hardware devices efficiently remains a challenge which requires very different design patterns, development tools and algorithms, in order to be efficient. Not all problems are suitable for GPUs and as we shall see in this chapter many of the tasks performed in medical image processing can efficiently be solved on these devices.

The primary aim of this chapter is to *a*) give the reader an understanding of which types of problems can efficiently be solved on GPUs; and *b*) to introduce the reader to methods for implementing medical image processing algorithms on GPUs. The rest of the chapter is organized as follows. Section 2 introduces the background and related work regarding algorithms and GPGPU processing technologies. Section 3 elaborates on the methodologies behind designing parallel algorithms for *a*) computing convolutions; *b*) performing adapting filtering; and *c*) detecting lines using volumetric datasets. Section 4 presents the corresponding applications which use the methods described in Section 3, while Section 5 concludes with several performance and precision issues when designing parallel algorithms on the GPU.

---

[1] http://www.gpgpu.org

2. Background

Typically a series of processing steps are required so as to achieve better accuracy and more coherent representation of volumetric structures when visualizing volumetric data. These steps include combinations of filtering, reconstruction, possibly segmentation and rendering, before the data can be visualized. In clinical applications, where time is perhaps the most important aspect when it comes to visualising volume data, the computational complexity behind these processing operations is increasing due to the high dimensional nature of the data, even though in several clinical applications real-time performance in processing and rendering is expected.

One of the major challenges with new volumetric image modalities are the low signal to noise ratio and poor spatial resolution, as compared to traditional 2D modalities. For example the computational complexity of the problem of 4D image de-noising, compared to 2D and 3D de-noising, increases by several orders of magnitude. On the other hand the trend of using GPUs can speed up the processing time in these computationally demanding tasks. Indeed this technique is well suited for processing large volumetric data sets, while there is already a handful of approaches (including our previous work [2]), which use GPUs in the context of 3D/4D ultrasound imaging and visualisation, thus increasing the processing speed typically many orders of magnitude, compared to conventional modern CPU's. In particular we have applied an adaptive filtering algorithm for 4D ultrasound data on the GPU. Filtering was done using multiple kernels implemented in OpenCL (Open Computing Language) working on multiple subsets of the data. Our results show a substantial speed increase of up to 74 times, resulting in a total filtering time less than 30 seconds on a common desktop computer. This implies that advanced adaptive image processing can be accomplished in conjunction with a clinical examination while GPUs undertake the demanding adaptive image filtering techniques that in turn enhance 4D echocardiographc data sets. The presented general methodology of implementing parallelism using GPUs is also applicable for other medical modalities that generate high-dimensional data.

Other examples which take advantage of the parallel processing power of GPUs to speed up the reconstruction time to fractions of a second while increasing the quality of the displayed volume include [6] and [16]. In [16] the results reported include real-time incremental reconstruction producing high-quality results based on advanced interpolation techniques. Their GPU implementation indicates a performance speedup of 14× for pixel-based methods, an impressive 51× for voxel-based methods, and speedup of 6-8× for the incremental methods, compared with single-threaded CPU implementations.

Another important aspect in medical imaging applications, in which GPUs can be particularly useful, concerns de-noising of the data. In this context work by [5] examine the problem of 4D image de-noising where they describe a novel algorithm for true 4D image de-noising, based on local adaptive filtering which was implemented on the GPU. Their algorithm was applied to 4D heart CT-data, reporting considerable decreases in computational time (25 minutes versus several days)[2] [5].

Finally a particularly interesting aspect of clinical applicability which we also consider in our approach is the preoperative assessment. Work by Yang et al [26] suggest that volume rendering of 3D anatomical and medical data can be particularly valuable in medical diagnosis and surgical planning. Indeed, this can be one way which the reconstructed volumetric data can be used so as to give the physician the opportunity to examine and possibly interact with, before an operation [11].

Catheters are being used extensively in interventional procedures, where for example fast needle segmentation and tracking are crucial in surgery, biopsy and therapy [4]. The position of the needle has to be determined accurately and quickly and 3D ultrasound image-guided interventional operation is an efficient technique used to perform this task. 3D ultrasound imaging aids physicians in observing the structures and shapes of the objects as well as the anatomical site from different viewpoints. Especially when used as a continuous imaging device, it conveys the distances clearly in 3D space, allowing, easier measurement of the positions of the intervention instruments. Real-time image analysis is a prerequisite for this concept while the desired accuracy should be in the range of 2-3mm [19].

2.1. *GPU parallel architectures*

Modern GPUs have a computational hardware that has evolved quite far from the traditional von Neumann architecture. Although the specifics of the hardware is dependant on the manufacturer and even the specific generation of GPUs, a few points that make a notable contrast from traditional CPU hardware can be generalized: Each GPU contains a number of units (compute units) that are able to execute compute kernels which in turn have access to a private local memory; each compute unit contains one or more processing elements that can execute instructions for a specific instance of a compute kernel.

The compute unit typically ranges from a SIMD (Single Instruction Multiple Data) to a MIMD (Multiple Instruction Multiple Data) with varying degrees of capabilities of executing different instructions concurrently depending on the specific GPU. As such, branch divergence should be avoided whenever possible in algorithms designed for GPUs. Recursive algorithms are obviously not supported under these conditions. The processing elements of modern GPUs typically contain vector register and vector operations or VLIW instructions (Very Large Instruction Word) for a further level concurrency that is exploited by the compiler/optimiser. Furthermore, GPUs of today typically have a significantly higher rate of floating point capacity as compared to the speed with which data can be fetched from global memory.

---

[2]Note that the CT data have greater resolution and less noise, and thus are not directly comparable with processing ultrasound data. However the performance increase due to the GPU is comparable with ultrasound GPU based techniques.

Typically up to a few dozen or hundreds arithmetic operations can be performed at the same cost as a single fetch from memory. When implementing GPU based algorithms the two major choices of languages and tool-sets are between CUDA and OpenCL.

2.1.1. *CUDA*

CUDA is a language specific tool-kit developed by NVidia that allows the programmer to perform general purpose computations on NVidia cards. Since CUDA was one of the first widespread tool-kits dedicated to GPGPU computations it has a large adoption in the high-performance computing community and there exists many GPU cluster machines that perform computationally heavy tasks.

However, one of the drawbacks of CUDA is that it restricts the user to NVidia specific platforms, and that it lacks support for some of the features of OpenCL. Some of the advantages include the ease of use coming from the mature tool-kit and the integration into the programming language itself. Additionally it supports dynamic parallelism which can be exploited for a limited form of recursion – something which is (at the time of writing) not supported by OpenCL.

2.1.2. *OpenCL*

OpenCL [13] is an open standard maintained by Khronos, a consortium consisting of representatives from different industrial groups including for example AMD, NVidia, Microsoft and IBM. The standard is younger and not as well established in the high performance computing community as CUDA, but due to the platform independence it is growing in popularity. The standard is focused on performing computations on any massively parallel hardware such as modern GPUs, multi-core CPUs and other future processing platforms. It is primarily targeted for efficiency in performing large amounts of floating point computations in parallel, and as such it is a very potent candidate for writing image processing algorithms.

The main features of OpenCL that allows for efficiency in computation is the focus around computational *kernels* that each compute outputs for *work items* with little or no data dependency between each work item. The scheduling between work items and actual processors or processing elements to perform the computation on is automatic and ensures that a very high degree of parallelism can be exploited. One of the advantages of OpenCL is that is an Open Standard that works with a wide range of devices and that is (host) language agnostic.

Although OpenCL is a less mature technology than CUDA we have in this chapter opted to make code examples in OpenCL and to use terminology from the OpenCL community since this allows the readers to exploit the code on a much wider range of devices. In the following sections only terms from the OpenCL terminology will be used and all code examples are for OpenCL.

2.2. *Standard mathematical building blocks*

A common element of many image processing algorithms includes standard mathematical operations for which many efficient implementations have always existed, such as LINPACK, BLAS [15] which are the de-facto standards for linear algebra operations. However these are implementations for the CPU and when one develops algorithms for the GPU which use advanced mathematical functions, there is no need to reimplement these routines as there exist several libraries for OpenCL.

For example, AMD APPML includes two libraries of mathematics routines with efficient OpenCL implementations. The first of these AmdBlas implements the full set of L2&L3 BLAS routines (Support for L1 is trivial in OpenCL) while the second, AmdFFT, implements several discrete Fast Fourier Transforms.

Although neither LINPACK or LAPACK can run directly on OpenCL devices there exists an implementation, MAGMA [10], that acts as a complement to LAPACK and which can perform many of the LAPACK task accelerated on GPUs. The interfaces allows for a CPU sided interface (source and results are stored in host memory) as well as GPU interfaces (source and results remain in GPU memory). In the latest release MAGMA accelerates several of LAPACK's operations such as factorizations and Eigen and singular value problem solvers in both real and complex arithmetic.

3. Methods

To help the reader develop new algorithms that can be parallelized on GPU hardware we will in this section take a look at a very simple problem, performing image convolutions. We will analyse why the straight forward implementation is not sufficient and walk through the steps needed to optimize it in a generic way. That is, even though convolutions can be optimized with problem specific methods (e.g. expressing it in the Fourier domain) we will here focus on the general steps and gain a 74 times performance increase by eliminating the bottlenecks.

For many problems, the task of parallelising algorithms in such a way that can be executed efficiently on modern GPU hardware, requires varying degrees of complexities. For many data-level parallel problems, a *trivially parallelisable* algorithm, is the one which requires an identical computation to be performed on each element of a large set with no inter-computation dependencies. This can be contrasted with the case when the algorithms have *non-local* dependencies in the performed computations. An example of the former would be to compute an image (of two or more dimensions), whose elements consists of the sum of corresponding elements in two source images. For a similar example of the later, consider a computation of a single sum of all elements in an image – a problem that can be solved in a number of parallel kernel executions using a *reduce* algorithm.

Fortunately, when implementing medical image processing algorithms, many of the problems that occur are either of the trivially parallelisable nature, or can be solved using established techniques such as using reduce operators. Nonetheless,

```
out[ p⃗ ]  ←  0
for j₁  =  0  ...  k₁  do
    ...
    for jₙ  =  0  ...  kₙ  do
        out[ p⃗ ]  ←  out[ p⃗ ] + f[ j⃗ ]·M[ p⃗ + j⃗ ]
```

Fig. 1.   An initial simple approach to implementing convolutions.

while implementing even trivially paralellisable algorithms, some care needs to be taken in order to maximize performance.

3.1. *Convolutions*

As a first real example of OpenCL code we will consider a basic convolution operation performed in the spatial domain – a problem that is trivially parallelizable. For this discussion we will assume that the size of the convolution filter size is significantly smaller than the image size. To avoid confusion we will call convolution kernels as convolution filters as to avoid a confusion with the notion of kernels from OpenCL

Assume that we have the convolution filter f of size $\vec{k}$, an image M and want to calculate the convolution $f * M$. A typical approach to this would be to launch one OpenCL kernel for each output point $\vec{p}$.

For a practical code example, see Listing 1 where we make the assumptions:

- The input image is a 3D dataset expressed as unsigned char intensity values.
- The filter size is given as an OpenCL compile time variable (`ksize`) and a set of N kernels (`nkernels`) to perform convolution upon is given to the kernel as a packed array of floats in K,X,Y,Z order (K for Kernel, XYZ for the 3 dimensions).

Note that the result is only defined in the area defined by $[0...(imagesize - kernsize)]$. This means that the filters are not centered around the input pixel but rather offsets the output image slightly.

3.1.1. *Analysing the performance of a kernel*

In order to determine how efficient an image processing algorithm is once implemented in OpenCL while being executed on a specific set of GPUs, a first approach is to measure the total execution time. For example, when we run the kernel in Listing 1 with an input size of 256^3 intensities and a filter size of 7^3 we see the corresponding mean execution times which are reported in the first row of Table 1 and also a negligible standard deviation. However, when looking at the execution times alone, we do not get answers as to whether the implementation is making efficient use of the hardware or if it can be made faster.

```
1   kernel void convolute(int4 imagesize, global unsigned char *input,
2           global unsigned char *output, global float *filter) {
3     int4 gid = (int4)(get_global_id(0),  get_global_id(1),
4                     get_global_id(2),  0);
5     int4 lid = (int4)(get_local_id(0), get_local_id(1), get_local_id(2), 0);
6     int4 group = (int4)(get_group_id(0), get_group_id(1), get_group_id(2), 0);
7     int4 pixelid = gid;
8
9     int imoffset=pixelid.s0+imagesize.s0*(pixelid.s1+imagesize.s1*pixelid.s2);
10    int i, dx, dy, dz;
11
12    if(gid.s0 + ksize > imagesize.s0 ||
13       gid.s1 + ksize > imagesize.s1 ||
14       gid.s2 + ksize > imagesize.s2) return;
15
16    float val[nkernels];
17    for(i=0;i<nkernels;i++) val[i]=0.0;
18    for(dz=0;dz<ksize;dz++)
19      for(dy=0;dy<ksize;dy++)
20        for(dx=0;dx<ksize;dx++) {
21          unsigned char raw = input[imoffset+dx+dy*imagesize.s0 +
22                              dz*imagesize.s0*imagesize.s1];
23          for(i=0;i<nkernels;i++) {
24            val[i] += raw * filter[i+nkernels*(dx+ksize*(dy+ksize*dz))];
25          }
26        }
27
28    for(i=0;i<nkernels;i++)
29      output[imoffset*nkernels+i] = val[i];
30  }
```

Listing 1. Example implementation of the naive convolution algorithm in OpenCL.

For the designer of a GPU based algorithm, we need further information before making an informed choice of optimising the algorithm or accepting the resulting execution times. Fortunately there exists tools[3] developed by the hardware manufacturers that give access to the *performance counters* of the hardware. These counters give profiling statistics on the execution status of the different units of the hardware and can tell us, for instance, if the implementation makes full use of the arithmetic logic units (ALUs) that perform the actual computations.

In Table 1 we list a subset of the performance counters for the executions of the naive implementation above. We note that the number of vector generic registers (VGRPs) that are consumed by the compiled kernel give a limitation to the number of wavefronts that can be executed. The limitation in number of wavefronts is presented as a kernel occupancy computed as a percentage of the theoretical maximum number of wavefronts on the given hardware[4]. Since the number of wavefronts are used for latency hiding the utilization of memory fetch operations and ALU

---

[3] For AMD there exists CodeXL while respectively for NVidia PerfKit.
[4] The AMD 5870M hardware allows for 248 registers and 24 wavefronts maximum, thus 10 registers per wavefront or less give full occupancy

Table 1. Execution time and performance counters for the naive implementation of a convolution operation, running on an AMD 5870M card.

nfilters	1	2	3	4	8	16
μ-time/filter	0.632	0.200	0.266	0.100	0.075	0.062
Registers	21	10	14	12	15	17
Kernel occupancy	33.3%	100%	67%	83.3%	67%	50%
ALU / Fetch	4.39	1.71	1.18	1.98	1.70	1.65
ALU busy	69.3%	42.7%	29.4%	49.4%	42.5%	41.1%
ALU packing	47.6%	94.7%	90.0%	92.1%	95.0%	89.6%
Fetch busy	62.16%	98.3%	98.3%	98.3%	98.3%	98.3%

operations are restricted by lower kernel occupancy rates as is evident by the *Fetch busy* and *ALU busy* in Table 1.

The next, and more important analysis to check is to see if the given algorithm makes full use of the ALU hardware and/or of the memory fetch hardware. Since modern GPUs have a significantly higher ALU performance than memory fetch performance we want to make full use of the ALU hardware and avoid the ALUs from being *memory bound*.

The two most important statistics are the occupancy of the ALU unit, as well as the percentage of possible parallel ALU operations that are executed each time the ALU unit is run. The former is given by the ALU *busy* percentage and should ideally approach 100% for a non-memory bound problem. The later is given by the *packing* of the ALU and represent the number of floating point operations that are performed in parallel. For reference each ALU hardware unit used here can perform up to five floating-point operations in a single clock cycle. As we can see the given algorithm makes poor use of the ALU hardware, with the ALU hardware operating either at a very low rate ($< 50\%$) and/or with a low utilization of parallel operations. Another clear sign that our implementation is memory bound is given by looking at the ALU / Fetch ratio, which shows that on average less than two ALU operation are performed for each memory fetch. To summarise the analysis we see that:

- The implementation is heavily *memory bound*.
- By computing multiple filter kernels at the same time the memory fetch from the input image can be reused for the different filters, thus giving a relative speed advantage.

3.1.2. *Reworking a memory bound algorithm*

Looking back at the initial formulation of the convolution algorithm in Section 3.1 we see that it needs to perform at least $n \prod_i k_i$ multiplications and additions, as well as the same number of *memory fetch* operations reading from the input image M. Thus it is hardly surprising that the analysis above showed an ALU / Fetch ratio of slightly less than two. Since memory fetches are either not cached or have very small caches on most modern GPU hardware, this low utilization of the ALU gives the performance problems described in Section 3.1.1.

$$\text{out}[\,\vec{p} + \overrightarrow{(0,...,0,0)}\,] \;\leftarrow\; 0$$

$$\cdots$$

$$\text{out}[\,\vec{p} + \overrightarrow{(0,...,0,k_o)}\,] \;\leftarrow\; 0$$

$$\text{for } j_1 \;=\; 0 \;\ldots\; k_1 \text{ do}$$

$$\qquad \cdots$$

$$\quad \text{for } j_{n-1} \;=\; 0 \;\ldots\; k_{n-1} \text{ do}$$

$$\qquad \text{for } j_n \;=\; 0 \;\ldots\; k_n + k_o - 1 \text{ do}$$

$$\qquad\quad v \;\leftarrow\; M[\,\vec{p} + \vec{j}\,]$$

$$\qquad\quad \text{out}[\,\vec{p} + \overrightarrow{(0,...,0,0)}\,] \;\leftarrow\; \text{out}[\,\vec{p} + \overrightarrow{(0,...,0,0)}\,] + v \cdot f[\,\vec{j} - \overrightarrow{(0,...,0,0)}\,]$$

$$\qquad\quad \cdots$$

$$\qquad\quad \text{out}[\,\vec{p} + \overrightarrow{(0,...,0,k_o)}\,] \;\leftarrow\; \text{out}[\,\vec{p} + \overrightarrow{(0,...,0,k_o)}\,] + v \cdot f[\,\vec{j} - \overrightarrow{(0,...,0,k_o)}\,]$$

Fig. 2.   A reworked algorithm that reuses memory fetches for multiple outputs.

Although modern GPUs have high bandwidth to on-board memory[5] they have even higher floating points capacities[6]. Assuming that the *out* and f variables are stored in on-board memory the naive; algorithm above would be capable of *at most* 6.4×10^{10} steps of the innermost loop and thus only utilize 1% of the theoretical computational capacity. In order to optimize on this and gain better performance we note that the same input image samples will contribute to many different output values, but will be multiplied with different filter coefficients before doing so. An obvious idea is thus to *re-use* the same input image values and use them to compute multiple output values.

The extreme case of this would be to load the whole image into high-speed memory (GPU registers or shared memory) – but this would obviously not be possible for anything but trivial image sizes. However, we can do this by redesigning our compute kernels to compute k_o number of outputs for each kernel and to re-use the same input image values for multiple output computations. We extend here the convolution filter f to contain zeroes at all points outside the original convolution filter. See Figure 2 for the unrolled algorithm.

The above code requires $k_1...k_n - 1(k_n + k_o - 1)$ memory accesses to compute k_o number of outputs. We thus gain a (theoretical) speed-up of a factor of $k_n k_o/(k_n k_o - 1)$ times. Then the obvious question remains: can we really implement the algorithm to give such a large speed-up and what would be its upper limit. The short answer to this is: it depends on the number of available hardware registers. With larger values of k_o we will exhaust the number of available hardware registers and the GPU will schedule fewer wavefronts. For the practical implementation of the algorithm we need to perform the following steps:

- Maximize ALU packing by utilizing multiple arithmetic instructions with no (control flow) dependencies between.

---

[5] 64 GB/s for the example 5870M, up to 288 GB/s for single GPU cards (AMD 7970, NVidia GTX Titan).

[6] 1.12×10^{12} FLOPS for the example hardware

- Store the filters in fast local memory, thus limiting the total filter size to less than 32K byte (for OpenCL) or 64K byte (for CUDA).
- Implement the algorithm that reuses the fetched input image

In order to simplify the code we will express the general loop unrolling, by using a number of macro expansions. The first of these are to generalize data-types for manipulating vectors with a size corresponding to the number of filters to be processed, see Listing 2. This will assist in keeping the ALU packing as high as possible.

Finally we need to perform the actual loop unrolling in a way that can be expressed generically for different levels of loop unrolling and preferably without introducing any new looping mechanism.[7] We do this here by giving preprocessor macros that expand to every possible case of the loop unrolling, and rely on *if-statements* with only static expressions to allow the optimizer to discard the excess code that is non-reachable at compile time. See Listing 3.

```
1   #if nkernels == 1
2     typedef float kernf;
3     typedef uchar kernuc;
4   #define kernstore(val,offset,arr) arr[offset]=val
5   #define convert_kernuc convert_uchar
6   #elif nkernels == 2
7     typedef float2 kernf;
8     typedef uchar2 kernuc;
9   #define kernstore vstore2
10  #define convert_kernuc convert_uchar2
11  ...
12  #endif
```

Listing 2. Specifying data-types and memory operations to be optimised depending on number of filters. Using vector primitives rather than arrays assist in ALU packing.

```
1   #define mmad(x,y,z) (x+y*z)
2   #define MAD(ko,pos) {
3     if(CONV_UNROLL>ko) {
4       if(pos-ko >= 0 && pos-ko < ksize) {
5         val[ko] = mmad(val[ko],(kernf)(raw),filter[(pos-ko)+offset]);
6       }
7   }}
8   #define MADS(pos) {
9     if(pos<ksize) {
10      raw=input[imoffset2+pos];
11      MAD(0,pos); ... MAD(32,pos);
12  }}
```

Listing 3. Macro-expansion for loop unrolling the innermost loop, creating every possible expression for all possible loop unrolling values but guarded by compile-time static if-statements that will remove the redundant code during the optimisation stage.

---

[7]When testing, the used OpenCL compiler failed to perform unrolling when the expression is given in another loop construct.

```
1    kernel void convolute(int4 imagesize, global unsigned char *input,
2                          global unsigned char *output, global kernf *filterG) {
3      int4 gid = (int4)(get_global_id(0)*CONV_UNROLL,  get_global_id(1),
4                        get_global_id(2),  0);
5      int4 lid = (int4)(get_local_id(0), get_local_id(1), get_local_id(2), 0);
6      int4 group = (int4)(get_group_id(0), get_group_id(1), get_group_id(2), 0);
7
8      // Starting offset of the first pixel to process
9      int imoffset = gid.s0 + imagesize.s0*(gid.s1+imagesize.s1*gid.s2);
10     int i,j, dx,dy,dz;
11
12     kernf val[CONV_UNROLL+1];
13     for(j=0;j<CONV_UNROLL;j++)
14       val[j]=(kernf)(0.0);
15     int localSize = get_local_size(0) * get_local_size(1) * get_local_size(2);
16     local kernf filter[ksize*ksize*ksize];
17
18     /* Copy global filter to local memory */
19     event_t event = async_work_group_copy(filter,filterG,ksize*ksize*ksize,0);
20     wait_group_events(1, &event);
21
22     if(gid.s0 + ksize + CONV_UNROLL > imagesize.s0 ||
23        gid.s1 + ksize > imagesize.s1 ||
24        gid.s2 + ksize > imagesize.s2) return;
25     for(dz=0;dz<ksize;dz++)
26       for(dy=0;dy<ksize;dy++)  {
27         int offset = dy*ksize*nkernels + dz*ksize*ksize*nkernels;
28         int imoffset2 = imoffset+dy*imagesize.s0 + dz*imagesize.s0*imagesize.s1;
29
30         /* Assumption: ksize<9, convolution_unroll<32 */
31         MADS(0); ... MADS(41);
32       }
33     for(j=0;j<CONV_UNROLL;j++) {
34       kernstore( convert_kernuc(val[j]), imoffset+j, output);
35     }
36   }
```

Listing 4. Final implementation of a convolution algorithm reducing the number of fetch operations per computed output value. Giving speeds up to 74 times faster than the naive implementation of convolutions.

For the remaining parts of the convolution code see Listing 4. After test running this code on the same hardware and input sizes as for the naive implementation we can see that the code gives significant performance increases. To understand why we gain these performance increases we take a look at the performance counters in Table 2. The first point to note here is the higher rates of ALU to Fetch operations as well as the lower rate of occupancy for the fetch unit. Secondly, we note that although the ALU packing is consistent it cannot reach 100% even with the large amount of arithmetic operations performed in the innermost loop[8]. Finally, we note that the execution times of the best convolution unroll and number of filters as

---

[8]The low packing of 5-VLIW was acknowledged as a problem in the 5000-series of ATI cards and was redesigned into 4-VLIW for the next generation of cards

Table 2. Execution time and performance counters for the rewritten convolution operation, running on an AMD 5870M platform.

One filter, total local shared memory used 1408 bytes.

loop unrolling	1	2	3	4	8	16	32
μ-time	0.226	0.123	0.096	0.072	0.036	0.019	0.020
Registers	9	14	13	12	12	24	13
Kernel occupancy	100%	67%	67%	83%	83%	33%	66.7%
ALU / Fetch	4.03	4.63	4.88	5.07	5.21	5.24	5.51%
ALU busy	88.7%	93.7%	95.5%	87.8%	90.1%	86.9%	87.3%
ALU packing	79.0%	73.0%	72.2%	72.2%	73.7%	73.7%	71.2%
Fetch busy	62.2%	78.5%	68.5%	69.4%	69.6%	66.3%	31.9%
ALU instructions	1336	1532	1605	1679	1726	1734.8	1824

Four filter, total local shared memory used 5504 bytes.

loop unrolling	1	2	3	4	8	16	32
μ-time/kernel	0.093	0.055	0.047	0.033	0.017	0.009	0.009
Registers	11	20	21	23	28	28	27
Kernel occupancy	83.3%	50%	33%	33%	33%	33%	33%
ALU / Fetch	7.06	8.35	9.06	9.8	10.5	10.5	10.6
ALU busy	94.3%	94.9%	91.3%	92.3%	94.1%	92.7%	92.3%
ALU packing	75.0%	73.7%	75.5%	72.4%	75.9%	75.9%	75.8%
Fetch busy	52.6%	44.0%	35.3%	37.5%	35.9%	35.3%	17.5%
ALU instructions	2331	2767	3000	3227	3470	3473	3500

compared to the simple implementation with only a single filter is a factor of 74 times faster (0.009 seconds per filter versus 0.663 seconds). We can thus summarize the main point of this section as follows:

> **Rewriting a memory bound algorithm to utilize ALUs fully is a necessity for fast GPU algorithms.**

3.2. *Multidimensional adaptive filtering*

Next, we see how we can implement an efficient data parallel version of an off-the-shelf adaptive filtering method for image *de-noising*. We apply this algorithm to 3D and 4D US data where we find that analysis of 3D and 4D volumetric data can be done in more practical time frames with the method presented here. In the multidimensional adaptive filtering, local filters are synthesized based on the signal orientation that is described by a tensor. This method can intuitively be seen as a linear combination of low pass and high pass filters, where the combination of the filters is spatially variant and relies on the orientation of the local structures surrounding each data sample. These orientation estimates adjust the filter to preserve the edges of surfaces while the low pass components remove the noise. The theory of this concept can be found in the literature [1, 9], only a concise introduction to the method is given here.

3.2.1. *Mathematical model*

At first the local orientation is determined by using a set of *quadrature filters* q_k [9, 14]. In a quadrature filter-set, the number of quadrature filters being used depends on the dimensionality of the data. In 3D six quadrature filters are used while twelve are used for 4D. Each quadrature filter has a specific orientation [9] and consists of a kernel pair, with even and odd convolution kernels that are sensitive for lines and edges respectively. The output of q_k is a complex number where the magnitude $|q_k|$ is an estimate of the certainty for identifying signal change corresponding to a line or an edge. Based on the response from the quadrature filters the local orientation tensor T is given by

$$T = \sum_k |q_k|(\alpha \hat{n}_k \hat{n}_k{}^T - \beta \mathbb{I}) \tag{1}$$

where $\hat{n}_k$ is the direction of the quadrature filter q_k, $\mathbb{I}$ the identity tensor and α, β are constants with the values $\alpha = 5/4$, $\beta = 1/4$ in 3D and $\alpha = 1$, $\beta = 1/6$ in 4D.

By calculating the eigenvalues and eigenvectors of T the local orientation is possible to interpret. If all eigenvalues are approximately equal, then T describes an isotropic neighbourhood with no dominant orientation, while in other cases, when there exists a differentiation in magnitude among the eigenvalues, neighbourhoods of, for example, planes and lines are described. Based on the intrinsic information in T regarding the orientation of the local neighbourhood, an adaptive filter synthesis is performed where the resulting adaptive filter s_ap is given by a weighted sum of fixed filters:

$$s_\text{ap} = s_\text{lp} + a_\text{hp} \sum_k c_k s_k \tag{2}$$

where s_lp is the result from a low pass filter, a_hp is the high-pass amplification factor which gives a trade-off between filtering quality and a risk for introducing high-pass filtering artefacts exaggerating edges and lines, s_k is the output from a high-pass filter with the same direction as the quadrature filter and c_k is the weighting coefficient below:

$$c_k = C \cdot (\alpha \hat{n}_k \hat{n}_k{}^T - \beta \mathbb{I}) \tag{3}$$

where C is the control tensor and $\cdot$ symbolizes the scalar product between tensors. The control tensor is used to control the degree of anisotropy in the adaptive filter. When determining C a low-pass filtered version of the local orientation tensor, T_lp, is being used [25]. Calculating the weighted outer product of the eigenvectors of T_lp gives the control tensor according to [1]

$$C = \frac{\lambda_1}{\lambda_1^2 + \alpha^2} \sum_{k=1}^{N} \lambda_k \hat{e}_k \hat{e}_k{}^T \tag{4}$$

where λ_k is the eigenvalue of T_lp with $\lambda_i \leq \lambda_{i+1}$ for all $i = 1 \ldots M$, α is "resolution parameter" ranging from zero to one and $\hat{e}_k$ is the eigenvector of T_lp corresponding to λ_k.

3.2.2. *GPU implementation*

To analyse the trade-off between execution times and quality of filtering we implement both 3D and 4D based filtering of the datasets. In the first case, we apply our filtering method on a volume of ultrasound data for each time frame of the dataset. For the latter case, we instead consider the whole dataset as a four dimensional array of data and perform filtering also along the fourth dimension.

In the standard way of describing the adaptive filtering method one typically constructs the orientation tensor for each data sample and apply a low pass filter component-wise to the tensors. We note that performing the low pass filtering before the tensor construction gives an equivalent result, but with fewer operations, since the constructed orientation tensors are a linear product of the quadrature filter responses.

$$ T \otimes f_{\mathrm{lp}} = (\sum_k (q_k \hat{e}_k \hat{e}_k{}^T)) \otimes f_{\mathrm{lp}} = \sum_k (q_k \otimes f_{\mathrm{lp}}) \hat{e}_k \hat{e}_k{}^T) $$

Thus, for the 3D and 4D filtering case we require only 6 or 12 low-pass filtering operations since q_k only contains the magnitude of the complex quadrature filter responses. We pre-compute the convolution kernels for line and edge detection as per Knutsson [9] for a given radius r_c and give a Gaussian low-pass kernel of radius r_g, as measured in data samples. The filter q_k could be computed by a combined kernel of e.g. size $(2r_c + 1 + 2r_g + 1)^3$ for the 3D filtering. However, we observe that we gain the same result by performing convolutions with the high-pass filters of $(2r_c + 1)^3$ followed by three (respectively four) convolutions with a 1D Gaussian filter of size $(2r_g + 1)$ consecutively. By performing this sequence of convolutions with smaller kernels fewer convolution operations are needed. Obviously, the same observation holds also for the case of 4D filtering.

As can be seen, the full filtering algorithm could be implemented in a naively data-parallel fashion where each work item would require convolutions with the larger kernels followed by the construction of control tensors and final filtering. Such approach would require no intermediate storage of values and thus require no communication between different work items. However, since the convolutions with the smaller quadrature filters and 1D low-pass filters give a significant reduction in the number of computations, we have elected to split the computation into a series of kernels. The intermediate value from the different kernel computations are here stored on-board the GPU.

1. Compute the quadrature filter q_k' for each data point as a combination of the line and edge detection filter kernels
2. Let $s_k = |q_k'|$ for each data point.
3. Perform a convolution of q_k' by applying three 1D low pass Gaussian filters oriented around each of the first three dimensions consecutively forming q_k. Apply the same convolutions to form the low pass filtered data s_{lp}.
4. Form the orientation tensor T (Eq. 1) using q_k and the corresponding directions $\vec{e}_k$.

5. Compute the eigenvalues λ_i of tensor T using the characteristic equation $\det(T - \lambda\mathbb{I}) = 0$ and find the corresponding eigenvectors $\vec{e}_i$ by Gauss Jordan elimination

6. Form the control tensor C (Eq. 4), and the weighting coefficients c_k (Eq. 3).

7. Compute the final output s_{lp} (Eq. 2) from the weighting coefficients, the low pass filtered data and the high pass filtered data.

We note that the only data dependencies between different data points occurs in step 3 above, and can thus implement the algorithm by the following three data parallel computation kernels, where the low pass filtering kernel is invoked once per dimension:

- The quadrature convolutions kernel which performs steps 1 - 2 of the algorithm.
- The low pass filtering kernel that performs filtering with a 1D Gaussian kernel.
- The adaptive filtering kernel that performs steps 4 - 7 of the algorithm.

A straightforward data-parallel implementation of these kernels that runs on one or more processor cores on a desktop machine that processes frame by frame the data can easily be implemented. To store the intermediate results for q_k we require two floating-point values per filter and data sample, in at least two copies during the low-pass convolutions. For the considered data sets this consumes at least 1536 MiB of data for the 3D filtering data sets and $(2r_g + 1)$ times that for the 4D filtering case since multiple frames need to be stored. Since the GPUs of today cannot handle the computations with such large temporary data we have split up the computational task into the consecutive filtering of a number of *sub volumes*, each responsible to compute N^3 data points of the filtered data on each frame.

For step 4 - 7 of the algorithm above, we require the corresponding N^3 values of T, s_{lp} and s_k to compute s_{ap}. For the multiple executions of step 3, however, we require between N^3 and $(N + 2r_g)^3$ values of q'_k to correctly handle the low-pass filtering of the overlap between sub-volumes. This gives a computational cost of $((N + 2r_g)/N)^3$ times higher than if all the intermediate calculations could be saved. In our implementation we have used $r_g = 4$ and $N = 64$ which results in 142% computational cost but ensures that the intermediate data sets can fit within the on-board RAM of the GPUs.

For an illustration of the split-up between kernel executions and the intermediate datasets that are stored see Figure 3. With the above value for N, the five kernel executions per sub volume will be performed 64 times per frame of the data set. Low-pass filtering was not performed along the time dimension for 4D filtering. This is due to the requirement of storing a four dimensional q'_k, requiring $(2r_g + 1)$ times as much memory for intermediate calculations and either storing the computed q'_k between the different invocations for different frames (requiring too much on-board memory or swapping to the CPUs RAM memory) or by the corresponding $(2r_g + 1)$ multiplied cost by recomputing the values for each new frame. However, since the input datasets are of considerably smaller sizes, the individual values of q_k for the a N^3 subset can be computed along the fourth dimension for reasonable sizes of r_c.

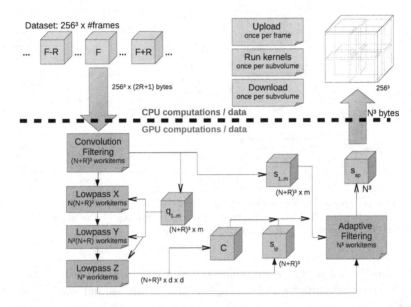

Fig. 3. Illustration of kernel invocations and data flow between CPU/GPU and GPU/GPU. Data on CPU side stored with one byte per volumetric sample, temporary data on GPU side stored as floating point vectors/tensors per sample. R is the radius of convolution kernels, $N = 64$ the size of each sub volume for which filtering is performed.

3.2.3. *Computational performance*

The computationally most expensive steps in the algorithm above is the convolution with the quadrature filters and with the low-pass filters. For the later, we have already seen how it can be changed from using 3D or 4D convolution kernels to a sequence of 1D kernels, giving a speed-up of e.g. $(2r_g + 1)^3/(3(2r_g + 1))$ which for $r_g = 11$ gives 40 respectively 332 times less computations needed. For the former, we cannot in an easy way reduce the problem to lower dimensions. Due to the relatively small size of the convolution kernels and the large number of convolutions to perform, we have used spatial domain convolutions on the GPU [8] using the method described in Section 3.1. In Figure 4 we compare the overall speed when using different values for the filter kernels and the convolution unroll parameter. As we can see the optimal values for unrolling the kernels vary with the different convolution sizes and need to be optimized for the specific radius used in the application.

3.3. *Line detection*

Another example of a GPU based algorithm which was recently used by the authors, concerns a data parallel method for catheter detection in noisy 3D images, and was applied in detecting needles in 3D ultrasound images in dose planning during prostate brachytherapy treatment.

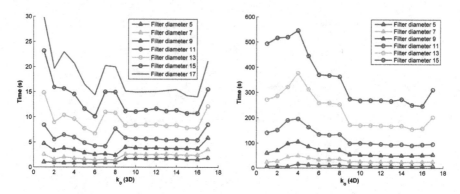

Fig. 4. Timing comparison for different kernel sizes and values of the optimization parameter k_o when performing 3D (left) respectively 4D (right) filtering of the aortic valve data set (116x200x117x36 samples) for different filter diameters r_g.

The Hough Transform, one of the most well known line-detection techniques, is particularly well suited for detecting needles in ultrasound images due to its robustness to the extraneous noise. Unfortunately, its high computational needs often prevent it from being applied in real-time applications – but fast variations [4, 19, 22] thereof have been successfully applied in clinical settings.

When implementing a traditional hough transform on CPUs a typical approach is to consider each voxel and transform it's coordinates into a subset of the corresponding hough space. The voxel intensities of each such subset is summed in a number of accumulator cells sampling the hough space and the highest accumulator cells determine the recognized lines/shapes. Implementing this algorithm directly on OpenCL is not a good idea since this would imply work items that corresponds to voxels, each of which would write into the hough-space accumulators simultaneously. The later part would either require a large number of atomic operations which is slow on GPUs, or other synchronization methods such as exploiting local memory, or writing to multiple copies of the hough-space accumulators. Similarly, by parallelising the work load on the hough space accumulators and checking the corresponding voxels imply a brute-force approach that will visit the source image for each voxel on each considered line. A more efficient approach [24] is to exploit the rasterisation hardware of the GPUs which already is capable of handling the atomic updates of target samples – or pixels when considering the hough space as a target image. Although the authors approach here has a sampling problem due to the non-linear nature of the corresponding shape in the hough space of a line and the lack of true non-linear rasterisation functionalities their approach makes good use of the GPU hardware albeit with a trade-off in precision.

However, before we implement a rasterisation based approach or an approach that utilizes atomic counters, shared memory or other more advanced algorithms it is worth to consider the main question of the application – is it fast enough for the given purpose? In Listing 5 we implement a hough transform in a straight forward

```
1   kernel void needleDetect(global float *rawIn, global float *lines) {
2       int2 id = (int2)(get_global_id(0),get_global_id(1));
3       int dx, dy, dz, index = id.s0 + id.s1 * HS0;
4       float bdx = 0.f, bdy = 0.f, best = 0.f;
5
6       for(dy=-R;dy<=R;dy++) for(dx=-R;dx<=R;dx++) {
7           float thisval = 0.f;
8           for(z=0;z<HS2;z++) {
9               int x=id.x + (dx*z+HS2/2)/HS2;
10              int y=id.y + (dy*z+HS2/2)/HS2;
11              if(x >= 0 && x < HS0 && y >= 0 && y < HS1) {
12                  thisval +=rawIn[x+y*HS0+(HS2-z)*HS0*HS1];
13              }
14          }
15          if(thisval > best) {
16              best=thisval;
17              bdx=(float) dx;
18              bdy=(float)
19          }
20      }
21      lines[index*3+0] = bdx; lines[index*3+1] = bdy; lines[index*3+2] = best;
22  }
```

Listing 5. Brute force implementation of line detection. HS0, HS1 and HS2 are compile time defines with the input image sizes. R is a compile time define that defines the maximum deviation of needle angle (measured in pixels corresponding to $HS2 \times \tan\phi$).

approach that considers every possible combination of lines that are known to start in the base plane of the image. We instantiate work items for each XY pixel in the base plane of the image and letting the kernels consider each neighbourhood $\Delta x, \Delta y$ of XY in the opposite side of the image volume and summing the intensities of the source image along the corresponding lines. This gives an equivalent algorithm for detecting only the subset of lines in the hough-space that corresponds to needles deviating at most by the angle given by the maximum values of the Δx, Δy. Although this approach may seem overly simplistic and not as efficient as the rasterisation based approach, a first trial demonstrates that all the needles in the considered brachytherapy dataset could be identifies within a few seconds. As such there is no need for further optimizations in our application and we conclude:

> **Sometimes a brute force algorithm is fast enough on GPUs.**

4. Applications

Here we illustrate two applications which use the algorithms presented in the previous section. The first concerns image de-noising in 4D volume datasets using the convolution and adaptive filtering algorithms. The second application concerns automatic detection of needles in 3D ultrasound images during brachytherapy treatments.

4.1. *Image de-noising in 4D echocardiography using adaptive filters*

For the purpose of validating the filtering algorithms presented here, we have used volumetric data sets collected from a healthy volunteer using a GE VingMed Vivid E9 cardiovascular ultrasound system. We have sampled the heart of the volunteer from multiple projections, most importantly a parasternal basal short-axis view at the level of the aortic valve and an apical four-chamber view. Volume data was acquired using four consecutive cardiac cycles (multibeat). These recordings were exported as envelope data sets from the proprietary system to DICOM format which was read using a custom program running on standard laptops and desktops.

4.1.1. *Hardware & Software*

For the implementation of the above algorithm we have evaluated it on a modern desktop PC computer and an off-the-shelf laptop computer. The former consists of a 3.33GHz AMD Phenom II SixCore processor, 4GB DDR3 RAM, with an AMD 6950 graphic card. The later is an Asus G73JH laptop containing an Intel Core i7 720QM (4 hyper threaded CPU cores at 1.6GHz), 8GB DDR3 RAM and a AMD 5870 Mobility Radeon graphic card. For reference, the graphic cards above contain 1408 and 800 individual stream processors operating at 800 and 700MHz, respectively. As we see in the results these numbers reflect almost linearly on the performance of the algorithm. Parsing of the volumetric data files of 40-700MB each was performed onboard the CPU following the standard DICOM specification with the VolDICOM extension as specified by the manufacturer of the ultrasound machines. In order to perform the computations we have used OpenCL 1.2 [13].

4.1.2. *Handling border data*

Due to the nature of the sampled data, there is an artificial cut off of the data outside the pyramid that can be sampled by the ultrasound probe. This change between inside and outside data sets requires a special treatment of the quadrature filter convolution kernels to avoid creating an artificial edge. We have performed this correction of the convolutions by counting the number of data samples c_i that are non-zero (falls within the pyramid of data) during the convolutions and comparing this to the total size of the convolutions c_t. By scaling the quadrature responses by c_i/c_t we avoid creating false borders that affect the adaptive filtering adversely.

4.1.3. *Results*

We provide timing results both for applying the filtering based on using a 3D orientation estimate as well as a 4D orientation estimate and investigate how the timing scales on a GPU and/or CPU cores. The measurement for CPU cores have been performed using an identical OpenCL implementation, exploiting vectorization and

Table 3. Relative computational time per kernel for filter size 7

	3D/cpu	3D/gpu	4D/cpu	4D/gpu
Quadrature convolutions	61.8%	23.0%	96.2%	69.9%
Lowpass filtering	12.3%	20.6%	1.0%	12.5%
Adaptive filtering	18.0%	34.5%	2.4%	7.7%
Post Processing	7.9%	21.9%	0.4%	9.9%

with a manual fine tuning of the work group sizes to optimize speed. As such the relative numbers between GPU and CPU performance should reflect the true difference in computational speed between these types of devices.

We saw in Section 3.2.3 that the optimal convolution unroll factor was dependent on the hardware and the given input radius. During the application runs we note that the optimal convolution unroll parameter is invariant to the specific dataset since the control flow is independent on the actual data-values. The total execution times when performing 3D filtering of a dataset consisting of 116x200x117x36 samples on the CPU is 133.2s (desktop) and 205.8s (laptop), respectively. When running the same dataset on the GPUs the total running times of 4.6 (desktop) and 10.5 seconds demonstrate a significant speed improvement. Similarly, when performing 4D filtering on the CPU we have running times of 1522.8s (desktop) and 2467.8s (laptop) which can be contrasted to the GPU running times of 20.6s (desktop) and 63.7s (laptop). As we can see both the 3D and 4D filtering can be performed on-board GPUs, for the given data set size, within a time span suitable for analysis immediately after and in conjunction with the physical examination.

In Table 3 we present the total fractions of computational time spent in the different computational kernels for a filter size of 7. As we can see, the CPU based computations are dominated by the cost of performing convolutions. Although the convolutions are one of the more expensive operations also for the GPU, we see that for the smaller 3D convolution problem it is of the same magnitude as the other kernels while for the 4D case it scales up and takes a larger share of the computational cost. The post processing column kernel here contains all the eigen value computation and assembly of final convolution filter.

To illustrate the effect of 3D and 4D adaptive filtering on the considered echocardiography data set we present a 2D slice at one time frame for the data sets (Figure 5) before filtering and after 3D/4D filtering, respectively. In this figure we present the original, 3D filtered and the 4D filtered data taken from one frame of the aortic valve view data set.

Visual assessment of the adaptive filtering indicate, according to a clinician with over 15 years of experience of echocardiography and cardiology, an improvement of image quality in both the 3D and 4D filtered data set. When comparing the 4D and 3D filtered images further improvements, according to the same clinician, are noticed in the 4D filtered images where for instance the atrioventricular valves are more distinctly visualized which makes the interpretation of the image even easier.

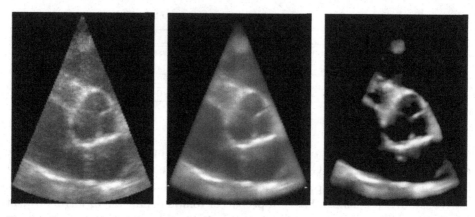

Fig. 5. Cross sections of the aortic valve in basal short axis view using the original, 3D filtered and 4D filtered signal.

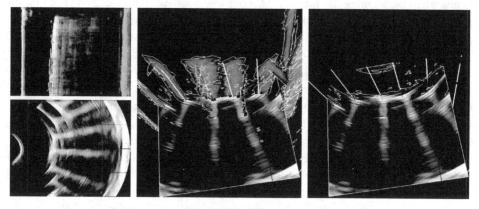

Fig. 6. Example of in-vitro ultrasound data-set for brachy therapy. On the left side the the traditional side and top 2D views, in the middle a volumetric rendering of thresholded data and on the right side the automatically detected needles.

4.2. *Automatic needle detection for image guided HDR prostate brachytherapy treatment*

In trans-rectal ultrasound (TRUS) prostate brachytherapy the needle-tip position is critical for treatment planning and delivery. Currently, needle-tip identification on ultrasound images can be subject to large uncertainty and errors due to the quality of ultrasound images as well as imaging artefacts. One particular approach considers measurements of the residual needle length and an off-line pre-established coordinate transformation factor to calculate the needle-tip position in TRUS-based prostate brachytherapy [27].

For the second application example we will therefore consider the use of the GPU accelerated hough-transform inspired algorithm from Section 3.3. We have run this algorithm on in-vitro and on in-vivo datasets and visualize the needle tip positions over-imposed on the raw ultrasound data.

Together with the department of medical physics we have computed the deviations between measured positions and true position for in-vitro datasets – giving standard deviations less than 0.5mm. Furthermore, preliminary results on in-vivo datasets demonstrate a similar deviation between the needle position estimated by clinical experts observers and the algorithm. This standard deviation is of the same magnitude as the intra-observer deviations and thus we conclude that the simplified hough-transformed inspired algorithm is suitable for clinical needs.

5. Discussion

When implementing image processing algorithms on GPUs we have seen methods for improving the performance of computations to around 10 - 100 times faster than ordinary CPUs. While this advantage in computational speed translates into a possibility of performing on-line image processing on much larger datasets than before, required to cope with the even higher dimensions of modern medial imaging sensors, it also requires additional care from the algorithm designer. We have seen in the previous sections that minimizing the required memory bandwidth is necessary to achieve full usage of the arithmetic units and that efficient algorithms can require close knowledge of the performance of the hardware. As such, for many time consuming algorithmic building blocks it is better to reuse existing software libraries. Fortunately several such libraries for GPUs, including most of BLAS and LAPACK are available. With the speed advantages of GPU based processing we have seen a number of applications that was consider infeasible before.

5.1. *Applications*

We have presented a general method for fast local orientation estimation and filtering of 4D echocardiographic data sets using GPU hardware. This specific combination of 3D and 4D filtering show promising results that require further studies to determine suitability in echocardiographic examinations. Such a clinical evaluation would preferably be performed as a double blind study involving several data sets and clinicians. This specific application of filtering of ultrasound data should be seen as an example of applications that can be implemented on large 4D data sets using the GPU based quadrature filtering approach. We believe that this method as well as any other technique requiring local orientation estimates on large data sets, seem quite promising.

When looking at recent development of computational hardware we have seen an exponential growth of the number of parallel processing elements matching Moore's law [23] on the GPU side [21]. With the advent of Accelerated Processing Units (APUs) where GPU and CPU processors are combined on the same chip, this exponential growth in number of processing elements can be expected to continue in the near future. Given the performances of the algorithms on modern hardware, it is not unreasonable to assume that real-time interactive filtering can be performed during clinical examinations within a few years.

In conclusion, GPUs facilitate the use of demanding adaptive image filtering techniques that enhance 4D echocardiographic data sets. This may open up for an improvement in diagnosis and pre- and even per-surgical examinations using 4D echocardiograms. This general methodology of implementing parallelism is also applicable for other medical multidimensional data sets, such as MRI and CT, that would benefit from fast adaptive image processing.

Additionally, we have seen an application of needle detection using a brute force approach on GPUs. While this problem could be solved with less computational hardware using other algorithms, the possibility of using brute force computations opens up for fast prototyping and tuning of algorithm parameters (e.g. adding curvature to the parameter space, median filtering along the needles, position dependent weighting of intensities).

5.2. *Numerical precision of arithmetic operations*

When implementing image processing algorithms there have traditionally been a trade-off between utilizing single precision (32 bit), double precision (64 bit) or even higher precision floating point numbers for the computations. While certain algorithms are quite sensitive to numerical rounding errors the cost for higher precision can be quite significant for GPUs.

On first generation GPU hardware capable of general purpose computations, there often did not exist any double floating-point ALU units at all. In more recent hardware the ALUs often support double floating-point precision – but at a significantly higher cost. As for example, the 5000-series hardware used in Section 3.1 where each ALU unit is capable of performing either five single floating point operations or one double floating point operation. The ratio of the number of single precision point operations that can be performed in the same time as a double precision point operation varies widely between different cards and manufacturers, for example with only 1/16 for NVidia GTX 680 and up to 1/2 for NVidia Tesla cards.

An algorithm should only use the higher requirements on precision in the instances where they are needed. If we return to the Adaptive filtering example of Section 3.2 we note that the eigen value computation requires a solver for complex roots. These computations are very sensitive to numerical precision and yields incorrect results when using single precision arithmetic.However, since the amount of time spent in this kernel is relatively low ($< 1\%$ for the 4D case) we elected to use 64 bit (double precision) floating point numbers for these computations and only 32 bit (single precision) floating point numbers for the convolution operations that are much less sensitive to numerical precision. This has shown to cause no detectable effect to the filtered data while giving a speed-up of 5.8 times on the target ATI 5000-series hardware, as compared to using double precision point operations for all of the computations.

```
1  #define mmad(x,y,z) fma(x,y,z)
2  #define mmad(x,y,z) (x+y*z)
3  #define mmad(x,y,z) mad(x,y,z)
```

Listing 6. Selection of operator for floatingpoint multiply-add operation.

A common low level operation performed in various image processing operations is that of a floating point multiplication followed by an addition, commonly used for computing the sum of a number of products. When performing this operation as two distinct operations we have a higher rounding error as compared to utilizing the built-in floating-point multiply-add operations of modern hardware (FMA). When the precision is not of consideration the OpenCL standard function multiply-add (MAD) that relaxes the requirements of precision in favour of possible compiler optimizations can be used. If we return to the examples in Listings 3 we see that this choice was made by one of the possible selections in Listing 6.

We have here a choice of three different functions with varying trade-off between speed and guaranteed precision. The first uses the FMA which guarantees infinite precision in the multiplication followed by standard IEEE 754 precision after addition. The second option uses distinct operators for addition and multiplication which gives a slight performance increase on some hardware to either be as good as the FMA operation (if optimized) or come in as the second most exact operator. Finally, the third operator has no guarantees what so ever for precision but allows the hardware to optimize for speed.

References

[1] I. Bankman. *Handbook of Medical Imaging: Processing and Analysis*. Academic Press, 2000.

[2] M. Broxvall, K. Emilsson, and P. Thunberg. Fast gpu based adaptive filtering of 4d echocardiography. *IEEE Trans Med Imaging*, 2011.

[3] B. Cabral, N. Cam, and J. Foran. Accelerated volume rendering and tomographic reconstruction using texture mapping hardware. In *Proceedings of the 1994 symposium on Volume visualization*, VVS '94, pages 91–98, New York, NY, USA, 1994. ACM.

[4] M. Ding and A. Fenster. A real-time biopsy needle segmentation technique using hough transform. *Medical Physics*, 30(8):2222–2233, 2003.

[5] A. Eklund, M. Andersson, and H. Knutsson. True 4d image denoising on the gpu. *International Journal of Biomedical Imaging*, 2011, 2011.

[6] A. F. Elnokrashy, A. A. Elmalky, T. M. Hosny, M. A. Ellah, A. Megawer, A. Elsebai, A. B. M. Youssef, and Y. M. Kadah. *GPU-based reconstruction and display for 4D ultrasound data*, pages 189–192. 2009.

[7] G. Gao, G. Penney, Y. Ma, N. Gogin, P. Cathier, A. Arujuna, G. Morton, D. Caulfield, J. Gill, R. Aldo, et al. Registration of 3d trans-esophageal echocardiography to x-ray fluoroscopy using image-based probe tracking. *Medical image analysis*, 2011.

[8] B. Gaster, D. Kaeli, L. Howes, and P. Mistry. *Heterogeneous Computing with OpenCL*. Morgan Kaufmann Pub, 2011.

[9] G. H. Granlund and H. Knutsson. *Signal Processing for Computer Vision*. Kluwer Academic, 1994.

[10] M. Horton, S. Tomov, and J. Dongarra. A class of hybrid lapack algorithms for multicore and gpu architectures. In *Proceedings of the 2011 Symposium on Application Accelerators in High-Performance Computing*, SAAHPC '11, pages 150–158, Washington, DC, USA, 2011. IEEE Computer Society.

[11] S. Jacobs, R. Grunert, F. W. Mohr, and V. Falk. 3d-imaging of cardiac structures using 3d heart models for planning in heart surgery: a preliminary study. *Interactive CardioVascular and Thoracic Surgery*, 7(1):6–9, 2008.

[12] F. Jiang, D. Shi, and D. Liu. Fast adaptive ultrasound speckle reduction with bilateral filter on cuda. In *Proceedings of the 5th International Conference on Bioinformatics and Biomedical Engineering (iCBBE)*, pages 1–4. IEEE, 2011.

[13] Khronos OpenCL Working group. OpenCL 1.2 specification. Available online: www.khronos.org/opencl/. Document revision 15.

[14] H. Knutsson. Representing local structure using tensors. In *The 6th Scandinavian Conference on Image Analysis*, pages 244–251, 1989.

[15] C. L. Lawson, R. J. Hanson, D. R. Kincaid, and F. T. Krogh. Basic linear algebra subprograms for fortran usage. *ACM Trans. Math. Softw.*, 5(3):308–323, Sept. 1979.

[16] H. Ludvigsen. *Real-Time GPU-Based 3D Ultrasound Reconstruction and Visualization: Harnessing the power of the GPGPU*. LAP LAMBERT Academic Publishing, 2012.

[17] R. Narayanan, P. Werahera, A. Barqawi, E. Crawford, K. Shinohara, A. Simoneau, and J. Suri. Adaptation of a 3d prostate cancer atlas for transrectal ultrasound guided target-specific biopsy. *Physics in medicine and biology*, 53:N397, 2008.

[18] P. M. Novotny, J. A. Stoll, N. V. Vasilyev, P. J. Del Nido, P. E. Dupont, T. E. Zickler, and R. D. Howe. Gpu based real-time instrument tracking with three-dimensional ultrasound. *Medical image analysis*, 11(5):458–464, 2007.

[19] H. M. Overhoff and S. B. mann. Online detection of straight lines in 3-d ultrasound image volumes for image-guided needle navigation. In *Workshop Bildverarbeitung fr der Medizin*, Berlin, Germany, March 2010.

[20] F. Palhano Xavier De Fontes, G. Andrade Barroso, P. Coupé, and P. Hellier. Real time ultrasound image denoising. *Journal of Real-Time Image Processing*, 6(1):15–22, 2011.

[21] G. Pratx and L. Xing. Gpu computing in medical physics: A review. *Medical Physics*, 38:2685, 2011.

[22] W. Qiu, M. Ding, and M. Yuchi. Needle segmentation using 3d quick randomized hough transform. *2008 First International Conference on Intelligent Networks and Intelligent Systems*, 17(6):449–452, 2008.

[23] R. Schaller. Moore's law: past, present and future. *Spectrum, IEEE*, 34(6):52–59, 1997.

[24] M. Ujaldón, A. Ruiz, and N. Guil. On the computation of the circle hough transform by a gpu rasterizer. *Pattern Recognition Letters*, 29(3):309–318, 2008.

[25] C. Westin, L. Wigström, T. Loock, L. Sjöqvist, R. Kikinis, and H. Knutsson. Three-dimensional adaptive filtering in magnetic resonance angiography. *Journal of Magnetic Resonance Imaging*, 14(1):63–71, 2001.

[26] F. Yang, W. Zuo, K. Q. Wang, and H. Zhang. Visualization of segmented cardiac anatomy with accelerated rendering method. In *Computers in Cardiology, 2009*, pages 789–792, 2009.

[27] D. Zheng and D. A. Todor. A novel method for accurate needle-tip identification in trans-rectal ultrasound-based high-dose-rate prostate brachytherapy. *Brachytherapy*, 10(6):466(8), 2011-11-01.

Part 3

Specific Image Processing and Computer Vision Methods for Different Imaging Modalities Including IVUS, MRI, etc.

CHAPTER 15

COMPUTER VISION IN INTERVENTIONAL CARDIOLOGY

Kendall R. Waters

ACIST Medical Systems
47697 Westinghouse Dr., Fremont, California 94539
E-mail: kendall.waters@acistmedical.com

The role of computer vision in the field of interventional cardiology continues to advance the role of image guidance during treatment. This chapter reviews a selection of minimally invasive imaging and sensing technologies used in the treatment of patients with coronary artery and valvular heart diseases.

1. Introduction

The role of computer vision in the field of interventional cardiology has grown steadily in recent years. Minimally invasive treatment of cardiovascular disease has expanded from coronary balloon angioplasty and stenting to aortic valve replacements and mitral valve repairs. Imaging and physiology guidance, including related computer vision techniques, has long played a role in percutaneous coronary intervention (PCI) and is playing an increasingly critical role in transcatheter valve repairs. This chapter will review the role of computer vision in percutaneous coronary and valvular heart interventions. For the present context computer vision is characterized by the extraction of information from image data to guide an intervention.

2. Coronary Artery Disease

Coronary artery disease (CAD) is estimated to affect more than 16 million adults in the United States. Of this population, approximately 785,000 Americans are estimated to have a first heart attack each year, another 470,000 Americans estimated to have a recurrent heart attack. An estimated 618,000 PCIs (i.e., balloon angioplasty) were performed in 2007 to treat CAD patients. In addition, an estimated 560,000 stenting procedures were also performed.[1]

While statistics reported here are for the United States, prevalence rates are expected to be similar in other Westernized nations. Imaging and physiology guidance help answer two critical questions: 1) Should the physician treat; and 2) Has the physician optimized treatment? Clinical trials have shown that certain technologies are more appropriate to address certain clinical questions.

2.1. *To Treat or Not To Treat*

The heart muscle (myocardium) requires oxygen to enable physiological processes. Ischemia may occur when there is a restriction of blood flow due to epicardial (stenosis) and/or microvascular resistance. The reduced blood flow may lead to a shortage of oxygen as well as chest pain (angina). If the ischemia persists for a sufficient length of time, a heart attack (myocardial infarction) may result from heart muscle that is damaged or dies.

Not all stenotic lesions are equal. Intermediate lesions that are characterized (angiographic) stenoses >40 % and <70 % of the coronary lumen diameter may or may not be functionally significant. It is not apparent from angiography alone whether an atherosclerotic lesion restricts blood flow sufficient to cause ischemia.

In recent years, pressure wires have been used to measure fractional flow reserve (FFR) to determine whether revascularization can be deferred. The increasing role of FFR follows the FAME I trial that demonstrated FFR-guidance of PCI reduced major adverse cardiac events compared to angiographic-guidance of PCI.[2]

Pressure wires are designed to be similar to standard 0.014" guide wires that are used to deliver coronary catheters.[3] The pressure wires include a piezoresistive sensor at the distal end of the wire for measuring the coronary artery pressure that is used to calculate the FFR value. Briefly, the FFR value is the ratio of the pressure distal to a lesion to the pressure proximal to a lesion. A FFR value of 1 represents a normal healthy artery. A FFR value >0.80 indicates that a lesion is not functionally significant. Correspondingly, a physician will generally treat a lesion with a FFR value ≤0.80.

While there is no imaging performed or computer vision for FFR measurements using pressure wires, the use of FFR for PCI guidance is relevant to emerging technologies that do involve computer vision as described below in Sec. 2.3.1.

2.2. *Optimizing the Intervention*

Once the decision to treat the CAD patient is made there are multiple imaging modalities available to the physician that aim to optimize the intervention. In particular, clinically available adjunctive imaging technologies have recently expanded beyond intravascular ultrasound (IVUS) technologies to include two optical technologies.

2.2.1. *Angiography*

X-ray angiography during PCI is the *workhorse* image guidance tool for interventional cardiologists. Fig. 1 shows an illustration of a representative cardiac catheterization suite. The biplane angiography system includes two imaging chains: two generators, two fluoroscopy detectors, and two x-ray tubes. Biplane angiography systems are designed to reduce the amount of injected contrast agent by near-simultaneous acquisition of different views.

The patient is generally under conscious sedation. A 6 F (or 7 F) guide catheter (approx. 2 mm inner diameter) is introduced into the arterial system through a femoral or radial artery. The guide catheter is delivered to either the left or right coronary artery. A radio-opaque contrast agent is injected manually or by means of a power injector. Radio-opaque contrast agents attenuate x-ray energy substantially more than soft tissue and serve as an image contrast mechanism. Imaging during contrast injection enables real-time visualization of the lumen of a coronary artery and interventional devices.

Angiograms provide the physician with an interventional roadmap. An exemplary angiogram of a right coronary artery (RCA) is shown in Fig. 2. The guide catheter (GC) is seated at the ostium of the RCA. Balloon angioplasty was performed in the proximal section of the RCA prior to acquiring this image. The guide wire (GW) is visible in the distal section of the vessel. Contrast agent reflux into the aorta is visible below the guide catheter.

Limitations of angiography have long been recognized.[4] The angiogram is a two-dimensional projection of the lumen and may not adequately represent the coronary anatomy. There may be significant variability in visual interpretation. Furthermore, severity of an angiographic stenosis does not indicate functional severity as may be assessed with FFR measurements. Quantitative coronary angiography (QCA) was developed to enable objective assessment of lesion length and reference vessel diameter measurements. While QCA has reduced interobserver variability, the accuracy of angiography to assess coronary lesion severity has not improved.[5]

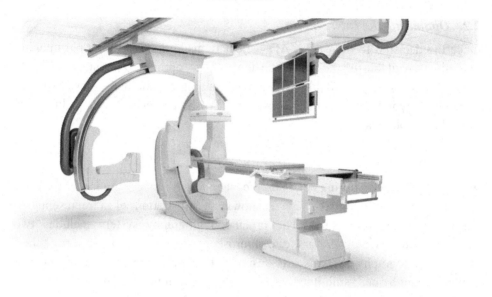

Fig. 1. Photo-realistic illustration of a cardiac catheterization suite, including a biplane angiography system, patient table with bedside controller, and six-panel monitor boom.

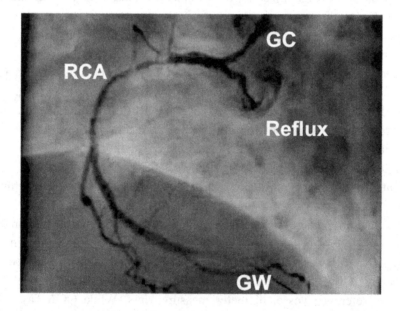

Fig. 2. Angiogram of right coronary artery (RCA) with diffuse disease during contrast injection following balloon angioplasty. Reflux of contrast into the aorta is visible below the guide catheter. (GC = Guide Catheter, GW = Guide Wire)

2.2.2. *Intravascular Ultrasound*

Intravascular ultrasound (IVUS) is the *grand daddy* of adjunctive imaging technologies. IVUS technology has been clinically available since the early 1990s. Clinical applications of IVUS include measuring vessel dimensions to select stent size and length, optimizing stent expansion, insuring full lesion coverage, and guiding strategies to manage procedural complications. The most common use of IVUS is optimizing stent expansion.[1]

Despite IVUS being a mature technology with compelling clinical data, penetration (i.e., percent of PCI cases) is relatively low. Several reasons for the low penetration include the time and cost to perform IVUS, difficulties with image interpretation and relevance of the information, and the perspective that IVUS is more for learning than day-to-day use. The exception to this rule is IVUS use in Japan where penetration is estimated to be >75 % and catheter costs are reimbursed.

IVUS imaging catheters are available in two different designs: a single-element mechanical rotation design and a synthetic aperture array design. Table 1 compares a small selection of catheter design features. Both catheter designs are delivered over a 0.014" guide wire.

The mechanically rotating catheter includes an imaging core that is housed within the catheter sheath. The imaging core includes a single element transducer connected to a torque coil that extends the length of the catheter that can both rotate and translate within the catheter sheath. The transducer transmits a short-time ultrasound pulse and receives the ultrasound backscatter as the imaging core rotates. The array catheter includes 64 transducer elements that are effectively embedded in the catheter sheath. Because of size constraints, a limited number of transmission lines are connected to the transducers. A synthetic aperture algorithm reconstructs an image from a sequence of transmit and receive events.

Table 1. Comparison list of IVUS imaging catheter design features relevant to imaging performance.

Feature	Mechanical Rotation	Array
Transducer	Single Element	64 Elements
Imaging Frequency	40 MHz or 45 MHz	20 MHz
Axial Resolution	Approx. 80 μm	Approx. 150 μm
Image Artifacts	Guide Wire Non-Uniform Rotational Distortion	Grating Lobe Ringdown

Mechanically rotating catheters operate at higher frequencies (40 MHz or 45 MHz) compared to the array catheter (20 MHz). The higher frequency leads to better spatial resolution at the cost of reduced penetration depth. Both catheter designs provide penetration depth sufficient to visualize total plaque burden of coronary arteries. An advantage that array catheters provide by imaging at a lower frequency is an increased contrast between blood (in the lumen) and the vessel wall. This can facilitate image interpretation and dimensional measurements.

Each catheter design has particular image artifacts. Images from mechanically rotating catheters include a guide wire artifact that can potentially obscure details behind the guide wire. Mechanically rotating catheters may also produce images with an artifact known as non-uniform rotational distortion (NURD) that occurs if the imaging core rotates at a non-uniform rate. Array catheter images may have grating lobe artifacts due to the transducer element spacing and array-based image reconstruction technique. Array catheter images may also have a ringdown artifact caused by the location of the transducers close to the outer diameter of the catheter sheath.

A strength of IVUS for guiding PCI is the ability to provide structural detail of the diseased coronary artery. This enables segmentation of the atherosclerotic plaque from the blood in the vessel lumen and vessel adventitia. Measurement of vessel dimensions, such as minimum lumen diameter and minimum lumen area, and detection of stent malapposition provide useful information to the physician. The physician or IVUS technician rather than an algorithm generally determines these image features. This type of post-acquisition analysis of standard grayscale IVUS images would generally not be considered to involve computer vision.

The role of computer vision in IVUS imaging is best exemplified in the image maps of plaque composition. Plaque classification based on IVUS spectral characterization has generated considerable clinical research interest in recent years,[6] but remains controversial for clinical decision making. There are three commercially available IVUS-based plaque classification tools: VH® IVUS,[7] iMAP™,[8] and IB-IVUS.[9] The clinical availability of these plaque classification tools vary from country to country.

The three plaque classification technologies are similar in technical approach. Each technology aims to classify a region of atherosclerotic plaque as one of four plaque component types. The four plaque components vary between technologies and generally include lipidic plaque, fibrous plaque, necrotic core, and dense calcification. Classification algorithms are based on spectral analysis of the pre-processed backscatter IVUS data. The spectral characteristics of a particular plaque type are determined by matching of IVUS images to histology images from diseased cadaver coronary arteries. A training data set of IVUS images, histology images, and spectral data are used to train each classification algorithm. VH IVUS and iMAP use statistical classification techniques whereas IB-IVUS determines ranges of a single spectral parameter (integrated backscatter) that correlate with specific plaque components. Each classified region of the IVUS image is mapped to one of four colors based on the plaque composition. The color scales vary between each plaque classification technology.

The PROSPECT study has been the largest study to date that examined the role of IVUS-based plaque classification (VH IVUS) for guiding treatment decisions.[10] A conclusion of the PROSPECT study is that prospective use of IVUS and IVUS-based plaque classification is not sufficient to predict which lesions will progress and potentially lead to an adverse event. It is not clear at this time how much additional effort medical device companies will invest in IVUS-based plaque classification technologies.

2.2.3. *Intracoronary Optical Coherence Technology*

Optical technology plays an increasingly key role in medical imaging and sensing applications. Intracoronary optical coherence tomography (OCT) is sometimes referred to as the *new kid on the block* and has had a significant impact on adjunctive imaging technologies for guiding PCI. OCT images are rich in detail and provide real-time, microscale resolution of coronary artery disease.

Intracoronary OCT catheters are similar in some ways to mechanically rotating IVUS catheters. The OCT catheters include an imaging core with a side-looking device that rotates and translates, has a short monorail tip that rides on an 0.014" guide wire, and interfaces to an interface module that in part performs calibrated pullbacks of the imaging core. The OCT catheter imaging core includes a fiber optic wire and a microlens assembly that couples light from the system into the tissue in contrast to IVUS catheters that have a transmission line and piezoelectric transducer. OCT catheters also have slightly smaller profiles than IVUS catheters (2.7 F vs. 3.2 F).

Intracoronary OCT systems have a tunable near-infrared (NIR) light source that can be swept over wavelengths of approximately 1250 nm to 1370 nm. A so-called imaging engine includes an interferometer that uses a beamsplitter to split the source light into a reference arm and a tissue arm. The interference of the two light beams enables provides amplitude and frequency data that enables visualization of tissue structures at different depths. The system also includes an interface module to which the catheter connects and enables both rotation and translation of the imaging core. The imaging core rotates at rates between 6,000 and 9,600 revolutions per minute and translates at speeds between 20 mm/s and 40 mm/s. Because NIR light does not transmit through blood, the vessel lumen is cleared of blood, generally by injection of a (transparent) contrast agent, during imaging.

The corresponding axial resolution is <20 µm whereas the lateral resolution is between 20 µm and 40 µm. The rapid pullback speed minimizes the duration to <10 s for which the vessel lumen must be cleared of blood. (This is incredibly fast compared to convention pullback rates for IVUS at 0.5 mm/s or 1.0 mm/s.) The rapid pullback speed further minimizes the amount of contrast that is required to be injected, which is of particular relevance for concerns about contrast-induced nephropathy. The high frame rate (between 100 and 160 frames per second) reduces the frame spacing (distance between the start of each image) which is important to insure maximal imaging coverage of the tissue. One limitation of intracoronary OCT images is a penetration depth of only 1 mm to 3 mm which in many cases is insufficient to visualize total plaque burden. More complete descriptions of OCT technology are available elsewhere.[11]

Fig. 3 shows a screen shot of an intracoronary OCT system that includes a cross-sectional image (top right), a longitudinal image (bottom), and a perspective view image of a diseased coronary artery with fresh (red) thrombus in the artery lumen. This is an impressive image for the fact that OCT not only enables detection of thrombus, but further enables distinguishing red (or fresh) thrombus from white thrombus. The ability to visualize thrombus has led to increasing interest and awareness for thrombus management. While consensus documents[1] indicate that intracoronary OCT is a research tool, early adopters have already incorporated OCT into clinical practice for optimizing stent deployment, understanding stent failure, and detailed analysis of coronary artery disease, including thrombosis.

Intracoronary OCT is a relatively new technology to the interventional cardiology field. Consequently, the role of computer vision in intracoronary OCT is currently limited. The perspective view of the coronary artery in Fig. 3 hints at possibilities for 3D imaging. Potential 3D applications include improved guidance of PCI involving bifurcations.[12] Plaque composition maps, based on image texture or optical attenuation,[13] may also be feasible.

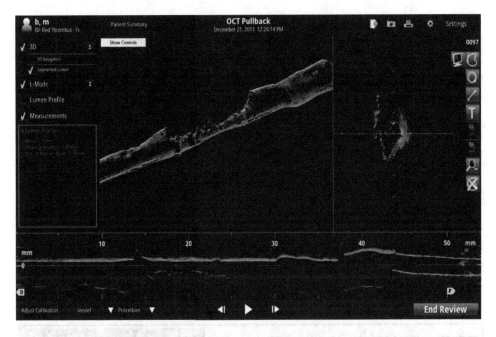

Fig. 3. Screen shot of an intracoronary optical coherence tomography (OCT) system (St. Jude Medical, C7-XR System) showing a perspective view, cross-sectional image, and longitudinal image of a coronary artery with fresh thrombus present in the artery lumen. (Image courtesy of Dr. Joseph Schmitt, PhD.)

2.2.4. *Intravascular Near-Infrared Spectroscopy*

Near-infrared spectroscopy (NIRS) is a second optical adjunctive imaging technology that has recently become available to interventional cardiologists for CAD assessment. It is noteworthy that this is the only medical device that has been cleared by the United States Food and Drug Administration for the detection of lipid core plaques,[14] a key plaque component associated with PCI procedural complications and heart attacks.

The NIRS/IVUS catheter and system is the most complex of the intracoronary adjunctive devices reviewed here. The catheter is similar in ways to mechanically rotating IVUS catheters wherein the profile at the distal section is approximately 3.2F, a catheter imaging core rotates and translates, a short monorail tip rides on an 0.014" guide wire, and the catheter interfaces to an interface module that in part performs calibrated pullbacks of the imaging core. The imaging core includes a NIRS delivery fiber and mirror, a NIRS collection fiber and mirror, and a 40 MHz ultrasound transducer.

A strength of the NIRS technology for lipid plaque detection is that cholesterols have characteristic NIRS signatures which enable reliable detection of lipid plaque. The credibility of this technology stems from a combination of the rigorous physics basis for NIRS identification of lipid plaque and a careful approach to the ex vivo cadaver studies for algorithm training.

Fig. 4 shows a screen shot of the NIRS/IVUS system that includes a cross-sectional IVUS image and lipid core plaque estimate (left), a chemogram (top right), and a longitudinal IVUS image with a block chemogram (bottom right). The cross-sectional, co-registered NIRS/IVUS image depicts a suspected intermediate lesion with dense calcification (bright reflection with acoustic shadowing between 9 o'clock and 11 o'clock) and a lipid-rich plaque from 8 o'clock to 10 o'clock (bright yellow). The chemogram indicates the presence of lipid-rich plaque at multiple sections along the vessel (horizontal axis). The block chemogram is co-registered with the longitudinal IVUS image and facilitates location of lipid rich regions of a lesion.

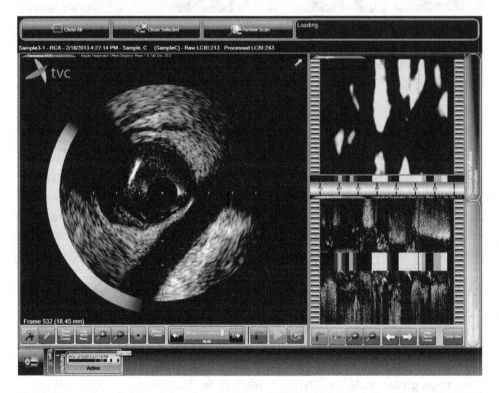

Fig. 4. Screen shot of a near-infrared spectroscopy (NIRS) and intravascular ultrasound (IVUS) system showing a cross-sectional image, longitudinal chemogram, and longitudinal IVUS image with block chemogram. (Image courtesy of Dr. Sean Madden, PhD and Michael Hendricks.)

A potential clinical application for the NIRS/IVUS technology is to identify high-risk cases of periprocedural heart attacks. The hypothesis of the COLOR registry is that stenting and/or high-pressure post-dilation of lesions with high lipid core burdens may lead to distal embolization in turn leading to procedural complications such as no reflow and heart attacks.[15] Results to date have been encouraging.

2.3. *Emerging Technologies*

Image guidance technologies for PCI continue to push the technology envelope. Two technologies that are briefly examined here include a (non-invasive) computed tomographic technique to visualize FFR throughout the coronary system and an intracoronary photoacoustic technique to visualize structure and composition of an atherosclerotic lesion, similar in aim to NIRS/IVUS.

2.3.1. *FFR_{CT}*

The use of a multi-row detector computed tomography (MDCT) enables non-invasive visualization of the coronary artery system. The combined advances in coronary computed tomography angiography (CCTA) and computational fluid dynamics applied to coronary blood flow have led to the development of a CT-derived FFR (FFR_{CT}) technique.[16] Anatomical structure alone is generally considered insufficient to evaluate the functional severity of a lesion. Initial comparisons of FFR_{CT} and FFR (from pressure wire) in patients provide are encouraging, but additional research and development is required to better understand the differences of FFR_{CT} and FFR. Nevertheless, FFR_{CT} technology represents a potentially dramatic change in clinical workflow if the use of FFR_{CT} is one day considered appropriate for determining whether to treat a patient.

2.3.2. *Intravascular Photoacoustics*

The combination of ultrasound and optical imaging technologies are a compelling approach to respectively provide structural detail and specify chemical composition of coronary atherosclerotic lesions. In recent years intravascular photoacoustics (IVPA) technology has been developed for potential application to intracoronary imaging.[17] Photoacoustics imaging involves absorption of near-infrared optical energy that leads to local thermal expansion of tissues. The thermal expansion subsequently generates a pressure wave that can be detected and localized by an ultrasound transducer. The contrast between different tissue components is determined in part by wavelength-dependent optical absorption characteristics that vary with chemical composition. The optical contrast enables differentiation of plaque composition based on unique spectral characteristics of tissues (or of contrast agents) within plaques. An IVUS/IVPA imaging system and catheter is potentially capable of visualizing total plaque burden and simultaneously improving the ability to differentiate plaque composition.

Fig. 5 shows ex vivo IVUS/IVPA images of the aorta of a balloon-injured rabbit model. Figs. 5A and 5B respectively show IVUS images of the aorta having a perspective view and a section cut-away view. Figs. 5C and 5D demonstrate localization of the gold nanorod contrast agent that selectively label atherosclerotic plaque. The contrast agent was systemically injected into the rabbit model prior to animal sacrifice. Further details of the experimental study are described elsewhere.[18]

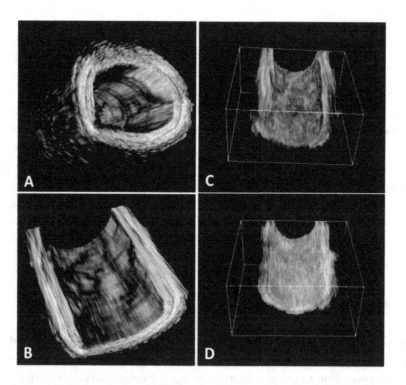

Fig. 5. IVUS and IVUS/IVPA images of an aorta of a balloon-injured rabbit model: (A) perspective view of IVUS image of aorta, (B) section cut-away view of IVUS image of section cut-away view of aorta, (C) section cut-away view of IVUS/IVPA image of aorta labeled with a gold nanorod contrast agent and imaged through saline, and (D) section cut-away view of IVUS/IVPA image of aorta labeled with a gold nanorod contrast agent and imaged through blood. The gold nanorods are co-localized with the atherosclerotic plaque. (Images courtesy of Dr. Stanislav Emelianov, PhD and Doug Yeager.)

3. Valvular Heart Disease

The final example of computer vision examined in this chapter involves ultrasound image guidance of transcatheter valve therapies.

3.1. *Prevalence and Treatment*

Valvular heart disease is estimated to affect 2.5 % of the United States population with mitral regurgitation being the most common disorder (1.7 %).[19] The prevalence of valve disease increases dramatically with age. Greater than 10 % of individuals that are 75 years or older are expected to have some form of valve disease. Heart valve surgery has traditionally been the approach in treatment of valvular heart disease.[20] Nevertheless, some patients may not be offered the option of surgery and will continue to be treated only medically, because they are not eligible candidates for surgery due to high-risk comorbidities. Catheter-based treatment of valvular heart disease is an option that is becoming increasingly available to such patients. The role of imaging has had and will continue to have a critical role in the screening of patients and image guidance of the treatment. Transesophogeal echocardiography (TEE) is one particularly relevant technology for assessing the structure and function of diseased native valves and prosthetic valves or valve implants.[21,22]

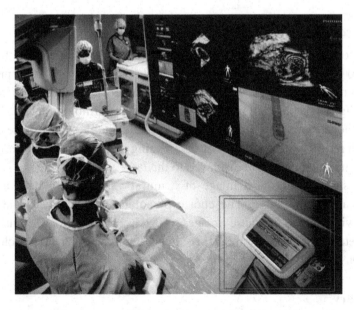

Fig. 6. Photograph of an interventional cardiology laboratory with a 3D transesopheal echocardiographic imaging system. (Image courtesy of Dr. Christopher Hall, PhD and Robert Burnham.)

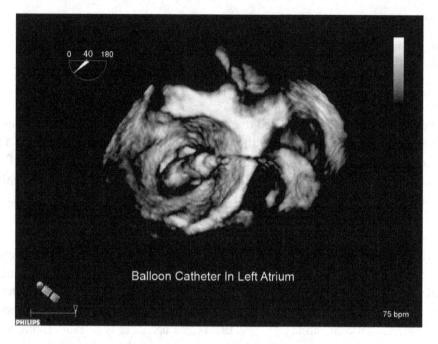

Fig. 7. Three-dimensional transesophogeal echocardiographic image for guidance of a valvuloplasty procedure. A balloon catheter crosses a stenosed mitral valve. (Image courtesy of Dr. Christopher Hall, PhD and Robert Burnham.)

3.2. *Echocardiographic Guidance and Computer Vision*

Transesophogeal echocardiographic probes having fully-sampled matrix arrays with >2500 transducer elements are remarkable technology.[23] These probes and corresponding 3D-capable imaging systems enable 3D visualization of cardiac anatomy. Fig. 6 is a photograph of an interventional cardiology laboratory with a portable echocardiography system (at head of patient table). A bedside controller (outlined in red) facilitates control of the imaging technologies. Fluoroscopic and echocardiographic images are displayed to the large monitor.

Fig. 7 shows a 3D TEE image of a mitral valve with a balloon catheter positioned across the valve. The choice of color scale facilitates the viewer's ability to view depth in these images. This exemplary image illustrates the type of detail available for real-time image guidance for these challenging interventions.

4. Summary

The role of computer vision in the field of interventional cardiology has grown steadily in recent years. Ultrasound and optical based catheters and probes provide structural and physiological detail that is key to improved assessment of coronary artery and valvular heart diseases. The clinical role of these technologies will be refined as their impact on clinical outcomes continues to be evaluated.

References

1. GN Levine et al., J Am Coll Cardiol. 2011;58(24):e44-e122.
2. PAL Tonino et al., N Engl J Med 2009;360:213-24.
3. S Watson and KA Gorski, *Invasive Cardiology: A Manual for Cath Lab Personnel* (Jones & Bartlett Publishers, 2010), pp. 202-206.
4. EJ Topol and SE Nissen, Circulation. 1995;92:2333-2342.
5. J Tobis et al., J Am Coll Cardiol 2007;49:839-48.
6. AN Demaria et al., J Am Coll Cardiol. 2006 Apr 18;47(8 Suppl):C32-9.
7. A Nair et al., EuroIntervention 2007;3:113-120.
8. S. Sathyanarayan et al., EuroIntervention 2009;5:133-139.
9. M Kawasaki (2012). *Integrated Backscatter Intravascular Ultrasound, Intravascular Ultrasound*, Dr. Yasuhiro Honda (Ed.), ISBN: 978-953-307-900-4, InTech.
10. GW Stone et al., N Engl J Med 2011;364:226-35.
11. HG Bezerra et al., J Am Coll Cardiol Intv 2009;2:1035-46.
12. V Farooq et al., Eur Heart J (2013) 34(12): 875-885. doi: 10.1093/eurheartj/ehr409
13. G van Soest et al., Journal of Biomedical Optics 15.1 (2010): 011105-9.
14. U.S. Food and Drug Administration, Center for Devices and Radiological Health. LipiScan IVUS Imaging System K093993 June 30, 2010. Retrieved April 7, 2012 from www.accessdata.fda.gov/cdrh_docs/pdf9/K093993.pdf.
15. JA Goldstein et al., Circ Cardiovasc Interv 2011;4;429-437.
16. JK Min et al., JAMA. 2012;308(12):1237-1245.
17. S. Sethuraman et al., IEEE Trans. Ultrasonics, Ferroelectr. Freq. Control 54(5), 978-986 (2007).
18. D Yeager et al., J Biomed Opt. 2012 Oct;17(10):106016.
19. VL Roger et al., Circulation 2011;123;e18-e209.
20. DR Holmes and MJ Mack, J Am Coll Cardiol 2011;58:445-55.
21. H Baumgartner et al., Eur J Echocardiogr 2009 Jan;10(1):1-25.
22. WA Zoghbi et al., J Am Soc Echocardiogr 2009 Sep;22(9):975-1014.
23. J Balzer et al., Eur J Echocardiogr (2009) 10, 341-349.

CHAPTER 16

PATTERN CLASSIFICATION OF BRAIN DIFFUSION MRI: APPLICATION TO SCHIZOPHRENIA DIAGNOSIS

Ali Tabesh[1,*], Matthew J. Hoptman[2,3], Debra D'Angelo[2], and Babak A. Ardekani[2,3]

[1]*Center for Biomedical Imaging, Department of Radiology and Radiological Science*
Medical University of South Carolina, Charleston, SC 29425 USA
[2]*The Nathan S. Kline Institute for Psychiatric Research, Orangeburg, NY 10962 USA*
[3]*Department of Psychiatry, New York University School of Medicine*
New York, NY 10016 USA
[*]E-mail: ali.tabesh@ieee.org

Pattern recognition (PR) applied to neuroimaging data may enable accurate and objective diagnosis of brain disorders. Several design choices (e.g., features and classifiers) must be made in the development of a PR system for disease detection. In this chapter, we investigate the impact of the classification method on the accuracy of diagnosing schizophrenia based on diffusion magnetic resonance imaging scans. We compared the performance of seven classical and state-of-the-art classifiers. Classifier training and testing using leave-one-out cross-validation were performed on a cohort of 43 patients with schizophrenia and 43 matched control subjects. The nonlinear support vector classifier (SVC) achieved slightly higher classification accuracy (88.4%) than the other classifiers. We also present a method for extracting the approximate discriminant pattern of the nonlinear SVC.

1. Introduction

Quantitative neuroimaging studies typically rely on univariate statistical tests to assess region- and/or voxel-wise structural or functional differences between groups of subjects. While the univariate approach is beneficial when large, region-specific differences are of interest, it overlooks the correlations between these differences across brain regions. This shortcoming is addressed by multivariate techniques, which allow for whole-brain group comparisons. Multivariate methods offer the additional benefit of being able to detect more subtle global differences between the groups.

Pattern recognition methods are a group of multivariate techniques that construct statistical models based on observations drawn from classes of patterns and utilize those models to assign previously unseen patterns to the predefined classes. The classification approach is different than conventional univariate and multivariate statistical tests in an important aspect: classification algorithms seek generalizable group differences that can be used to classify new subjects on a prospective case-by-case basis, whereas statistical tests are not explicitly designed for detecting such group differences. This distinction allows pattern classifiers to enable objective and possibly more accurate diagnosis of neurological and psychiatric disorders. Moreover, the multivariate nature of pattern classifiers allows for extraction of complex spatial patterns of structural and/or functional abnormalities characterizing brain disorders, which may elucidate the interaction between different brain regions in the disease process.

In the context of schizophrenia, a few studies in recent years have applied classification algorithms to T_1-weighted structural magnetic resonance imaging (MRI) scans to distinguish patients from healthy control subjects.[1-4] Generally, studies utilizing T_1-weighted images have been most effective in characterizing gray matter abnormalities.[5] Functional MRI has also been used alone or in conjunction with structural images to classify patients and healthy subjects.[6-8]

Growing evidence suggests that abnormalities in the white matter fiber tracts connecting different brain regions account for many clinical and cognitive manifestations of schizophrenia.[5] Diffusion tensor imaging (DTI)[9] is an MRI technique that characterizes the magnitude and orientation of water diffusion in the brain, thus providing a powerful means for noninvasive characterization of the organization and integrity of white matter fiber tracts. The importance of DTI is recognized considering that it provides unique information regarding white matter structure that is inaccessible with conventional structural MRI.

The diffusion information provided by DTI at each voxel is represented by a symmetric matrix, referred to as the diffusion tensor. The eigenvalues and eigenvectors of the diffusion tensor characterize the magnitude and orientation of water diffusion. Scalar measures derived from the diffusion tensor eigenvalues are used to evaluate white matter integrity. The most common of these measures is fractional anisotropy (FA), which is a normalized measure of deviation from isotropic diffusion.[10]

Region- and voxel-based analyses of DTI in schizophrenia have shown FA abnormalities in a number of brain regions.[5,11] These findings provide ample evidence in support of the value of DTI as a biomarker for schizophrenia.

A few studies to date have applied classification methods to demonstrate the feasibility of schizophrenia diagnosis based on DTI.[12-16] Several of these studies[12-14] have used a combination of principal component analysis and Fisher's linear discriminant analysis (FLDA) to accomplish classification. In another study,[15] support vector classifiers (SVCs) were used for schizophrenia diagnosis. Rathi *et al.*[16] investigated three classification methods for diagnosis of first-episode schizophrenia with an alternate diffusion MRI technique. We note that classification may be based on the spatial pattern of DTI measures in the brain[12-15] or it may be based on the whole-brain histogram of diffusion measures.[16] Our focus in this chapter will be on the former group of methods.[12-15]

It is unknown whether the choice of the classification technique affects the accuracy of schizophrenia diagnosis with DTI. In this chapter, we aim to address this question by performing a comprehensive comparison of several classification techniques. Specifically, we will consider the linear Gaussian classifier (LGC) (which is closely related to FLDA), naïve linear Gaussian classifier (NLGC), the *k*-nearest neighbor classifier (*k*NNC) with two different distance metrics, the linear and nonlinear SVCs, and L_1-regularized logistic regression (L1LR). While Gaussian classifiers and *k*NNC are regarded as classical techniques, the SVC and L1LR have emerged recently as state-of-the-art methods. We use leave-one-out (LOO) cross-validation (CV) to assess the performance of the above methods.

We also present a scheme for extracting discriminant patterns from nonlinear classifiers to enable the visualization of the spatial pattern of the contribution of image voxels to classification. We will demonstrate the application of this scheme to extraction of the discriminant pattern of the nonlinear SVC.

2. Review of Pattern Classification

2.1. *Standardization and Dimensionality Reduction*

Let $\mathbf{X} = [x_1 \ x_2 \ ... \ x_p]^T$ denote the FA image for a subject re-arranged as a $p \times 1$ vector, where p denotes the number of brain voxels in the image. Also, let $(\mathbf{X}_i, c_i) \in \mathbf{R}^p \times \{0, 1\}$, $i = 1, ..., n$, be pairs of FA images and class labels associated with them, where n is the number of training samples from patients and controls. We considered applying two preprocessing steps to $\mathbf{X}$, namely, standardization and dimensionality reduction. Standardization was applied to the inputs to all classifiers, whereas dimensionality reduction was used for the LGC and *k*NNC. Note that the estimation of the preprocessing transformations is part of classifier training and is thus carried out for each LOO training set separately. For a new test case, the estimated preprocessing transformations determined from the training set are applied to the test case, and then the resulting observation vector is presented to the classifier.

Standardization is known to make a significant impact on the performance of many classifiers in some classification tasks.[17] Classifiers such as the *k*NNC and

SVC are sensitive to the relative scale of the predictor variables. Standardization also accounts for inter-subject variability of DTI images. The two standardization steps applied to the images were between-subject standardization followed by within-subject standardization. Our observation was that the order of the standardization steps had very little impact on the classification results.

In the between-subject standardization step, each voxel was standardized to zero mean and unit within-class variance across subjects. For voxel j of subject i, denoted as x_{ij}, this transformation is given by

$$y_{ij} = \frac{x_{ij} - m_j^v}{s_j^v}, \tag{1}$$

where y_{ij} is the standardized voxel value, and m_j^v and s_j^v are the sample mean and standard deviation of voxel j across subjects. Superscript v indicates that the statistics were taken within voxels and across subjects.

In the within-subject standardization step, each image was standardized to zero mean and unit variance. This transformation is given by

$$y_{ij} = \frac{x_{ij} - m_i^s}{s_i^s}, \tag{2}$$

where y_{ij} is the standardized voxel value, and m_i^s and s_i^s are the sample mean and standard deviation of FA across brain voxels. Superscript s indicates that the means and standard deviations were taken within subjects and across voxels.

The second preprocessing step was dimensionality reduction. Dimensionality reduction has two aims. The first aim is to tackle the *curse of dimensionality*, which refers to the exponential increase in the number of training samples needed to train a classifier as the number of features increases.[17,18] The second goal of dimensionality reduction is to make the classification problem computationally tractable. Here, we applied whitening for dimensionality reduction.

Whitening summarizes the information in p-dimensional observation vector $\mathbf{X}$ as an r-dimensional vector $\mathbf{Y}$, $r \le p$, and standardizes the elements of $\mathbf{Y}$ to unit variance. The whitening procedure can be represented as $\mathbf{Y} = \mathbf{AX}$, where whitening transform $\mathbf{A}$ is given by $\mathbf{A} = \mathbf{\Lambda}^{-1/2}\mathbf{U}^T$. Matrix $\mathbf{\Lambda}$ is a diagonal $r \times r$ matrix and $\mathbf{\Lambda}_{ii}$ is the i-th largest eigenvalue of $\mathbf{C}$, the covariance matrix of $\mathbf{X}$. Column i of $p \times r$ matrix $\mathbf{U}$ is the eigenvector corresponding to the i-th largest eigenvalue of $\mathbf{C}$ (i.e., $\mathbf{\Lambda}_{ii}$). When $n \le p$, $\mathbf{C}$ is rank-deficient, as only $n-1$ eigenvalues of $\mathbf{C}$ are nonzero. In this case, $r = n-1$ components of $\mathbf{Y}$ encompass all the information in the training set $\{\mathbf{X}_i, i = 1, ..., n\}$. We refer to the space spanned by these $n-1$ components as the $\mathbf{Y}$ space.

2.2. *Pattern Classifiers*

Statistical classifiers fall into two broad categories of parametric and non-parametric methods. Parametric methods assume that the functional form of the class-conditional distributions or the decision boundary separating them is known, whereas non-parametric methods make minimal assumptions about the distributions or decision boundary. Gaussian classifiers, logistic regression and linear SVCs are parametric methods, whereas kNNCs and nonlinear SVCs are non-parametric algorithms.

Statistical classifiers can also be categorized as being *generative* or *discriminative*. The goal in statistical classification is to find a mapping from the observation vector $\mathbf{X}$ to the class label c. Generative classifiers accomplish this *indirectly* by estimating the joint probability of c and $\mathbf{X}$ as $p(c,\mathbf{X}) = p(c)p(\mathbf{X}|c)$, where $p(c)$ denotes the prior probability of class c, and $p(\mathbf{X}|c)$ is the probability of $\mathbf{X}$ given c. On the contrary, discriminative classifiers *directly* estimate $p(c|\mathbf{X})$ or find a mapping from $\mathbf{X}$ to c. Discriminative classifiers exploit the available training data more efficiently than generative classifiers, as they attempt to only answer the question of predicting c from $\mathbf{X}$ rather than estimating the joint distribution of all variables. Gaussian classifiers are generative methods, whereas logistic regression, kNNCs and SVCs are discriminative approaches.

The choice of the best classifier for a classification task depends on the sample size and prior knowledge about the class-conditional distributions. For small sample sizes and high-dimensional data, parametric and generative classifiers often outperform non-parametric and discriminative classifiers,[19,20] particularly if the assumptions regarding $p(\mathbf{X}|c)$ are valid. However, the choice is also highly dependent on the dataset at hand and must ultimately be made based on the empirical performance of the candidate classifiers. In this study, we considered candidate classifiers in all of the above categories.

The classifiers considered here can be represented in generic form as discriminant function $f(\mathbf{X})$, which may be a linear or nonlinear function of $\mathbf{X}$. The decision rule is to assign $\mathbf{X}$ to class 0 if $f(\mathbf{X}) < 0$, class 1 if $f(\mathbf{X}) > 0$, and a random class if $f(\mathbf{X}) = 0$.

In the following description of the linear Gaussian classifier, L1LR, and linear SVC, $f(\mathbf{X})$ will be represented as

$$f(\mathbf{X}) = \mathbf{w}^T \mathbf{X} + b . \tag{3}$$

The above equation defines a hyperplane and the decision rule comparing $f(\mathbf{X})$ to zero simply determines the side of the hyperplane that observation $\mathbf{X}$ falls on.

2.2.1. *Linear Gaussian Classifier*

For Gaussian class-conditional distributions having a common covariance matrix, the Bayes optimal $f(\mathbf{X})$ is given by (3), where $\mathbf{w} = \mathbf{W}^{-1}(\mathbf{m}_1 - \mathbf{m}_0)$ and $b = (1/2)(\mathbf{m}_0^T \mathbf{W}^{-1} \mathbf{m}_0 - \mathbf{m}_1^T \mathbf{W}^{-1} \mathbf{m}_1) - \ln(P_0/P_1)$. Parameters P_i, and $\mathbf{m}_i$ are the prior probability and mean of class $i = 0, 1$, respectively, and $\mathbf{W}$ is the within-class covariance matrix common to both classes given by

$$\mathbf{W} = \frac{P_0}{n_0 - 1} \sum_{i=1}^{n_0} (\mathbf{X}_i - \mathbf{m}_0)(\mathbf{X}_i - \mathbf{m}_0)^T + \frac{P_1}{n_1 - 1} \sum_{i=n_0+1}^{n} (\mathbf{X}_i - \mathbf{m}_1)(\mathbf{X}_i - \mathbf{m}_1)^T . \tag{4}$$

Note that $\mathbf{w}$ in the linear Gaussian classifier is identical to the projection characterizing FLDA. However, maximizing the cost function that yields FLDA does not specify b. Typically, to define a classifier based on FLDA, the mid-point between the means of the two classes after projection is used as the threshold, that is, $b_{\text{FLDA}} = -(1/2)\mathbf{w}^T(m_0 + m_1)$.[21] Comparing b_{FLDA} and b_{LGC} yields $b_{\text{LGC}} = b_{\text{FLDA}} - \ln(P_0/P_1)$. Thus, the FLDA classifier becomes equivalent to the LGC for equal class prior probabilities.

For $n < p + 2$, $\text{rank}(\mathbf{W}) = n - 2$; therefore, $\mathbf{W}^{-1}$ does not exist. Thus, the linear Gaussian classifier as described above cannot be defined in the $\mathbf{X}$ or $\mathbf{Y}$ space. We addressed this issue by considering two alternatives. The first alternative was a regularized version of $\mathbf{W}$ in the $\mathbf{Y}$ space. The regularized within-class covariance matrix,[21] denoted as $\tilde{\mathbf{W}}$, is given by

$$\tilde{\mathbf{W}} = (1 - \delta)\mathbf{W} + \delta c \mathbf{I}, \tag{5}$$

where $c = [1/(n-1)]\,\text{tr}(\mathbf{W})$ is the average of the eigenvalues of $\mathbf{W}$ and δ is the regularization parameter. Parameter δ is typically set to a small value to ensure the invertibility of $\tilde{\mathbf{W}}$. In our classification problem, we found that $\delta = 10^{-5}$ yielded invertible $\tilde{\mathbf{W}}$'s in all of the LOO training iterations.

The second alternative that we considered was in the $\mathbf{X}$ space. In this case, the diagonal elements of $\tilde{\mathbf{W}}$ were set to those of $\mathbf{W}$, and its off-diagonal elements were set to zero. This choice of $\tilde{\mathbf{W}}$ is equivalent to making the *naïve* assumption that the elements of $\mathbf{X}$ conditioned on c are statistically independent. The resulting classifier is thus referred to as the naïve linear Gaussian classifier (NLGC). Note that this classifier differs from the typical naïve Gaussian classifier in that here the class variances are assumed to be identical. Both variations of the linear Gaussian classifier were realized in the MATLAB environment (http://www.mathworks.com).

2.2.2. L_1-*Regularized Logistic Regression*

For the L1LR, $f(\mathbf{X})$ is also given by (3). In this case, parameters $\mathbf{w}$ and b minimize the convex cost function

$$J_{\text{L1LR}}(\mathbf{w},b) = L(\mathbf{w},b) + \lambda \sum_{i=1}^{p} |w_i|, \qquad (6)$$

where λ is a user-defined parameter.[22] Function $L(\mathbf{w},b)$ is the average logistic loss given by

$$L(\mathbf{w},b) = \frac{1}{n}\sum_{i=1}^{n} l(d_i f(\mathbf{X}_i)), \qquad (7)$$

where $l(u) = \log[1 + \exp(-u)]$ is the logistic loss and $d_i = -1$ and $+1$ for $c_i = 0$ and 1, respectively.

The average logistic loss (first term) in (6) controls how well the model fits the data, while the L_1 complexity (second term) constrains the flexibility of the model. Parameter λ controls the trade-off between the two terms.

The L_1 model complexity term above has attracted significant interest recently.[22] The primary advantage of this measure of complexity over alternatives, such as L_2 complexity ($\sum |w_i|^2$) used in classifiers such as SVC, is that L_1 complexity yields a *sparse* $\mathbf{w}$, i.e., a $\mathbf{w}$ with relatively few nonzero elements. This results in a compact classifier utilizing only a few elements of $\mathbf{X}$, corresponding to the nonzero elements of $\mathbf{w}$. Classifier compactness has two benefits. First, it improves the generalization ability of the classifier on future observations. Second, the classification rule is easier to understand and analyze.

Parameter λ was selected such that the 3-fold CV classification accuracy on the training set was maximized. Values considered for λ were of the form $\lambda = \alpha\lambda_{\text{max}}$, where λ_{max} was the largest regularization parameter that yielded a nonzero $\mathbf{w}$, and $\alpha \in \{10^{-11}, 2\times10^{-11}, 5\times10^{-11}, 10^{-10},..., 10^{-5}\}$. If two or more classifiers corresponding to different λ values were tied for the maximum 3-fold CV accuracy, the more heavily regularized classifier corresponding to the larger λ was selected. We used the implementation of Koh *et al.*[23] in the MATLAB environment, which uses a variation on the interior-point method to minimize (6) for large n and/or p. We applied the classifier in the $\mathbf{X}$ space.

2.2.3. k-*Nearest Neighbor Classifier*

For the *k*NNC, $f(\mathbf{X})$ is given by

$$f(\mathbf{X}) = \log(\frac{n_1}{n_0}), \qquad (8)$$

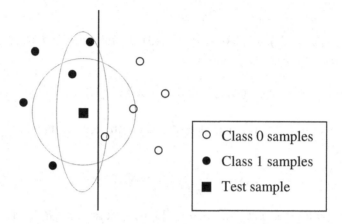

Fig. 1. An instance of classification with the *k*NNC in a two-dimensional space with $k = 3$ and the Mahalanobis distance. The vertical line separates the two classes. With $\mathbf{S} = \mathbf{I}$ corresponding to the circle, the test sample is classified to class 0, as two out of its three nearest neighbors, i.e., samples falling within the circle, belong to class 1. With $\mathbf{S} = \mathrm{diag}(9, 1)$ corresponding to the ellipse, the sample is classified to class 1. The sample actually belongs to class 1.

where n_i is the number of samples belonging to class i that fall within the set of k nearest neighbors of $\mathbf{X}$. Note that $n_0 + n_1 = k$.

Nearness is defined based on a distance measure $d(.,.)$ between $\mathbf{X}$ and samples $\mathbf{X}_i$ in the training set. A common choice for $d(.,.)$ is the Mahalanobis distance given by

$$d(\mathbf{X}, \mathbf{X}_i) = (\mathbf{X} - \mathbf{X}_i)^T \mathbf{S}(\mathbf{X} - \mathbf{X}_i), \qquad (9)$$

where $\mathbf{S}$ is usually a positive semi-definite matrix. The choice of $\mathbf{S}$ can significantly impact the performance of the *k*NNC as demonstrated by the example in Fig. 1. We considered two choices for $\mathbf{S}$ as described below.

Discriminant adaptive nearest neighbor (DANN): The first choice of $\mathbf{S}$ that we considered corresponds to a simple and effective *k*NNC referred to as the DANN classification rule.[24] This choice of $\mathbf{S}$ is based on Fisher's linear discriminant analysis and is given by

$$\mathbf{S} = \mathbf{W}^{-1/2}(\mathbf{W}^{-1/2}\mathbf{B}\mathbf{W}^{-1/2} + \varepsilon\mathbf{I})\mathbf{W}^{-1/2}, \qquad (10)$$

where $\mathbf{B}$ and $\mathbf{W}$ are the between- and with-class covariance matrices, respectively, $\mathbf{I}$ is the identity matrix and ε is a user-defined parameter. This choice of $\mathbf{S}$ gives larger weights to features with larger discriminative power and smaller weights to the less powerful ones. Increasing ε diminishes the difference between the weights. We set $\varepsilon = 1$ and the off-diagonal elements of $\mathbf{W}$ to zero.[24]

Note that Hastie and Tibshirani[24] determined $\mathbf{S}$ adaptively for each local neighborhood based on the training samples in that neighborhood, whereas we used a global $\mathbf{S}$ obtained from all training samples.

Large margin nearest neighbor (LMNN): The second choice of $\mathbf{S}$ that we considered corresponds to the LMNN classification rule.[25] The LMNN cost function, J_{LMNN}, minimization of which yields $\mathbf{S}$, consists of two terms. The first term penalizes large distances between each sample and its target neighbors. The target neighbors of a sample are defined as the k nearest neighbors of the sample that have the same class labels. The second term penalizes small distances between each sample and all other samples that have different labels. Specifically, J_{LMNN} is the convex cost function given by

$$J_{\text{LMNN}} = \sum_{i,j=1}^{n} \eta_{ij} d(\mathbf{X}_i, \mathbf{X}_j) + C \sum_{i,j,l=1}^{n} \eta_{ij}(1 - y_{il})\left[1 + d(\mathbf{X}_i, \mathbf{X}_j) - d(\mathbf{X}_i, \mathbf{X}_l)\right]_+, \qquad (11)$$

where $d(.,.)$ is defined in (9). Parameter η_{ij} is set to 1 when $\mathbf{X}_j$ is a target neighbor of $\mathbf{X}_i$ and 0 otherwise. Parameter y_{il} is set to 1 if class labels of $\mathbf{X}_i$ and $\mathbf{X}_l$ are identical, i.e., $c_i = c_l$, and 0 otherwise. Function $[z]_+$ is defined as $[z]_+ = \max(z, 0)$. This function is set to zero when the distance between the current sample i and non-target sample l is greater than the distance between the current sample i and target sample j by more than 1, thus incurring a zero penalty. Otherwise, a penalty equal to $1 + d(\mathbf{X}_i, \mathbf{X}_j) - d(\mathbf{X}_i, \mathbf{X}_l)$ is incurred. Parameter C is a positive constant that controls the trade-off between the first and second terms and is typically set by CV.

Another parameter of the kNNC is the number of neighbors k commonly found via CV. In our experiments we noted that for our choices of $\mathbf{S}$, most choices of k resulted in perfect separation of the training set samples in LOO CV. The only other guideline for choosing k is that to ensure convergence to the Bayes rule as $n \to \infty$, k must satisfy $k \to \infty$ and $k/n \to 0$.[18] Unfortunately, this guideline does not provide much information about the choice of k for a finite sample size. Thus, we opted for a preset choice of $k = 15$. This choice provides a moderately smooth decision boundary, while somewhat departing from the linear boundary. Note that an odd k helps avoid voting ties.

While the kNNC can in principle be directly applied in the $\mathbf{X}$ space, due to computational limitations we applied the classifier in the $\mathbf{Y}$ space. We realized the kNNC using MATLAB. To determine $\mathbf{S}$ for LMNN, we used Weinberger's implementation[25] with $k = 15$. In this implementation, the minimization of J_{LMNN} is cast as a semi-definite programming problem and is solved via an alternating projections algorithm.

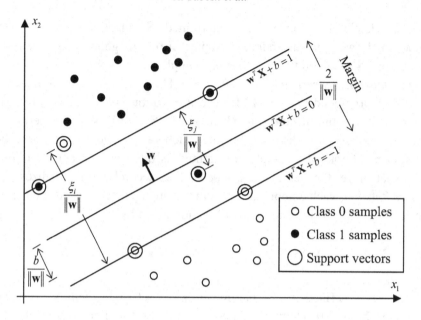

Fig. 2. The soft-margin linear SVC in a two-dimensional space.

2.2.4. *Support Vector Classifier*

The SVC[20] is given by

$$f(\mathbf{X}) = \mathbf{w}^T \mathbf{\Phi}(\mathbf{X}) + b , \qquad (12)$$

where $\mathbf{\Phi}(.)$ is a linear or nonlinear function. Parameters $\mathbf{w}$ and b are determined from the training set via solving the quadratic programming problem given by

$$J_{\text{SVC}}(\mathbf{w}, \xi) = \frac{1}{2}\mathbf{w}^T\mathbf{w} + C\sum_{i=1}^{n} \xi_i , \qquad (13)$$

subject to $d_i f(\mathbf{X}_i) \geq 1 - \xi_i$ and $\xi_i \geq 0$, $i = 1, ..., n$, where C is a user-specified positive parameter, $\mathbf{X}_i$ are training samples, ξ_i are slack variables, and $d_i = -1$ and $+1$ for $c_i = 0$ and 1, respectively.

Fig. 2 provides a graphical representation of the cost function in (13) for the linear SVC, i.e., for $\mathbf{\Phi}(\mathbf{X}) = \mathbf{X}$. The classifier attempts to separate the two classes by as large of a margin as possible (first term), while allowing for some misclassifications through the slack variables ξ_i (second term). The tradeoff between maximizing the margin and minimizing the misclassifications is controlled by C. The first term in (13) can also be viewed as model complexity aiming to avoid overfitting the model to the training data.

The dual representation of (13) yields an equivalent form of (12) as

$$f(\mathbf{X}) = \sum_{i=1}^{n_s} d_i \alpha_i K(\mathbf{S}_i, \mathbf{X}) + b, \tag{14}$$

where α_i denote the Lagrange multipliers associated with the constraints $d_i f(\mathbf{X}) \geq 1 - \xi_i$, $\mathbf{S}_i$ are support vectors, n_s is the number of support vectors, and $K(\mathbf{S}_i, \mathbf{X}) = \Phi(\mathbf{S}_i)^T \Phi(\mathbf{X})$ is the kernel function. Support vectors $\mathbf{S}_i$ are the samples from the training set for which the constraints $d_i f(\mathbf{X}) \geq 1 - \xi_i$ are active. Note that support vectors are the only training samples that characterize $f(\mathbf{X})$.

Typical choices for $K(.,.)$ are the linear and Gaussian kernels. The linear kernel is given by

$$K(\mathbf{S}_i, \mathbf{X}) = \mathbf{S}_i^T \mathbf{X}, \tag{15}$$

and the Gaussian kernel is given by

$$K(\mathbf{S}_i, \mathbf{X}) = \exp(-\gamma \|\mathbf{X} - \mathbf{S}_i\|^2), \tag{16}$$

where γ denotes the inverse of the kernel width. Note that (15) yields a linear $f(\mathbf{X})$, whereas (16) produces a nonlinear $f(\mathbf{X})$.

Parameters C and γ are jointly selected using a grid search such that the LOO classification accuracy on the training set is maximized. As the range of parameters varies substantially from one classification problem to another, a two-stage grid search is typically used to reduce the computational complexity. In the first stage, a coarse-grain grid search is carried out to narrow down the range of parameters to a small neighborhood and then a fine-grain search finds better approximations to the parameters. For the linear kernel, values considered for the coarse grid search for C were $\{2^{-30}, 2^{-28}, ..., 2^8, 2^{10}\}$. Then the search was narrowed down to the range $\{2^{-19}, 2^{-18.75}, 2^{-18.5}, ..., 2^{-15.25}, 2^{-15}\}$.

For the Gaussian kernel, values considered for C and γ in the coarse-grain search were $\{2^{10}, 2^{12}, 2^{14}, ..., 2^{30}\}$ and $\{2^{-45}, 2^{-42}, 2^{-39}, ..., 2^{-20}\}$, and for the fine-grain search they were $\{2^{19}, 2^{19.25}, ..., 2^{21}\}$ and $\{2^{-39}, 2^{-38.75}, ..., 2^{-33}\}$, respectively. If more than one choice of C maximized the LOO accuracy, the smallest C corresponding to the largest degree of regularization was used. If multiple γ values were tied for maximum LOO accuracy, the smallest γ, corresponding to the smoothest decision boundary, was selected. We used the LIBSVM (http://www.csie.ntu.edu.tw/~cjlin/libsvm) implementation of the SVC in the MATLAB environment, which solves (13) via a sequential minimal optimization-type algorithm. The classifier was applied in the $\mathbf{X}$ space.

2.3. *Discriminant Pattern*

Assessing the contribution of voxels to classification is crucial to understanding how the differences between patients and healthy individuals in various brain regions affect classification. The contribution of voxel x_i to $f(\mathbf{X})$ may be defined as the sensitivity of $f(\mathbf{X})$ to changes in x_i, $i = 1, ..., p$. When $f(\mathbf{X})$ is differentiable, its sensitivity to x_i is given by $\partial f(\mathbf{X}) / \partial x_i$, the partial derivative of $f(\mathbf{X})$ with respect to x_i. More compactly, the sensitivity of $f(\mathbf{X})$ to $\mathbf{X}$ is given by the gradient of $f(\mathbf{X})$ defined as $\nabla f(\mathbf{X}) = [\partial f(\mathbf{X})/\partial x_1 \quad ... \quad \partial f(\mathbf{X})/\partial x_p]^T$.

Voxel contributions can be straightforwardly computed when the dimensionality reduction algorithm and the classifier are both linear. For dimensionality reduction transform $\mathbf{A}$ and classifier weight vector $\mathbf{w}$, the overall linear discriminant function is given as $f(\mathbf{X}) = \mathbf{g}^T \mathbf{X} + b$, where $\mathbf{g} = \mathbf{A}^T \mathbf{w}$, yielding $\nabla f(\mathbf{X}) = \mathbf{g}$. The magnitude of g_i signifies the degree of contribution of x_i to the decision, whereas the sign of g_i signifies whether an increase in x_i tilts the decision towards class 0 or 1.

Note that in the linear scenario, $\nabla f(\mathbf{X})$ is a constant vector and does not depend on the image $\mathbf{X}$ being classified. Unfortunately, this is not the case for nonlinear classifiers such as the SVC with the Gaussian kernel. This problem may be addressed by taking the average of $\nabla f(\mathbf{X})$ over multiple $\mathbf{X}$ values on or close to the decision boundary. Thus, the overall sensitivity of $f(\mathbf{X})$ to $\mathbf{X}$, denoted as vector $\mathbf{g}$, becomes

$$\mathbf{g} = \frac{1}{J} \sum_{j=1}^{J} [\nabla f(\mathbf{X})]_{\mathbf{X}_j}, \qquad (17)$$

where $\mathbf{X}_j$, $j = 1, ..., J$, is the set of images situated near or on the decision boundary. For the nonlinear SVC, we used the support vectors $\mathbf{S}_j$, $j = 1, ..., n_s$, as they are the images in the training set closest to the decision boundary. For the Gaussian kernel in (16), the gradient of (14) becomes

$$\nabla f(\mathbf{X}) = -2\gamma \sum_{i=1}^{n_s} d_i \alpha_i \exp\left(-\gamma \|\mathbf{X} - \mathbf{S}_i\|^2\right)(\mathbf{X} - \mathbf{S}_i). \qquad (18)$$

Contribution vector $\mathbf{g}$ can then be obtained by plugging (18) into (17).

It should be recognized that the above scheme is useful only when the nonlinear discriminant function is differentiable and nearly linear (as was the case in our problem). For a highly nonlinear classifier, care must be taken in combining the contributions, particularly when the sign of the contribution changes in different regions of the image space.

2.4. *Error Estimation*

Estimating the performance of a classifier is needed for classifier design as well as for predicting the classification performance of a designed classifier on previously unseen data. A common method for error estimation is K-fold CV, where the available dataset is split into K subsets. Each subset is typically formed such that it contains roughly the same proportion of samples from each class as the entire dataset. Each fold of CV consists of using $K-1$ of the subsets for training a classifier and using the left-out subset for error estimation. The overall K-fold CV error is estimated as the average of the errors over the K subsets.

As mentioned above, classification error estimation is used for two different goals, namely, classifier design and classifier performance estimation on novel data. For the latter goal, we set K to the number of available samples, which is equivalent to the LOO method. Note that the left-out test sample should never be used for classifier design. Failure to do so introduces a bias into the LOO estimate causing it to underestimate the actual classification error.

Classifier design involves selecting design parameters, such as C for the SVC and λ for the L1LR, as well as parameter estimation for the preprocessing steps (i.e., standardization and whitening). The design parameters are selected via minimizing the K-fold CV error on the given training set. To clarify the procedure, let the total number of samples in the dataset be n. In each LOO iteration for generalization performance estimation, $n-1$ samples are used for training and the remaining sample is set aside for error estimation. The optimal design parameters are found as those that minimize the K-fold CV error on the $n-1$-sample training set. Then, a classifier is trained on the $n-1$-sample training set using the optimal parameters. Finally, the classifier is tested on the left-out sample. The above steps are repeated for all left-out samples. Note that the preprocessing steps are part of training and thus are repeated for each $n-1$-sample training set separately. For classifier design, we used LOO for all classifiers except for the L1LR, where we used $K=3$ due to computational limitations. Note that this should not be confused with classifier performance estimation, where LOO was used for evaluating all classifiers.

3. Application to Schizophrenia Diagnosis

3.1. *Participants*

Forty-three patients with schizophrenia were recruited from ongoing clinical research studies at the Nathan S. Kline Institute for Psychiatric Research. Diagnoses were based on the Structured Clinical Interview for DSM-IV Axis I Disorders, Patient Edition (SCID-I/P)[26] supplemented by information from family members and clinicians. All patients met DSM-IV criteria for schizophrenia or schizoaffective disorder. In addition, 43 healthy control subjects were recruited from the community. The groups were matched by gender, age, handedness, and parental socio-economic status. Exclusion criteria for control subjects included any major Axis I psychiatric disorder as determined from the SCID-I Non-patient Edition (SCID-I/NP).[27] Exclusion criteria for all study participants included history of seizures, head trauma, loss of consciousness for more than 30 minutes, major medical conditions, magnetic resonance contraindications, and history of alcohol or other drug dependence. This study was approved by the local Institutional Review Board and written informed consent was obtained from all study participants.

3.2. *Image Acquisition*

MRI scans were acquired on a 1.5 T Siemens Vision system (Erlangen, Germany). Diffusion-weighted images (DWIs) were acquired with a pulsed gradient, double spin echo, echo planar imaging sequence. Imaging parameters were: repetition time (TR) = 6000 ms, echo time (TE) = 100 ms, matrix = 128×128, field-of-view (FOV) = 320×320 mm^2, number of excitations (NEX) = 7, 19 slices, slice thickness = 5 mm, no gap. For each subject, eight volumes were acquired along noncollinear diffusion sensitizing gradient directions with $b = 1000$ s/mm^2, together with a volume without diffusion weighting ($b = 0$). A magnetization prepared rapidly acquired gradient echo (MPRAGE) T$_1$-weighted scan was also acquired to serve as a high-resolution anatomical reference. Imaging parameters were: TR = 11.6 ms, TE = 4.9 ms, matrix = 256×256, FOV = 256×256 mm, NEX = 1, 190 slices, slice thickness = 1 mm, no gap. In addition, a turbo dual spin echo proton density/T$_2$-weighted scan (TR = 5000 ms, TE = 22/90 ms, matrix = 256×256, FOV = 240 mm, 26 slices, slice thickness = 5 mm, no gap) was acquired at the same slice positions and orientation as the DWIs to aid in the co-registration process.

3.3. *Image Processing*

FA images for all participants were obtained from the DWIs using AFNI's 3dDWItoDT module (http://afni.nimh.nih.gov/afni) prior to image registration. FA images were then transformed into standard space using the steps described in detail elsewhere[28,29] and outlined below.

First, non-brain regions were removed from the MPRAGE images using FreeSurfer (http://surfer.nmr.mgh.harvard.edu). The skull-stripped MPRAGE images of all subjects were spatially normalized to the Montreal Neurologic Institute's

'Colin27' MRI volume[30] using the nonlinear registration module (3dwarper) of the Automatic Registration Toolbox (ART)[28] (http://nitrc.org/projects/art). For each subject, the MPRAGE volume was also registered to their T_2-weighted volume using a rigid-body 6-parameter linear transformation obtained from ART's multimodality image registration module.[31] This transformation was applied to the skull-stripped MPRAGE mask created above, which was then used to skull-strip the T_2-weighted volume.

To correct for the spatial distortion in the DWIs, the $b = 0$ image was registered to the skull-stripped T_2-weighted volume using ART's distortion correction module (unwarp2d). Finally, the FA volume for each subject was transformed into the stereotactic space of the 'Colin27' template by mathematically combining and applying the transformations obtained from the three registration steps outlined above: (1) nonlinear within-subject mapping of the $b = 0$ volume to the T_2-weighted volume for distortion correction; (2) rigid-body within-subject mapping of the T_2-weighted volume to MPRAGE volume; and (3) nonlinear between-subject mapping of the MPRAGE volume to the 'Colin27' reference volume. The resulting spatially normalized FA volumes were sampled to an isotropic voxel size of $2 \times 2 \times 2$ mm^3.

4. Results and Discussion

Table 1 summarizes the classification results for different algorithms. The table indicates that the SVC with the Gaussian kernel achieved a higher accuracy than the other classifiers, followed by the linear SVC, LGC, and kNNC. The L1LR and NLGC had the lowest performance. Among the linear classifiers, the linear SVC was slightly more accurate than the other classifiers. Moreover, for five out of seven classifiers, the specificity of the classifier was higher than its sensitivity.

Table 1. LOO classification accuracy for different classifiers. Sensitivity is measured with respect to the class of schizophrenia patients.

Classifier		Accuracy / Sensitivity / Specificity (%)
LGC		83.7 / 83.7 / 83.7
NLGC		77.9 / 74.4 / 81.4
SVC	Linear	84.9 / 83.7 / 86.0
	Gaussian	88.4 / 83.7 / 93.0
kNNC ($k = 15$)	DANN	82.6 / 83.7 / 81.4
	LMNN	84.9 / 83.7 / 86.0
L1LR		80.2 / 74.4 / 86.0

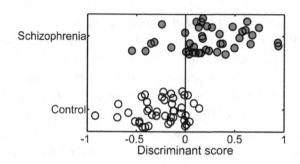

Fig. 3. Discriminant scores for the left-out test subjects in LOO obtained from the nonlinear SVC.

Fig. 3 shows the discriminant scores of the left-out test subjects in LOO obtained with the nonlinear SVC. Fig. 4(a) shows an axial slice of the image obtained by averaging the spatially normalized FA maps of all control subjects. Fig. 4(b)-(d) show the discriminant patterns for the same image slice.

Our results with the LGC showed a slight improvement in classification accuracy (83.7%) compared to those achieved by Caan et al.[13] (75%) and Caprihan et al.[14] (80%), and lower accuracy compared to that reported by Ardekani et al.[12] The differences in the reported accuracies may be attributed to variations in many factors such as cohort demographics, DTI acquisition protocol, inter-subject registration method, as well as differences in the dimensionality reduction algorithm.

The LGC as a linear generative classifier was competitive with the linear SVC as a linear discriminative classifier. This observation is consistent with previous results indicating that for high-dimensional data and small sample sizes, generative classifiers can achieve comparable or even higher accuracy than discriminative classifiers.[19]

The competitive performance offered by the kNNC highlights the importance of the choice of the distance metric for this classifier. While the generalization performance of the kNNC with the Euclidean metric declines rapidly with the dimensionality of the observation vector, voxel weighting schemes such as the ones in DANN and LMNN enable the kNNC to compete with the state-of-the-art methods for the classification of high-dimensional data.

As Table 1 indicates, the classification accuracy of the NLGC was lower than that of the LGC. The NLGC offers the advantage of operating in the image space, simplifying the interpretation of the discriminant pattern. However, this comes at the expense of a substantially larger number of parameters than for the LGC, which may have caused the inferior performance of the NLGC.

Table 1 also indicates that most of the classifiers achieved higher specificity than sensitivity. This may be attributed to the higher degree of variation of

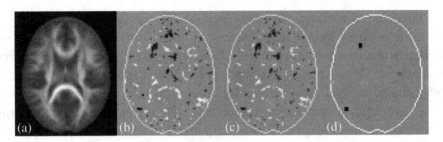

Fig. 4. (a) Average FA map across control subjects spatially normalized to standard space. (b)-(d) Discriminant patterns for the nonlinear SVC, LGC, and L1LR. The intensity of each voxel indicates the weight of that voxel in the discriminant function. For SVC and LGC, coefficients with the largest 10% absolute values are shown. For the L1LR, the nonzero coefficients have been dilated to improve visibility. Voxels with positive/negative weights are shown with lighter/darker shades of gray than the background.

patient images than those of controls, which in turn results in the higher variability of patient discriminant scores (Fig. 3).

The gradient of the nonlinear SVC evaluated at support vectors, $[\nabla f]_{s_j}$, $j = 1, ..., n_s$, yielded vectors pointing roughly in the same direction, indicating a nearly linear discriminant function. This enabled the visualization of the contribution of voxels to classification using (18) (Fig. 4(b)).

Fig. 4 indicates that the discriminant regions identified by the nonlinear SVC and the LGC are quite similar. This is notable considering that the two methods use different measures of class separation. The SVC maximizes the margin between the classes, whereas the LGC finds the largest ratio of between- to within-class variance.

Unlike the nonlinear SVC discriminant pattern in Fig. 4(b), the L1LR discriminant pattern in Fig. 4(d) was highly sparse. Interestingly, very few voxels from each of the larger regions in the SVC discriminant pattern contributed to the L1LR discriminant pattern. This is due to a characteristic property of the L_1 constraint. As pointed out by Zou and Hastie[32] in the context of L_1-regularized least squares, the constraint tends to force the classifier to select only one voxel from a group of highly correlated voxels, even though all those voxels may be strong predictors. This may be a limiting feature in neuroimaging studies for two reasons. First, clusters of voxels are preferred to individual voxels as they provide a higher degree of interpretability and reduced sensitivity to noise and inter-subject misregistration. Second, if the classification information is distributed among a large number of correlated voxels, the excessive sparseness of the discriminant pattern may diminish the classification accuracy. This limitation of L1LR may be addressed by using a combination of L_1 and L_2 constraints.[32]

A limitation of nonlinear SVCs (as well as other nonlinear classifiers) is that their corresponding discriminant pattern is more difficult to visualize and interpret. When interpretability is critical, the linear SVC may be preferred over the nonlinear SVC. Alternatively, the approximate method presented here or another similar method[33] may be used for interpretation.

The classification methods considered here were limited in that their resulting discriminant functions were either *overly* sparse (L1LR) or not sparse at all. The benefit of an *optimally* sparse classifier, such as a classifier using a sparse combination of clusters of voxels, is that its resulting discriminant pattern is more amenable to interpretation. Such a sparse classifier may potentially achieve better generalization performance. Future studies should investigate classifiers that are highly accurate and reasonably sparse at the same time. A potential contender is the combination of recursive feature elimination with SVC,[34] which has been observed to improve the classification accuracy in a functional MRI study.[35]

5. Conclusions

In this chapter, we reviewed several classical and state-of-the-art classifiers and compared their accuracy in schizophrenia diagnosis based on diffusion MRI. No previous study had determined the impact of the classifier on the accuracy of schizophrenia diagnosis. Our results based on a cohort of 43 patients and 43 controls suggest that the nonlinear SVC performed slightly better than the other classifiers, and may be the preferred classification method for schizophrenia diagnosis with DTI. Further studies with larger and more heterogeneous cohorts are needed to confirm this observation. Future work should also investigate whether alternative sparseness constraints and variable selection can further improve classifier performance in schizophrenia diagnosis.

Acknowledgments

This work was supported in part by National Institutes of Health grants R01 MH064783 to Matthew J. Hoptman, PhD, and R01 MH066374 to Pamela D. Butler, PhD.

References

1. C. Davatzikos, D. Shen, R. C. Gur, X. Wu, D. Liu, Y. Fan, P. Hughett, B. I. Turetsky and R. E. Gur, *Arch. Gen. Psychiatry* **62**, 1218 (2005).
2. Y. Fan, R. E. Gur, R. C. Gur, X. Wu, D. Shen, M. E. Calkins and C. Davatzikos, *Biol. Psychiatry* **63**, 118 (2008).
3. Y. Kawasaki, M. Suzuki, F. Kherif, T. Takahashi, S. Y. Zhou, K. Nakamura, M. Matsui, T. Sumiyoshi, H. Seto and M. Kurachi, *Neuroimage* **34**, 235 (2007).

4. Y. Liu, L. Teverovskiy, O. Carmichael, R. Kikinis, M. Shenton, C. S. Carter, V. A. Stenger, S. Davis, H. Aizenstein, J. Becker, O. Lopez and C. Meltzer, in *Proc. Int. Conf. Med. Image Comput. Comput. Assist. Interv.* (Saint-Malo, France, 2004), pp. 393-401.
5. M. Kubicki, R. McCarley, C. F. Westin, H. J. Park, S. Maier, R. Kikinis, F. A. Jolesz and M. E. Shenton, *J. Psychiatr. Res.* **41**, 15 (2007).
6. V. D. Calhoun, P. K. Maciejewski, G. D. Pearlson and K. A. Kiehl, *Hum. Brain Mapp.* **29**, 1265 (2008).
7. O. Demirci, V. Clark, V. Magnotta, N. Andreasen, J. Lauriello, K. Kiehl, G. Pearlson and V. Calhoun, *Brain Imaging Behav.* **2**, 207 (2008).
8. J. Ford, L. Shen, M. F, L. A. Flashman and A. J. Saykin, in *Proc. IEEE Joint EMBS/BMES Conf.* (Houston, TX, 2002), pp. 48-49.
9. P. J. Basser, J. Mattiello and D. LeBihan, *Biophys. J.* **66**, 259 (1994).
10. P. J. Basser and C. Pierpaoli, *J. Magn. Reson. B* **111**, 209 (1996).
11. I. Ellison-Wright and E. Bullmore, *Schizophr. Res.* **108**, 3 (2009).
12. B. A. Ardekani, A. Tabesh, S. Sevy, D. G. Robinson, R. M. Bilder and P. R. Szeszko, *Hum. Brain Mapp.* **32**, 1 (2011).
13. M. W. Caan, K. A. Vermeer, L. J. van Vliet, C. B. Majoie, B. D. Peters, G. J. den Heeten and F. M. Vos, *Med. Image Anal.* **10**, 841 (2006).
14. A. Caprihan, G. D. Pearlson and V. D. Calhoun, *Neuroimage* **42**, 675 (2008).
15. M. Ingalhalikar, S. Kanterakis, R. Gur, T. P. Roberts and R. Verma, in *Proc. Int. Conf. Med. Image Comput. Comput. Assist. Interv.* (Beijing, China, 2010), pp. 558-65.
16. Y. Rathi, J. Malcolm, O. Michailovich, J. Goldstein, L. Seidman, R. W. McCarley, C. F. Westin and M. E. Shenton, in *Proc. Int. Conf. Med. Image Comput. Comput. Assist. Interv.* (Beijing, China, 2010), pp. 657-65.
17. R. O. Duda, P. E. Hart and D. G. Stork, *Pattern Classification.* (Wiley, New York, ed. 2nd, 2001).
18. L. Devroye, L. Gyorfi and G. Lugosi, *A Probabilistic Theory of Pattern Recognition.* (Springer, New York, 1996).
19. A. Y. Ng and M. I. Jordan, in *Proc. Advances in Neural Information Processing Systems 14*, T. G. Dietterich, S. Becker, Z. Ghahramani, Eds. (MIT Press, Cambridge, MA, 2002), pp. 841-848.
20. V. Vapnik, *Statistical Learning Theory.* (Wiley, New York, 1998).
21. G. J. McLachlan, *Discriminant Analysis and Statistical Pattern Recognition.* (Wiley, New York, 1992).
22. A. Y. Ng, in *Proc. Int. Conf. Machine Learning.* (Banff, Canada, 2004), pp. 78-85.
23. K. Koh, S. J. Kim and S. Boyd, *J Mach. Learn. Res.* **8**, 1519 (2007).
24. T. Hastie and R. Tibshirani, *IEEE Trans. Pattern Anal. Machine Intell.* **18**, 607 (1996).
25. K. Q. Weinberger, J. Blitzer and L. K. Saul, in *Proc. Advances in Neural Information Processing Systems 18*, Y. Weiss, B. Scholkopf, J. Platt, Eds. (MIT Press, Cambridge, MA, 2006), pp. 1473-1480.
26. M. B. First, R. L. Spitzer, M. Gibbon and J. B. W. Williams, *Structured Clinical Interview for DSM-IV-TR Axis I Disorders, Research Version, Patient Edition (SCID-I/P).* (Biometrics Research, New York State Psychiatric Institute, New York, 2001).
27. M. B. First, R. L. Spitzer, M. Gibbon and J. B. W. Williams, *Structured Clinical Interview for DSM-IV-TR Axis I Disorders, Research Version, Non-patient Edition (SCID-I/NP).* (Biometrics Research, New York State Psychiatric Institute, New York, 2001).
28. B. A. Ardekani, S. Guckemus, A. Bachman, M. J. Hoptman, M. Wojtaszek and J. Nierenberg, *J. Neurosci. Methods* **142**, 67 (2005).
29. B. A. Ardekani, J. Nierenberg, M. J. Hoptman, D. C. Javitt and K. O. Lim, *Neuroreport* **14**, 2025 (2003).

30. C. J. Holmes, R. Hoge, L. Collins, R. Woods, A. W. Toga and A. C. Evans, *J. Comput. Assist. Tomogr.* **22**, 324 (1998).
31. B. A. Ardekani, M. Braun, B. F. Hutton, I. Kanno and H. Iida, *J. Comput. Assist. Tomogr.* **19**, 615 (1995).
32. H. Zou and T. Hastie, *J. Royal Stat. Soc. B* **67**, 301 (2005).
33. Z. Lao, D. Shen, Z. Xue, B. Karacali, S. M. Resnick and C. Davatzikos, *Neuroimage* **21**, 46 (2004).
34. I. Guyon, J. Weston, S. Barnhill and V. Vapnik, *Machine Learning* **46**, 389 (2002).
35. F. De Martino, G. Valente, N. Staeren, J. Ashburner, R. Goebel and E. Formisano, *Neuroimage* **43**, 44 (2008).

CHAPTER 17

ON COMPRESSED SENSING RECONSTRUCTION FOR MAGNETIC RESONANCE IMAGING

Benjamin Paul Berman, Sagar Mandava, and Ali Bilgin*

University of Arizona
Tucson, Arizona
*E-mail: bilgin@email.arizona.edu

Magnetic Resonance Imaging (MRI) is a medical imaging modality that generates images without subjecting the patient to ionizing radiation. Accelerating data acquisition in MRI is critical. The duration of the scan affects image quality and patient throughput but, perhaps more importantly, faster data acquisition also enables novel MRI applications which are infeasible under current data acquisition rates. Compressed Sensing (CS) is a recent undersampled data acquisition and reconstruction framework that has been shown to achieve significant acceleration in MRI. Sparse transformations and incoherent measurements are at the heart of CS. This chapter describes the basic principles of CS and how they apply to MRI, as well as the various optimization algorithms that are used for image reconstruction.

1. Introduction

Magnetic Resonance Imaging (MRI) is a non-invasive medical imaging technique that is based on the principles of nuclear magnetic resonance. Today, MRI is routinely used in the clinic to obtain highly detailed images of internal organs, blood vessels, muscle, joints, tumors, areas of infection, etc. MRI has several attributes that makes it a desirable medical imaging technique. Since MRI does not subject patients to harmful ionizing radiation, it is considered to be non-invasive. Thus, MRI is often used for longitudinal non-invasive monitoring of patients. MRI allows arbitrary orientation, two-dimensional and three-dimensional imaging, as well as dynamic and functional imaging. One of the most useful attributes of MRI is the flexible contrast mechanisms it provides. Despite all of these useful attributes, a fundamental problem associated with the use of MRI in a clinical or preclinical setting remains to be the lengthy examinations. Long data acquisition times lead to high healthcare costs and increase patient discomfort during the exam. In addition, long scans often lead to reduction in image quality due to patient motion during the scan. Perhaps most importantly, long data acquisition times prevent use of conventional MRI in new clinical applications that require large amounts of information to be acquired over very small periods of time.

Conventional MRI techniques are designed using the celebrated Nyquist–Shannon sampling theorem [39]. This theorem states the sampling requirements for bandlimited signals. Recently, a new theory of sampling, called Compressive Sampling or Compressed Sensing (CS) [6, 13], has emerged as an alternative to the Nyquist–Shannon sampling theory. In contrast to the Nyquist-Shannon theory, the CS theory relies on sparsity or compressibility of signals. The CS theory illustrates that a signal which has a sparse or compressible representation can be recovered from a small number of random linear measurements. In many cases, the number of measurements needed to recover a signal using the CS theory can be significantly smaller than the number of measurements suggested by the Nyquist–Shannon sampling theorem. This novel mathematical framework has received significant attention in the MRI community, because the CS theory promises to significantly accelerate data acquisition. The goal of this chapter is to provide a brief introduction to CS and its application to MRI.

Since its recent introduction to MRI [27, 28], applications of CS in MRI has exploded. CS has been used to accelerate dynamic MRI where the goal is to reconstruct a series of temporally varying images [16, 23, 32, 33]. There has also been great recent interest to use CS for quantitative MR parameter mapping [11, 4, 21]. MR parameter mapping requires multiple images with varying contrast to be acquired in succession which usually results in long acquisition times. CS has also been used for water-fat seperation [12], diffusion weighted MRI [34, 44]. It is clear that CS will greatly enhance the clinical utility of MRI.

This chapter is organized as follows: In Section 2, the basic principles of signal generation and detection in MRI are described. Section 3 introduces the CS theory. Sections 4 and 5 discuss sparsity and data acquisition in MRI, respectively, as these are the two key principles behind successful utilization of CS theory. Section 6 describes several algorithms that can be used to reconstruct MR images from compressive measurements.

2. Principles of Signal Generation and Detection in MRI

This section provides a brief introduction to signal generation and detection in MRI. The goal of this section is to provide sufficient description to enable comprehension of the discussion in subsequent sections. For more detailed description, the reader is referred to one of many excellent textbooks on MRI [2, 25, 31].

In MRI, the physical quantity being imaged is the transverse magnetization $\widetilde{M}_{xy}$ of excited protons. An object is placed in a strong static magnetic field $B_0\hat{z}$, and this causes the protons in the object to align with the field. The collective magnetization of these protons is disturbed from equilibrium by a radio frequency pulse oscillating at the Larmor frequency, which is proportional to the $B_0\hat{z}$ field. This perturbation generates a component of the magnetization in the transverse plane perpendicular to $B_0\hat{z}$. The precession of this component is a time varying signal $S(t)$ which is measured through induced current in receiver coils. The analog signal received by the coils is digitized so that the end result is a digital data vector.

In order to associate the transverse magnetization with spatial information, linear magnetic gradient fields $(G_x(t), G_y(t), G_z(t))$ are modulated in a controlled fashion. The time varying signal $S(t)$ can then be stated as

$$S(t) \propto \int \widetilde{M}_{xy}(x, y, z, t) e^{-i\gamma(x \int G_x(t)dt + y \int G_y(t)dt + z \int G_z(t)dt)} dx\, dy\, dz \qquad (1)$$

where $\widetilde{M}_{xy}(x, y, z, t)$ denotes the transverse magnetization that varies in space and time. γ denotes the gyromagnetic ratio. Simplifying Equation 1 using

$$k_i(t) = \frac{\gamma}{2\pi} \int G_i(t)dt \qquad (2)$$

where i denotes each spatial dimension x, y, and z, we can obtain

$$S(t) \propto \int \widetilde{M}_{xy}(x, y, z, t) e^{-2\pi i(x k_x(t) + y k_y(t) + z k_z(t))} dx\, dy\, dz \qquad (3)$$

and this equation illustrates the measured signal $S(t)$ is simply the spatial Fourier transform of the transverse magnetization $\widetilde{M}_{xy}(x, y, z, t)$. This Fourier formalism leads to a convenient representation of the measurement space called the k-space, where the coordinates k_x, k_y, k_z are the Fourier conjugate variables of x, y and z respectively. Thus, changing the gradient fields appropriately, one can cover the entire k-space and acquire Fourier coefficients of the object that is being imaged. In conventional MRI, the Fourier coefficients that are needed to reconstruct the object at the desired resolution without aliasing are acquired sequentially. Once all coefficients are acquired, the object of interest is reconstructed using an inverse Fourier transform.

One of the main challenges with the data acquisition process in MRI is that the transverse magnetization $\widetilde{M}_{xy}$ is characterized by an exponential decay, called the T_2 decay:

$$\widetilde{M}_{xy}(x, y, z, t) = M_{xy}(x, y, z, 0) e^{\frac{-t}{T2(x,y,z)}} \qquad (4)$$

As shown in Equation 4, the spatially-varying time constant T_2 describes the speed of decay of the transverse magnetization. In biological materials, this decay time can be quite short and this means that there is a finite amount of time before the signal decays to zero. Thus, the measurements must be performed within this finite amount of time. Unfortunately, the strength (and slew rates) of the gradients do not usually allow coverage of the entire k-space within this short period of time after just one excitation (i.e. one radio frequency pulse). Thus, many excitations are needed to measure the entire k-space. This repetition can be very time consuming and the sequential nature of such data acquisition is one of the main reasons for long examinations in MRI.

3. Compressed Sensing Theory

The idea behind CS comes from traditional signal and image compression. In conventional compression, transforms are used to exploit dependencies in the data. A signal is first transformed into a domain where the signal energy is concentrated into a small number of transform domain coefficients. During compression, the vast majority of the transform-domain coefficients that have small magnitude can be discarded to yield high compression ratios without significantly reducing fidelity of the decompressed signal.

CS asks the question: if we end up keeping only a small set of coefficients that can efficiently represent the signal during compression, why do we need to acquire so much information in the first place? In 2006, Emmanuel Candès, Justin Romberg, Terrance Tao, and David Donoho provided the answer [6, 13] , that in many cases, we don't need to acquire much data at all. In fact if an image of size N^2 can be compressed to S points using some known transform, then by using a particular measurement system, the image can be reconstructed not from $\sim N^2$ measurements, but from $\sim S \log(N)$ measurements [36].

To elaborate, CS relies on two fundamental assumptions:

(1) *Transform sparsity* – There exists a transformation Ψ such that for image x,

$$\alpha = \Psi x \tag{5}$$

  is sparse. In other words, for α the number of nonzero elements S is significantly less than its size.

(2) *Measurement incoherence* – The basis in which the measurements are made is uncorrelated to the basis in which the image is sparse. If Φ is the measurement basis, then $y = \Phi x$ is the data that is measured from the underlying image x. In order for these measurements to be considered incoherent to the sparse transform Ψ,

$$\mu(\Phi, \Psi) = \max_{i,j} \; |(\phi_i, \psi_j)| \tag{6}$$

  needs to be as small as possible. Here ϕ and ψ are the vectors that build the measurement and sparsity bases respectively.

Minimizing the mutual coherence μ guarantees that each measurement will lead to new and distinguishing information about the sparse coefficients α [7]. This relationship binds the two fundamental properties of CS, and can be formalized as the Restricted Isometry Property [37].

To better understand the measurement framework of CS, let us compare it to traditional Nyquist–Shannon sampling. In conventional signal processing, the sampling frequency in the spatial or temporal domain is determined by the bandwidth of the signal in Fourier space. Therefore in conventional MRI, the sampling frequency in k-space is determined by the field-of-view of the object in image space, while resolution requirements dictate the number of samples to be acquired. If the sampling is not fine enough, i.e. the Nyquist criterion is not satisfied, then the reconstructed image will contain aliasing.

CS data acquisition may be very different than Nyquist sampling. Firstly, CS takes place in a discrete setting. And secondly, the CS measurements can correspond to inner products between the object and any general function. Whereas for a traditional sampling scheme, measurements correspond to inner products between the underlying data and delta functions that are uniformly spaced. In fact, many of the analytical results of CS theory rely on the measurement basis being random Gaussian noise. That is, in the theoretical case, each data point is a linear projection of the image onto a random vector.

CS theory adopts the use of random measurements because they are universally incoherent with any sparsity basis. For most sensing schemes, including MRI, we do not have the luxury of generating data through such projections. MRI measurements are made based on the Fourier transform as shown in Equation 3, meaning linear projection of the image onto complex exponential functions with particular spatial frequencies. At first, this may seem like great news, because the Fourier basis is incoherent to the canonical pixel basis of an image. But we cannot forget about the first fundamental assumption of CS; it is very rare for a medical image to be sparse in the pixel basis!

Writing the forward problem in matrix form helps in generalizing the undersampled data acquisition problem into a simple system of linear equations. Equation 7 places this system of equations in matrix form for x the image and y the data.

$$y = \Phi x \tag{7}$$

In order to accelerate the scan, less data is acquired, meaning that this system is underdetermined, and simple reconstruction from the inverse is not possible. This problem is not new, and even before CS, accelerated reconstruction techniques have a long tradition in MRI. For example, one may utilize the Hermitian symmetry of the Fourier transform together with phase correction in order to reduce the amount of data being acquired by almost half [25]. Another example is called parallel imaging, which reconstructs the image using data that is simultaneously recorded in multiple coils, each with a unique spatial sensitivity profile [19]. The common feature between these methods is the use of additional prior information to build reconstructed images from fewer data points.

When the data is undersampled and the inverse transform is not well defined, image reconstruction is typically cast as an optimization problem.

$$\underset{x}{\operatorname{argmin}} \ ||\Phi x - y||_2 + R(x) \tag{8}$$

Equation 8 expresses the goal of minimizing the error between the reconstruction and the data that was originally collected, as well as minimizing a cost function $R(x)$ that incorporates additional information or assumptions that is anticipated for the reconstructed image. These terms are called data agreement and regularization, respectively. In the case of CS, image sparsity is used to regularize the reconstruction problem. Thus, the general reconstruction problem in Equation 8 turns into Equation 9

$$\underset{x}{\operatorname{argmin}} \ \|\Phi x - y\|_2 + \|\Psi x\|_0 \tag{9}$$

The notation $\|\cdot\|_0$ is a simple count of the number of nonzero entries — a direct measure of the sparsity. Though it is expressed as a norm, and even referred to as the "ℓ_0 norm", it is important to understand that it does not satisfy the conditions of a norm at all. The optimization problems seeks to pick the sparsest vector Ψx that can explain the measurements. In practice, it turns out to be an NP-hard combinatorial search with no solution expected in feasible times for even very small problems. A major breakthrough was to show that under certain conditions, convex relaxation to the ℓ_1 norm is equivalent to solving the ℓ_0 norm problem [6, 10, 13, 14]. Using this norm instead changes the optimization from a NP-hard combinatorial search, to a convex problem that may be iterated toward its minimizer using a variety of methods. Section 6 will highlight three examples of these reconstruction methods.

4. Sparsity in MRI

Most medical images, like natural images, are not sparse in the image domain, and they must be transformed into a domain in which they are. In this section we will examine the sparsifying effects of the wavelet transform, and the total variation operator.

4.1. *Wavelet sparsity*

The wavelet transform is commonly used in many signal and image processing applications [1, 9, 40, 42]. It forms the backbone of the popular image compression standard JPEG-2000 as it can generate very good sparse approximations of natural image content in the wavelet transform domain. An example of this is shown in Figure 1 where a representative brain MR image is first transformed into the wavelet domain. Figure 1(b) shows the wavelet coefficients in the transform domain. These coefficients can be sorted according to amplitude (Figure 1(c)) which shows that coefficients decay very rapidly, i.e. most of the signal energy has been compacted into few large coefficients. A simple thresholding operation that would set 80% of the smallest wavelet coefficients to zero would still yield an image with high perceptual quality (Figure 1(d)) upon applying the inverse wavelet transform to the thresholded coefficients. Hence MR images, like most natural images, can be highly compressed via wavelet transforms.

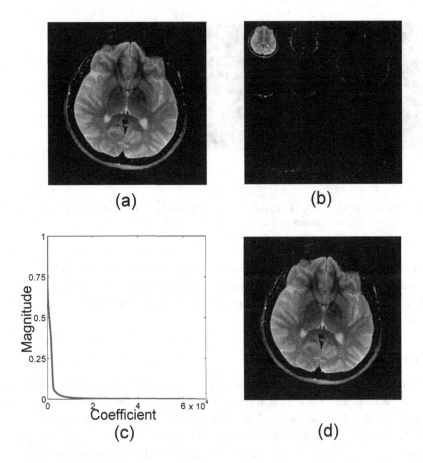

Fig. 1. Wavelet sparsity in MRI. (a) Representative MR image, (b) its wavelet decomposition, (c) wavelet coefficients sorted by magnitude and (d) sparse approximation with just the top 20% of the wavelet coefficients.

4.2. *Total Variation*

Total variation was first introduced within the context of image denoising [38]. Given an image $I(x, y)$, the total variation of the image is defined as

$$TV = \sum_{\forall x,y} \sqrt{(I(x+1, y) - I(x, y))^2 + (I(x, y+1) - I(x, y))^2} \qquad (10)$$

In other words, the total variation is defined as the sum of the absolute gradient of the image. Many natural images, including MR images, exhibit large smooth areas with relatively small number of edges. Such images have low total variation values compared to images with excessive, noise-like detail. This is illustrated in Figure 2 using a MR brain image. Figure 2(a) shows the original image and Figure 2(b) shows the absolute gradient of the image. It can be seen that the absolute gradient for this image is very sparse and this sparsity leads to a low total variation. The absolute

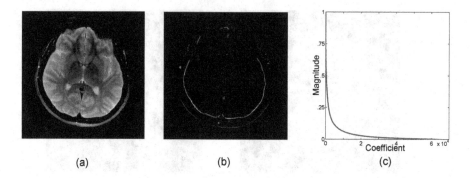

Fig. 2.   TV sparsity in MRI. (a) Representative MR image, (b) absolute gradient of the image and (c) absolute gradient values sorted according to magnitude.

gradient values sorted in decreasing order of magnitude are shown Figure 2(c). The plot confirms that only a very small fraction of the absolute gradient values are large. Hence, the TV operation can efficiently sparsify images that are approximately piecewise–smooth.

5. Data Acquisition in MRI

The standard MR experiment involves filling k-space with enough points to satisfy the field of view and resolution requirements. It is possible to fill arbitrary points in k-space, but this is impractical as movement in k-space is dependent on the area under the gradient functions as seen in Equation 3. Finite rise time and peak amplitudes of the gradients restrict us to acquire smooth and contiguous trajectories.

From a sampling perspective, acquiring less data in the Fourier space will create aliasing artifacts in the image space. From a CS standpoint, the undersampling pattern used should ideally create highly incoherent aliasing artifacts in the sparse domain. Incoherent in this context means that the artifacts are irregular and distinguishable from the object. Highly incoherent artifacts looks like additive random noise in the sparsity basis. The CS reconstruction will use the sparsity of the image to separate the actual signal above a certain noise level. Hence, the acquisition signal-to-noise ratio of the imaging experiment is also important in the success of CS.

Acquiring k-space data on Cartesian grid points is very popular and forms the vast majority of the present day clinical scans. Image reconstruction from these trajectories is simple because the fast Fourier transform can be applied to a fully-sampled uniformly-spaced grid. However, when this data is undersampled by uniformly skipping lines along one dimension of the grid, there is very coherent aliasing as the object folds over itself in the field of view. In terms of compressed sensing measurements, these artifacts are difficult to reduce due to their structure, intensity and similarity to the object of interest. This situation is shown in Figure 3.

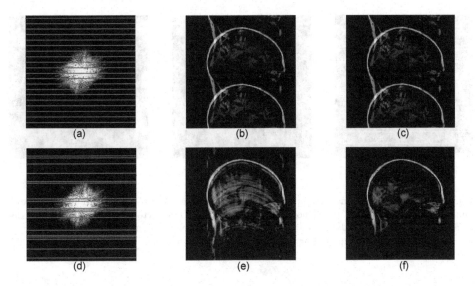

Fig. 3.   Uniform and random undersampling of Cartesian k-space lines and the associated minimum energy and minimum ℓ_1 norm reconstructions. (a)Uniformly undersampled Cartesian trajectory, (b) pseudo-inverse reconstruction for data acquired using the trajectory in (a), (c) reconstruction using ℓ_1 norm minimization exhibits no suppression of artifacts, (d)randomly undersampled Cartesian trajectory, (e) pseudo-inverse reconstruction for data acquired using the trajectory in (d), (f) reconstruction using ℓ_1 norm minimization exhibits residual aliasing artifacts.

Figure 3(a) shows the Fourier transform of the brain image shown in Figure 1(a). As shown in the figure, every other line of the Fourier transform has been skipped to achieve an undersampling factor of two. Figure 3(b) shows reconstructed image obtained using the minimum energy reconstruction (pseudo-inverse). As expected, the image exhibits the half field-of-view ghost artifact due to aliasing. The image reconstruction using ℓ_1 norm minimization is presented in Figure 3(c). It can be seen that the ghost artifacts are also present in this image. Due to the coherent nature of the aliasing artifacts, the CS reconstruction algorithm has not yielded significantly better results than the minimum energy reconstruction in this case.

Randomly skipping lines would on the face of it seem the best way to generate incoherent artifacts. An example of this scenario is shown in Figure 3(d) where half of the lines were randomly picked. Figure 3(e) shows reconstructed image obtained using the minimum energy reconstruction (pseudo-inverse). Clearly the artifacts here are incoherent when compared with the ones in Figure 3(b). The image reconstruction using ℓ_1 norm minimization is presented in Figure 3(f). Residual aliasing artifacts are still clearly visible in this case. In these reconstructions, the measurement basis Φ is the Fourier basis while a wavelet basis was used as the sparsity basis Ψ. It is well known that the Fourier-wavelet basis pair are not perfectly incoherent. Low frequency Fourier coefficients tend to be clustered around the coarse scale wavelet coefficients. For most MR images of interest, the Fourier coefficients at low

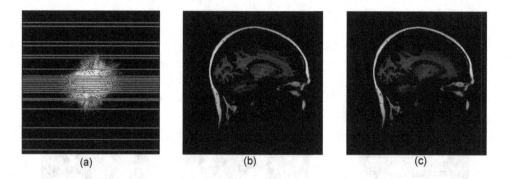

Fig. 4. Variable density undersampling (VDS) of Cartesian k-space lines and the associated minimum energy and minimum ℓ_1 norm reconstructions. a)VDS Cartesian trajectory, (b) pseudo-inverse reconstruction for data acquired using the trajectory in (a), (c) reconstruction using ℓ_1 norm minimization clear the aliasing artifacts clearly visible in (b).

frequencies contain most of the energy i.e most of the energy of images tends to be concentrated around the center of k-space. Uniform and random undersampling of the Cartesian lines generate artifacts that do not take into account this energy distribution. This is why the image reconstruction using ℓ_1 norm minimization fails in these cases.

To make the undersampling aliasing artifacts incoherent, a variable density sampling scheme may fully sample the low frequency region and undersample the higher frequencies [27, 29, 41]. This kind of undersampling helps in distributing the aliasing artifacts in a more incoherent fashion while accounting for the energy distribution in k-space. An example is shown in Figure 4. The Fourier domain undersampling pattern is shown in Figure 4(a). As can be seen in the figure, the center of k-space is sampled fully while the higher frequencies are undersampled according to a power law. The image obtained using the minimum energy reconstruction (pseudo-inverse) is shown in Figure 4(b). It can be seen that the aliasing artifacts are significantly incoherent compared to the image in Figure 3(b), although they are still noticeable. The image reconstruction using ℓ_1 norm minimization is presented in Figure 4(c). It can be seen that the aliasing artifacts were greatly reduced by the CS algorithm due to their incoherent nature.

Artifacts from non-Cartesian trajectories such as radial can be more incoherent compared to those from Cartesian trajectories. As seen in Figures 3–4, skipping k-space lines on the grid leads to artifacts that spread only in one direction. Figure 5(a) illustrates an undersampled radial trajectory where 68 lines and 256 samples along each radial line were used to sample the Fourier transform of a 256×256 image (this amounts to a 6-fold acceleration). Radial reconstruction cannot directly utilize the inverse fast Fourier transform (FFT) for reconstruction since the acquired data does not lie on a uniform Cartesian grid. A filtered backprojection can be used to transform the radial k-space data back to image domain. Alternatively,

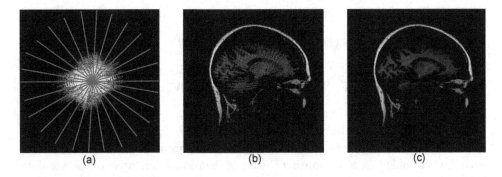

Fig. 5.   Six fold undersampled radial k-space, (b) the associated backprojection reconstruction and (c) minimum ℓ_1 norm reconstruction.

nonuniform fast Fourier transform (NUFFT) techniques which rely on interpolating the data onto a uniform Cartesian grid followed by a FFT can be used for reconstruction. In fact, NUFFT is a convenient method of reconstruction for any non-Cartesian trajectory [15]. Figure 5(b) illustrates the image obtained by using NUFFT on the undersampled data in Figure 5(a). The resulting streaking artifacts can be seen in the figure. Figure 5(c) illustrates the image obtained by using ℓ_1 norm minimization with the same data. It can be seen that the streaking artifacts were greatly reduced at the expense of some blurring.

6. Reconstruction Methods

So far we have introduced the compressed sensing MRI optimization problem, and various techniques for finding sparsity and optimizing measurements. But solving the optimization is another issue that often relies on computationally intensive iterative algorithms. Here we will highlight some of these methods that vary in their approach to the minimization problem. In terms of previous notation, the measurement basis Φ will be the undersampled Fourier transform $\mathcal{F}$. The sparsity bases Ψ may vary as wavelets or total variation, W or TV respectively.

6.1. *Nonlinear Conjugate Gradient (NLCG)*

NLCG is a useful method for solving optimization problems; it determines the minimum by using the derivative of the objective function. NLCG is based on the method for solving linear systems called conjugate gradient [20].

For CS MRI, it is useful to include sparse penalties for both wavelets and total variation. Thus, NLCG may be used to reconstruct images from the problem

$$\underset{x}{\mathrm{argmin}}\ \left\|\mathcal{F}x - y\right\|_2^2 + \lambda_1 \left\|Wx\right\|_1 + \lambda_2 \left\|TV(x)\right\|_1 \tag{11}$$

By solving the unconstrained problem, this method can be readily modified to include other types of regularization, with weights λ associated to each component.

The gradient of the objective function can be computed term by term as follows:

$$\nabla_x \left(||\mathcal{F}x - y||_2^2 \right) = 2\mathcal{F}^*(\mathcal{F}x - y) \tag{12}$$

$$\nabla_x \left(||Wx||_1 \right) \approx W^* D^{-1} W x \tag{13}$$

$$\nabla_x \left(||TV(x)||_1 \right) \approx TV^*(D^{-1}TV(x)) \tag{14}$$

The matrix D is diagonal such that $d_i = \sqrt{(\Psi x)_i^*(\Psi x)_i + \mu}$. The parameter μ is used to smooth the function near its minimum, and Ψ represents the either of the sparse transforms, wavelets or total variation as appropriate. Computing the ℓ_1 derivative is analogous to computing the one dimensional derivative of the absolute value.

$$\frac{d}{dx}(|x|) \approx \frac{d}{dx}(\sqrt{x^2 + \mu}) = \frac{x}{\sqrt{x^2 + \mu}} \tag{15}$$

Once the gradient is computed, it is rescaled using an iterative line-search, and then subtracted from the reconstructed image. This process repeats until it has converged to the minimizer.

The NLCG convergence rate, as well as the minimizer itself, depend on the value of the weighting parameters λ_i [17]. Furthermore, this value is dependent on the scale of the various terms in the objective function (data agreement, and degree of sparsity with various transformations). Techniques exist to optimize (L–curve method [18]) or to automate (maximum likelihood method [22]) the selection of these weights, but they are chosen empirically in many cases.

In 2007, Lustig *et al.* released a toolbox called sparseMRI that uses NLCG to reconstruct MR images [27]. Over the years, it has served as a benchmark and foundation for many projects in CS MRI ([27] has been cited over 1000 times as of the date of this publication).

Table 1. The nonlinear conjugate gradient procedure.

0	Initialize x_0, $\Delta x_0 = -\nabla_x f(x_0)$
1	Line search for $t = \underset{t>0}{\operatorname{argmin}} f(x_i + t\Delta x_i)$
2	Update reconstruction $x_{i+1} = x_i + t\Delta x_i$
3	Update gradient $\Delta x_{i+1} = -\nabla_x f(x_{i+1}) + \frac{||\nabla_x f(x_{i+1})||_2^2}{||\nabla_x f(x_i)||_2^2}\Delta x_i$
4	Iterate steps 1 through 3 until convergence
	$f(x) = ||\mathcal{F}x - y||_2^2 + \lambda_1 ||Wx||_1 + \lambda_2 ||TV(x)||_1$

6.2. *Projection Onto Convex Sets (POCS)*

POCS is an algorithm that does not rely on weights, and aims to solve the constrained optimization problem.

$$\underset{\alpha}{\operatorname{argmin}} ||\alpha||_1 \text{ such that } \mathcal{F}x = y, \Psi x = \alpha \tag{16}$$

Here we think of the set of reconstructed images where the data agrees, and the set where the sparse transform applies as a convex sets [45]. The objective function can be minimized iteratively, while it is projected onto these sets to incorporate the constraints. For an ℓ_1 problem, soft-thresholding is used to enforce sparsity: elements below the threshold are set to zero, while other elements are shifted toward zero [35].

$$\text{SoftThresh}(\alpha, \lambda) = \begin{cases} \alpha - \lambda, & \text{if } \alpha \geq \lambda \\ 0, & \text{if } |\alpha| < \lambda \\ \alpha + \lambda, & \text{if } \alpha \leq -\lambda \end{cases} \tag{17}$$

POCS may be less stable compared to the nonlinear conjugate gradient, but since its introduction in 1933 modifications have been made that may improve the algorithm depending on the applications [43, 24]. It has been used in MRI due to its computational simplicity and ability to account for additional constraints [8]. Recently, the parallel imaging technique called SPIRiT has used POCS with CS to reconstruct images from multiple receiver coils [26, 30].

Table 2. The projection onto convex sets procedure.

0	Initialize x_0
1	Let $\beta = \mathcal{F}x_i$, restrict β to y at acquired points
2	Let $\alpha = \Psi\mathcal{F}^{-1}\beta$
3	Threshold $\alpha = \text{SoftThresh}(\alpha, \lambda)$
4	Update $x_{i+1} = \Psi^{-1}\alpha$
5	Iterate steps 1 through 4 until convergence

6.3. *Iterative Hard Thresholding (IHT)*

In an alternative form of the imaging problem, the data agreement term is minimized under the constraint of the true sparsity.

$$\underset{x}{\text{argmin}} \; \|\mathcal{F}x - y\|_2^2 \text{ such that } \|\Psi x\|_0 \leq K \tag{18}$$

IHT combines gradient descent and thresholding to solve this problem. While soft-thresholding is used to minimize the ℓ_1 norm, hard-thresholding may be used to minimize the "ℓ_0" norm. The hard-thresholding operation is defined as

$$\text{HardThresh}(\alpha, \lambda) = \begin{cases} \alpha, & \text{if } |\alpha| \geq \lambda \\ 0, & \text{otherwise} \end{cases} \tag{19}$$

The convergence of this algorithm was proven in 2009 by Blumensath and Davies [5]. By the nature of this constrained optimization problem, IHT is a good choice when a certain level of sparsity is expected. It has been used in MR applications where the sparse transform is learned from a training data set [3].

Table 3.   The iterative hard thresholding procedure.

0	Initialize x_0
1	Compute $\Delta x_i = -\mu 2 \mathcal{F}^*(\mathcal{F} x_i - y)$
2	Let $\alpha = \Psi(x_i + \Delta x_i)$
3	Threshold $\alpha = \text{HardThresh}(\alpha, \lambda)$
4	Update $x_{i+1} = \Psi^{-1}\alpha$
5	Iterate steps 1 through 4 until convergence

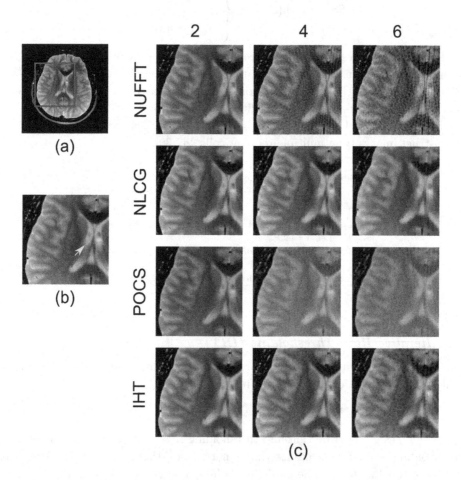

Fig. 6.   (a) The underlying brain image (b) The underlying region of interest, the arrows point to features that vary between each method and undersampling factor (c) Image reconstructions through various methods and undersampling factors. Data is acquired from radial sampling, the columns are undersampled by a factor of 2, 4, and 6. The first row of images are reconstructed using NUFFT, a pseudo-inverse of the data. The second row contains images reconstructed using NLCG (Table 1). Row three reconstructions utilized POCS (Table 2), and row four IHT (Table 3).

6.4. *Comparison*

Because these reconstruction methods vary in the optimization problems that they solve, the images to which they converge also vary. In the Figure 6, the three methods from this section are compared for different undersampling factors.

The first row of NUFFT reconstructions in Figure 6(c) do not use CS regularization, and lead to significant aliasing. Each reconstruction method detailed in this section solves a different reconstruction problem (Equations 11, 16, 18), but they each incorporate a sparse penalty. All three of the algorithms reduce aliasing. NLCG reconstructions appear to contain the least amount of sampling artifacts, but may also be over–smoothed, as is apparent in the 6-fold undersampling case. POCS seem to be less effective at removing artifacts and there is noticeable contrast loss with POCS. IHT remains somewhat noisy with 4 and 6-fold undersampling, but has good contrast.

7. Conclusion

This chapter has provided an overview of the requirements and the means for applying CS in MRI. CS will continue to play an important role in accelerating the data acquisition rates beyond the current state of art. This is vital in the pursuit of new applications that are currently constrained by scan times.

8. Acknowledgment

It has been a great honor and privilege to receive support from the ARCS Foundation and the Papadopoulos family.

References

1. A. N. Akansu and R. A. Haddad, *Multiresolution Signal Decomposition: Transforms, Subbands, and Wavelets*, (Academic Press, 1992).
2. M. A. Bernstein, K. F. King, and X. J. Zho, *Handbook of MRI Pulse Sequences*, (Academic Press, 2004).
3. A. Bilgin, Y. Kim, F. Liu, and M. Nadar, *Proc. Annual Meeting of ISMRM.* 4887 (2010).
4. K. T. Block, M. Uecker and J. Frahm, *IEEE Trans. Medical Imaging.* **28**, 1759 (2009).
5. T. Blumensath and M. E. Davies, *Appl. Comp. Harmonic Analysis.* **27**, 265 (2009).
6. E. Candès, J. Romberg, and T. Tao, *IEEE Trans. Information Theory.* **52**, 489 (2006).
7. E. Candès and J. Romberg, *Inverse Problems.* **23**, 969 (2007).
8. J. Chen, L. Zhang, H. Jian-Hua, and M. Y. Zhu, *Bioinf. and Biomed. Eng.* 1 (2009).
9. C. K. Chui, *An Introduction to Wavelets*, (Academic Press, 1992).
10. M. A. Davenport, M. F. Duarte, Y. C. Eldar, and G. Kutyniok, in *Compressed Sensing: Theory and Applications,* Eds. Y. Eldar and G. Kutyniok (Cambridge University Press, 2011), p. 1.
11. M. Doneva, P. Börnert, H. Eggers, C. Stehning, J. Sénégas, and A. Mertins, *Magn. Reson. Med.* **64**, 1114 (2010).
12. M. Doneva, P. Börnert, H. Eggers, A. Mertins, J. Pauly, and M. Lustig, *Magn. Reson. Med.* **64**, 1749 (2010).

13. D. Donoho, *IEEE Trans. Information Theory.* **52**, 1289 (2006).
14. D. Donoho, *Comm. Pure Appl. Math.* **59**, 797 (2006).
15. J. A. Fessler and B. P. Sutton, *IEEE Trans. Signal Processing.* **51**, 560 (2003).
16. U. Gamper, P. Boesiger, and S. Kozerke, *Magn. Reson. Med.* **59**, 365 (2008).
17. W. W. Hager and H. Zhang, *Pacific J. Optim.* **2**, 35 (2006).
18. P. C. Hansen and D. P. O'leary, *SIAM J. Sci. Comp.* **14**, 1487 (1993).
19. R. M. Heidemann, Ö. Özsarlak, P. M. Parizel, J. Michiels, B. Kiefer, V. Jellus, M. Müller, F. Breuer, M. Blaimer, M. A. Griswold, and P. M. Jakob, *European Radiology.* **13**, 2323 (2003).
20. M. R. Hestenes and E. Stiefel, *J. Research National Bureau of Standards.* **49**, 409 (1952).
21. C. Huang, C. G. Graff, E. W. Clarkson, M. I. Altbach, and A. Bilgin, *Magn. Reson. Med.* **67**, 1355 (2012).
22. F. Huang and Y. Chen, *Proc. Annual Meeting of ISMRM.* 4592 (2009).
23. H. Jung, K. Sung, K. S. Nayak, E. Y. Kim, and J. C. Ye, *Magn. Reson. Med.* **61**, 103 (2009).
24. A. S. Lewis and J. Malick, *Math. Operations Research.* **33**, 216 (2008).
25. Z. Liang and P. Lauterbur, *Principles of Magnetic Resonance Imaging: A Signal Processing Perspective*, (SPIE Press, 1999).
26. M. Lustig, M. Alley, S. Vasanawala, D. L. Donoho, and J. M. Pauly, *Proc. Annual Meeting of ISMRM.* 334 (2009).
27. M. Lustig, D. Donoho, and J. M. Pauly, *Magn. Reson. Med.* **58**, 1182 (2007).
28. M. Lustig, D. Donoho, J. M. Santos, and J. M. Pauly, *IEEE Signal Processing Mag.* **25**, 72 (2008).
29. G. J. Marsaille, R. de Beer, M. Fuderer, A. F. Mehlkopf, and D. van Ormondt, *J. Magn. Reson.* **B111**, 70 (1996).
30. M. Murphy, K. Keutzer, S. Vasanawala, and M. Lustig, *Proc. Annual Meeting of ISMRM.* 4854 (2010).
31. D. Nishimura, *Principles of Magnetic Resonance Imaging*, (Stanford University, 2010).
32. R. Otazo, D. Kim, L. Axel, and D. K. Sodickson, *Magn. Reson. Med.* **64**, 767 (2010).
33. Y-C Kim, S. S. Narayanan, and K. S. Nayak, *Magn. Reson. Med.* **61**, 1434 (2009).
34. L. Pu, T. P. Trouard, L. Ryan, C. Huang, M. I. Altbach, and A. Bilgin, *Biomed. Imaging: From Nano to Macro, 2011 IEEE Int. Symp.* 254 (2011).
35. X. Qu, W. Zhang, D. Guo, C. Cai, S. Cai, and Z. Chen, *Inverse Problems Sci. Eng.* **18**, 737 (2010).
36. J. K. Romberg, *IEEE Signal Processing Mag.* **25**, 14 (2008).
37. M. Rudelson and R. Vershynin, *Comm. Pure and Appl. Math.* **61**, 1025 (2008).
38. L. I. Rudin, S. Osher, and E. Fatemi, *Physica D: Nonlinear Phenomena.* **60**, 259 (1992).
39. C. E. Shannon, *Proc. Institute of Radio Engineers,* **37**, 10, (1949).
40. D. S. Taubman and M. W. Marcellin, *Kluwer Academic* (2002).
41. C. Tsai and D. G. Nishimura, *Magn. Reson. Med.* **43**, 452 (2000).
42. M. Vetterli and J. Kovačević, *Wavelets and Subband Coding*, (Prentice Hall, 1995).
43. J. von Neumann, *Functional Operators, Vol. II*, (Princeton University Press, 1950). (Reprint of lecture notes first distributed in 1933.)
44. Y. Wu, Y-J Zhu, Q-Y Tang, C. Zou, W. Liu, R-B Dai, X. Liu, E. X. Wu, L. Ying, and D. Liang, *Magn. Reson. Med.* (2013).
45. D. C. Youla and H. Webb, *IEEE Trans. Med. Imag.* **MI1**, 81 (1982).

CHAPTER 18

ON HIERARCHICAL STATISTICAL SHAPE MODELS WITH APPLICATION TO BRAIN MRI

Juan J. Cerrolaza*, Arantxa Villanueva, and Rafael Cabeza

Electrical and Electronic Engineering Department, Public University of Navarra
Campus Arrosadia 31006, Pamplona, Spain
*E-mail: juanjose.cerrolaza@unavarra.es

The accurate segmentation of subcortical brain structures in magnetic resonance (MR) images is of crucial importance in the interdisciplinary field of medical imaging. Although statistical approaches such as active shape models (ASMs) have proven to be particularly useful in the modeling of multi-object shapes, they are inefficient when facing challenging problems. Based on the wavelet transform, the fully generic multi-resolution framework presented in this paper allows us to decompose the inter-object relationships into different levels of detail. The aim of this hierarchical decomposition is twofold: to efficiently characterize the relationships between objects and their particular localities. Experiments performed on an 8-object structure defined in axial cross sectional MR brain images show that the new hierarchical segmentation significantly improves the accuracy of the segmentation, and while it exhibits a remarkable robustness with respect to the size of the training set.

1. Introduction

Together with CT, MRI is one of the most common ways to visualize the brain, providing ever more detailed anatomic images that allow an adequate study of the main cerebral structures, a key point in the interdisciplinary technologies of computer-aided detection, diagnosis and patient follow-up[1]. The need for an accurate segmentation step, which aims to partition the intra-cranial images into different regions of interest, is of crucial importance in this context[2]. The characterization of the brain morphology associated with a particular pathology such as Alzheimer's disease or autism[3] is one example.

The appearance of deformable shape models in the late eighties[4] represented an interesting alternative to the traditional bottom-up segmentation approaches, proven inadequate in the presence of noise, occlusion, or when faced with the anatomical complexity and variability intrinsic to biological structures such as the human brain. One of the segmentation methods that has been of considerable research interest since its inception in the early 1990s is the active shape models (ASMs) proposed by Cootes et al.[5]. Roughly speaking, ASMs consist of describing the population statistics from a set of examples via point distribution models (PDMs) and learning the particular patterns of variability of the points, called landmarks, used to describe the structures of interest. Over the years, these statistical shape models have proven very effective in addressing a number of applications in the field of medical imaging[6,7,8].

One of the most interesting properties of ASMs when faced with the segmentation of cerebral regions is their inherent capacity to deal with multi-object structures. In cases where multiple objects form a given anatomic region, the characterization of the relations between subparts provides valuable additional information compared to the single-object modeling approach. However it suffers from two major drawbacks. First, this global modeling does not consider object-based scale levels, lacking the ability to explicitly describe important local geometric information. Secondly, there is the high-dimension-low-sample-size (HDLSS) problem: the concatenation of the features of all objects directly implies a considerable increase in the dimensionality of the problem, requiring a large number of parameters to accurately describe the underlying geometry and a large number of training samples, which are of limited availability in most medical applications.

A few authors have investigated a third alternative to estimate probability distributions of multi-object anatomic geometry: the hierarchical approach. The work of Davatzikos et al.[9] was one of the first that proposed the use of a hierarchical scheme in the context of ASMs. Originally restricted to single-object structures and recently extended to the multi-object environment by Cerrolaza et al.[10], the scheme is based on the decomposition of the shape into small pieces of information via the wavelet transform. Although this strategy reduces the HDLSS problem, it does not allow explicit description the inter-object relationships because each piece of information is modeled independently, which also reduces the robustness of the model significantly.

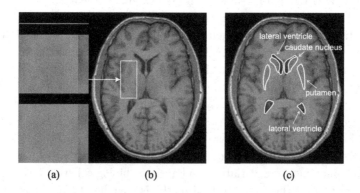

(a)   (b)   (c)

Fig. 1.   (a) Detail of the left putamen of an axial cross-section MR image of the brain. (b) Complete MR brain image. (c) Manual segmentation of the four subcortical brain structures.

The aim of this paper is to present a new hierarchical multi-shape segmentation framework that is able to characterize the different inter-object relationships, and to accurately model the particular local variations of each single object. To introduce the idea behind this new approach, it is interesting to consider how the human vision system faces this kind of situation[11]: Fig. 1(a) shows the specific region of the left putamen corresponding to the axial cross-section of the brain depicted in Fig. 1(b). With this single-object image and in the absence of any other spatial reference, even the experienced eye of a specialist and thus a single-object based algorithm may have some difficulties in defining the contour of the putamen. However, this task becomes more affordable if working with the whole composition (Fig. 1(b)). Firstly, the human vision system uses the prior knowledge about the spatial relationships of the subcortical brain structures to roughly locate them into the image. Being the easiest identifiable structure, the next step would probably be to locate the ventricle, using it as a reference to identify the caudate nucleus and the putamen, using prior knowledge about the variability of these structures and their dependencies to delineate their boundaries. This multi-level scheme of the human vision system provides an illustrative example of how statistical information previously learned is used to model both, the inter-object relationships and the single-object variability, resulting in an effective segmentation approach.

Based on wavelet theory, we provide a landmark-based multi-resolution framework to decompose the multi-object structure into levels with different degrees of detail. This multi-resolution decomposition of the objects allows us to establish different degrees of association between them and thus successfully model both the statistical inter-relationships between objects and the local variation of each object itself. The automatic segmentation of the set of subcortical brain structures depicted in Fig. 1(c) has a clear medical interest, providing us an excellent opportunity to illustrate the behavior and potential benefits of this new segmentation approach.

2. Active Shape Models

Basically, the ASMs[5] can be described as an iterative scheme in which two statistical models, of shape and appearance, are sequentially applied to drive the segmentation process. The statistical appearance model guides the matching process of the shape to a new image, whereas the shape model imposes shape constraints to guarantee that only plausible instances occur.

2.1. *Shape Model Construction using PDMs*

Suppose x_i represents the i-th shape of the training set, where $i = 1, \ldots, N$. Each of these shapes is described by a fixed number of K d-dimensional points ($d = 2$ or 3), called landmarks, distributed across the surface or contour of interest. The careful placement of these points is of crucial importance because each landmark corresponds to a defined part of the shape, establishing a point of correspondence between the training shapes. From this previously marked training set, the statistical shape model is built by computing the PDM as follows. Concatenating the coordinates of each landmark, x_i can be represented in vectorial form as

$$\mathbf{x}_{(i)} = (x_{1,1,i}, ..., x_{1,K,i}, ..., x_{d,1,i}, ..., x_{d,K,i})^T \qquad (1)$$

The statistical shape model is then built by Principal Component Analysis (PCA) of the N aligned training shapes. Any instance of the shape space can be approximated by the equation $\mathbf{x} = \bar{\mathbf{x}} + \mathbf{Pb}$, where $\bar{\mathbf{x}}$ is the mean shape, $\mathbf{P}$ is a matrix formed by the eigenvectors, and $\mathbf{b}$ is a vector defining the set of parameters of the statistical shape model. The number of modes of variation is commonly limited by the size of the training set, since in general $N << K$. That is, the capacity of the model to generate new shapes is strongly conditioned by the training set.

Although more sophisticated alternatives have been proposed[12], one of the simplest and most popular ways to guarantee that only legitimate instances are generated is to constraint $\mathbf{b}$ to lie inside an hyperrectangle by applying hard limits to each element: $\mid b_j \mid \leq \beta\sqrt{\lambda_j}$, where β is a constraint that determines the flexibility of the model, typically defined between 1 and 3.

The process described above is completely independent of the underlying number of contours that the K landmarks define in the image. This generality is one of the main advantages of the process and one of the most popular strategies when dealing with multi-object cases.

2.2. Appearance Model

During the segmentation process of a new image, any new shape instance generated is conveniently adjusted by means of equations presented in Section 2.1, guaranteeing that only plausible shapes are obtained. These new instances of the target shape are generated by a landmark update process during which each landmark seeks its optimal location according to a particular appearance model, which is also obtained from the set of training examples[5,13].

3. Multi-Resolution Representation of Composed Structures

The aim of this section is to present a new general framework able to provide a multi-resolution decomposition of composed structures such as those frequently observed in the context of medical imaging, e.g., MR brain images.

3.1. Matrix Notation in Wavelet Filtering

Although the origin of wavelet theory can be traced back to the early 20th century[14], the main contributions to its development are relatively recent[15]. Its usefulness has been proven in a wide variety of disciplines including biomedical engineering[16]. Basically, the wavelet transform is a computationally efficient mathematical tool that provides information in a space-frequency domain, unlike the Fourier transform, which only provides frequency information.

The matrix notation initially proposed by Lounsbery et al.[17] and extended by Finkelstein and Salesins[18] is of special interest in the field of computer graphics in general and to our purposes in particular. Let $\mathbf{c}_0$ be a generic discrete unidimensional signal composed of K_0 samples and expressed in vector form as $(c_0^0, c_1^0, \ldots, c_{K_0}^0)^T$. The wavelet filtering of this signal can be formulated in terms of simple matrix products:

$$\mathbf{c}^1 = \mathbf{A}^1 \mathbf{c}^0 = (c_1^1, c_2^1, \ldots, c_{K_1}^1)^T \tag{2}$$

$$\mathbf{d}^1 = \mathbf{B}^1 \mathbf{c}^0 = (d_1^1, d_2^1, \ldots, d_{K_0-K_1}^1)^T \tag{3}$$

where $\mathbf{A}^1$ and $\mathbf{B}^1$ are the so called analysis filters. Equation (2) implements the filtering and downsampling of $\mathbf{c}^0$, providing a lower resolution version of it ($K_0 > K_1$), while equation (3) captures the lost detail between $\mathbf{c}^1$ and $\mathbf{c}^0$. A proper selection of the filters $\mathbf{A}^1$ and $\mathbf{B}^1$ guarantees that no information is lost during the process, and it is possible to reverse the analysis process with the following synthesis equation:

$$\mathbf{c}^0 = \mathbf{F}^1 \mathbf{c}^1 + \mathbf{G}^1 \mathbf{d}^1 \tag{4}$$

where $\mathbf{F}^1$ and $\mathbf{G}^1$ are the corresponding synthesis filters. This filtering process can be applied iteratively over any of the new signals, $\mathbf{c}^1$ and $\mathbf{d}^1$, creating a filter bank that provides a multi-resolution representation of the original signal. One of the most typical decomposition schemes is the logarithmic tree 2-band wavelet packet, in which only the low-pass branch is filtered (Fig. 2). That is,

$$\mathbf{c}^r = \mathbf{A}^r \mathbf{c}^{r-1} \tag{5}$$

$$\mathbf{d}^r = \mathbf{B}^r \mathbf{c}^{r-1} \tag{6}$$

$$\mathbf{c}^{r-1} = \mathbf{F}^r \mathbf{c}^r + \mathbf{G}^r \mathbf{d}^r \tag{7}$$

where the index r ($r \in \mathbb{N}$) indicates the level of resolution, with $r = 0$ being the finest one. The synthesis and analysis matrices are defined by the choice of the particular wavelet basis and are related between them by the equation

$$\left(\frac{\mathbf{A}^r}{\mathbf{B}^r}\right) = (\mathbf{F}^r \mid \mathbf{G}^r)^{-1} \tag{8}$$

The selection of the wavelet basis tends to be conditioned by the particular context of use. Stollnitz et al.[19] provide a whole set of synthesis filters for the Haar and B-spline wavelet basis, which are of special interest in computer graphics.

3.2. *Wavelet Filtering of Multi-Object Structures*

Following the notation presented in Section 2.1, let $\mathbf{x}^0$ represents the vectorial expression of a single-object shape described with K_0 landmarks in a general d-dimensional space:

$$\mathbf{x}^0 = (x_{1,1}^0, \ldots, x_{1,K_0}^0, \ldots, x_{d,1}^0, \ldots, x_{d,K_0}^0)^T = (\mathbf{c}_1^0, \ldots \mathbf{c}_d^0)^T \tag{9}$$

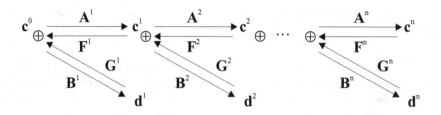

Fig. 2. Schematic representation of a common logarithmic tree 2-band wavelet packet.

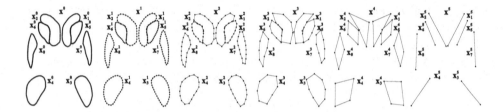

Fig. 3. Wavelet filtering of the 8-object 2-dimensional structure formed by the lateral ventricle, the putamen and the caudate nucleus, using a linear B-spline wavelet basis. The tree 2-band wavelet filtering bank provides a multi-resolution representation of the original shape, $\mathbf{x}^0$, by iteratively decomposing the low-frequency branch and creating coarser versions of it, $\mathbf{x}^r$ $(r = 1, \ldots, 5)$.

Considering $\mathbf{x}^0$ as the concatenation of d unidimensional signals, $(\mathbf{c}_1^0, \ldots, \mathbf{c}_d^0)$, the formulation presented in Section 3.1 can be easily adapted to the typical PDM matrix notation. Thereby, the $(dK_1 \times dK_0)$ analysis matrix, $\widehat{\mathbf{A}}^1$, that provides a lower resolution version of $\mathbf{x}^0$, $\mathbf{x}^1$, can be obtained as

$$\widehat{\mathbf{A}}^1 = \begin{pmatrix} \mathbf{A}^1 & \mathbf{0} & \cdots & \mathbf{0} \\ \mathbf{0} & \mathbf{A}^1 & \cdots & \mathbf{0} \\ & & \ddots & \\ \mathbf{0} & \mathbf{0} & \cdots & \mathbf{A}^1 \end{pmatrix} \tag{10}$$

where $\mathbf{A}^1$ is the analysis matrix in (2) and $\mathbf{0}$ represents a matrix of zeros. Proceeding in the same way, the original set of matrices, $\mathbf{B}^j$, $\mathbf{F}^j$ and $\mathbf{G}^j$, can be extended to obtain $\widehat{\mathbf{B}}^1$, $\widehat{\mathbf{F}}^1$ and $\widehat{\mathbf{G}}^1$, respectively. Due to the convenience of addressing the wavelet transform from a matrix point of view, this simple extension of the formulation allows us to directly address the multi-resolution decomposition of a d-dimensional single-object structure. Consider now a general shape composed of M single-object structures, whose vectorial form can be expressed as the concatenation of M vectors,

$\mathbf{x}_1^0, \mathbf{x}_2^0, ..., \mathbf{x}_M^0$, that is,

$$\mathbf{x}^0 = (\mathbf{x}_1^0; \ldots; \mathbf{x}_M^0) \tag{11}$$

$$= (x_{1,1,1}^0, \ldots, x_{1,K_0^1,1}^0, \ldots, x_{d,1,1}^0, \ldots, x_{d,K_0^1,1}^0, \cdots$$

$$x_{1,1,M}^0, \ldots, x_{1,K_0^M,M}^0, \ldots, x_{d,1,M}^0, \ldots, x_{d,K_0^M,M}^0)^T$$

where $K_0^1, \ldots, K_0^M$ are the original number of landmarks of each sub-shape. Proceeding in the same way as we did in 10, it is possible to use $\widehat{\mathbf{A}}^r$, $\widehat{\mathbf{B}}^r$, $\widehat{\mathbf{F}}^r$ and $\widehat{\mathbf{G}}^r$ to redefine the multi-object extension of the analysis and synthesis matrices: $\mathcal{A}^r$, $\mathcal{B}^r$, $\mathcal{F}^r$ and $\mathcal{G}^r$. The reformulation of the logarithmic tree 2-band wavelet packet (5)-(7) is as follows:

$$\mathbf{x}^i = \mathcal{A}^i \mathbf{x}^{i-1} \tag{12}$$

$$\mathbf{z}^i = \mathcal{B}^i \mathbf{x}^{i-1} \tag{13}$$

$$\mathbf{x}^{i-1} = \mathcal{F}^i \mathbf{x}^i + \mathcal{G}^i \mathbf{z}^i \tag{14}$$

Attending to the particular case of the subcortical brain regions illustrated in Fig. 1(c), this set of structures defines an 8-object 2-dimensional shape, whose wavelet filtering process is depicted in Fig. 3.

4. Hierarchical PDMs Using Wavelets

4.1. *Previous Approaches*

In the well-known hierarchical scheme of Davatzikos et al.[9], the shape is decomposed into different levels of resolution by means of a tree 2-band wavelet packet. The information contained at each resolution is then split into smaller equal-sized bands, which are modeled independently to reduce the HDLSS problem. However, two main drawbacks appear as a consequence of this decomposition strategy. First, the independent characterization of each band of information potentially reduces the robustness of the segmentation because no relationship between them is being modeled. Although many approaches to wavelet shrinkage consider the wavelet coefficients as independent, some studies[20] have pointed out the existence of important relationships between scales even separated by several levels of resolution. Second, the scheme does not provide the possibility to define those relationships between objects we want to explicitly model.

4.2. *General Description of the Algorithm*

Following the parallelism with the human vision system introduced in Section 1, the aim of the present algorithm is to characterize the inter-relationships between objects in a hierarchical multi-resolution fashion. By means of the general framework presented in Section 3.2 the multi-object structure of interest is decomposed into different levels of resolution. This decomposition allows us to create specific statistical shape models that characterize those inter-object associations defined at each scale.

Let us consider the particular case of the set of subcortical structures observed in axial cross sectional MR images of the brain (see Fig. 1(c)), whose multi-resolution decomposition is depicted in Fig. 3. As is often the case when dealing with multi-object anatomical structures, the relative spatial location of each object is usually defined by a certain general pattern that controls the whole set; i.e., the lateral ventricles delimit the top and bottom part of the composition, with the caudate nucleus and the putamen disposed across the laterals. These initial broad shape constraints can be efficiently imposed at the coarser resolution of the algorithm, building a global statistical shape model of the whole set, $(\mathbf{x}_1^5, \ldots, \mathbf{x}_8^5)$. However, new details and relationships between objects become relevant as we move forward to more detailed contours. Thus, once a coherent disposition of the elements is guaranteed by the above global model, we might be interested in modeling the subset defined by the lateral ventricles and the caudate nucleus $(\mathbf{x}_1^4, \ldots, \mathbf{x}_6^4)$ and the putamen $(\mathbf{x}_7^4, \mathbf{x}_8^4)$ separately. Following this philosophy as we move towards finer resolutions, the shape is gradually divided into smaller sets of objects, which are able to efficiently capture the new relevant details. To illustrate this new decomposition scheme, Fig. 4 shows one possible association between objects at each level of resolution.

4.3. *Mathematical Formulation*

Following the notation presented in Section 3.2, suppose $\mathbf{x}^r$ represents the vectorial expression of a generic d-dimensional multi-object shape composed by M different objects or contours at the r-th level of resolution. That is,

$$\mathbf{x}^r = (\mathbf{x}_1^r; \ldots; \mathbf{x}_M^r) \tag{15}$$

where $r = 0, \ldots, R$, and 0 and R the finest and coarsest scale, respectively. At each level of resolution, a specific division of the M objects into M_r disjoint subsets, $(S_1^r, \ldots, S_{M_r}^r)$ is established. Each of these subsets, S_s^r, where $s = 1, \ldots, M_r$, is formed by the indices of the objects that are modeled jointly at the r-th level of resolution, and therefore: $\bigcap_{s=1}^{M_r} S_s^r = \emptyset$ and $\bigcup_{s=1}^{M_r} S_s^r = (1, \ldots, M)$.

At lower resolutions it will be convenient to model all the objects collectively, imposing general restrictions on the relative positions between them. On the other hand, as the resolution and therefore the level of detail of the contours increases, the number of subsets increases and thus each object can be modeled in more detail. Attending to the example configuration depicted in Fig. 4, only one subset is defined at the coarsest resolution $(r = R)$, $M_R = 1$, which means that all objects are modeled jointly, that is, $S_1^R = (1, \ldots, M)$ (Fig. 4(a)). Moving to the next resolution $(r = R-1)$, the putamen is modeled separately from the rest creating two separate subsets $(M_{R-1} = 2)$, $S_1^{R-1} = (1, \ldots, 6)$ and $S_2^{R-1} = (7, 8)$ (Fig. 4(b)). Gradually

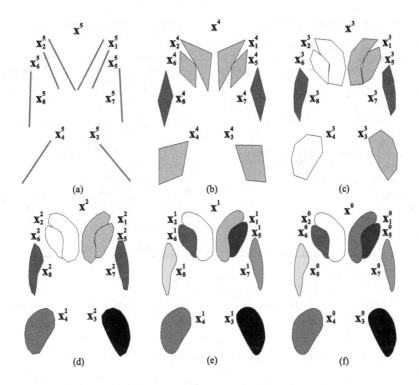

Fig. 4. Possible hierarchical configuration to model the inter-object relationships of the three subcortical brain structures. At each level of resolution, the objects depicted with the same color are modeled jointly via PDM.

separating the objects as we move towards finer resolutions, at $r = 0$ each object is modeled independently, i.e., $M_0 = M$.

Once the multi-resolution configuration has been defined, it is necessary to statistically model the underlying population of each subset via PDMs, as described in Section 2.1. The step by step description of the process is presented in *Algorithm 1* (Fig. 5(a)). The subscript (i) identifies the i-th shape in the training set; T_s^r (*Alg.1-line 11*) represents the training set for the s-th subset of objects at the r-th level or resolution, and Λ_s^r (*Alg.1-line 12*) is the set of eigenvalues obtained after applying PCA to T_s^r, that is, $\Lambda_s^r = \lambda_{s,1}^r, \ldots, \lambda_{s,t_s^r}^r$. As in Section 2.1, the rest of parameters, $\bar{\mathbf{x}}_s^r$, $\mathbf{P}_s^r$ and t_s^r, represent the average vector, the number of eigenvectors and the matrix created by the concatenation of these t_s^r eigenvectors, respectively.

Fig. 6(a) shows the shapes generated by the first mode of variation of a classical shape model, where the whole set of the object was modeled together at the finest resolution. It can be observed how this principal mode of variation controls the relative position between the objects. As Fig. 6(b) illustrates, these broad constraints on the set can be modeled more efficiently at lower resolutions ($r = 5$) to model the singularities of each object at higher levels (Fig. 6(c)).

Algorithm 1 Hierarchical Statistical Modeling

1: $\{\mathbf{x}_{(i)}\}, (i = 1, ... N)$ ▶ Set of training shapes;
2: **for** $r = 0$ **to** R **do**
3:      **for** $i = 1$ **to** N **do** ▶ Adapt the resolution of each training shape;
4:          **if** $r > 0$ **then**
5:              $\mathbf{x}_{(i)}^r = \mathcal{A}^r \mathbf{x}_{(i)}^{r-1}$;
6:          **else**
7:              $\mathbf{x}_{(i)}^0 = \mathbf{x}_{(i)}$;
8:          **end if**
9:      **end for**
10:     **for** $s = 1$ **to** M_r **do** ▶ Create the statistical shape model of each subset;
11:         $T_s^r = \{\mathbf{x}_{(i),j}^r : j \in S_s^r, \ \forall i\}$;
12:         $PCA(T_s^r) \rightarrow \{\bar{\mathbf{x}}_s^r, P_s^r, t_s^r, \Lambda_s^r\}$;
13:     **end for**
14: **end for**

Algorithm 2 Hierarchical Shape Constraint

1: $\mathbf{x} = \mathbf{y}$;
2: **while** (not convergence) **or** (not max. iterations) **do**
3:      $\mathbf{x} \rightarrow \{\mathbf{x}^R, \mathbf{z}^1, ..., \mathbf{z}^R\}$; ▶ MR decomposition using (17 and 18);
4:      **for** $\mathbf{r} = R$ **to** 0 **do**
5:          **if** $\mathbf{r} == R$ **then**
6:              $\tilde{\mathbf{x}}^R = \mathbf{x}^R$;
7:          **end if**
8:          **for** $s = 1$ **to** M_r **do**
9:              $\tilde{\mathbf{x}}_{(s)}^r = \{\tilde{\mathbf{x}}_j^r : j \in S_s^r\}$;
10:             $PDM_s^r(\tilde{\mathbf{x}}_{(s)}^r) = \hat{\mathbf{x}}_{(s)}^r$;
11:         **end for**
12:         $\hat{\mathbf{x}}^r = \bigcup_{s=1}^{M_r} \hat{\mathbf{x}}_{(s)}^r$;
13:         **if** $\mathbf{r} > 0$ **then**
14:             $\tilde{\mathbf{x}}^{r-1} = \mathcal{F}^r \hat{\mathbf{x}}^r + \mathcal{G}^r \mathbf{z}^r$; ▶ Resolution updating using (19);
15:         **end if**
16:     **end for**
17:     $\mathbf{x} = \hat{\mathbf{x}}$;
18: **end while**

(a)   (b)

Fig. 5.   (a) Algorithm for the hierarchical statistical modeling. (b) Algorithm for the hierarchical shape constraint procedure.

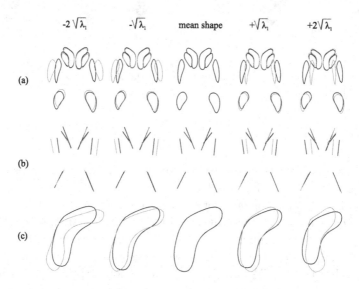

Fig. 6.   Shapes generated by the first mode of variation. (a) All objects modeled jointly at the higher resolution. (b) All objects modeled together at low resolution. (c) Detail of upper right ventricle modeled independently at high resolution. The mean shape is depicted in black.

Suppose that now we want to segment a new image using this new multi-resolution hierarchical decomposition of the shape space as an alternative to the classical PDM. Basically, as in the original ASMs, the segmentation algorithm is an iterative procedure in which the statistical appearance model guides the matching process to the target image, i.e., updating the landmarks, whereas the new statistical shape model guarantees that only plausible instances are generated. Let $\mathbf{y}$ represent the shape obtained after the landmark updating stage. *Algorithm 2* (Fig. 5(b)) details the hierarchical shape constraint process of $\mathbf{y}$ according to the statistical shape models previously built using *Algorithm 1* (Fig. 5(a)). Roughly speaking, the algorithm applies the corresponding constraints to each subset in which the shape has been divided at each level of resolution. The original shape, i.e., the unconstrained shape, at the r-th level of resolution is indicated by $\widetilde{\mathbf{x}}^r$, while $\widetilde{\mathbf{x}}^r_{\{s\}}$ represents the vector that forms the s-th subset of objects at this scale, S^r_s (Alg.2, line 9). Once $\widetilde{\mathbf{x}}^r_{\{s\}}$ has been properly corrected by the corresponding statistical model a new subset of constraint objects is obtained, $\widehat{\mathbf{x}}^r_{\{s\}}$, whose union determines $\widehat{\mathbf{x}}^r$ (Alg.2, lines 10 and 12). The transition from r to $r-1$, i.e., resolution upgrading, is performed by means of the synthesis equation (14), using the original high-frequency information, $\mathbf{z}^r$ and generating the new unconstrained shape $\widetilde{\mathbf{x}}^{r-1}$. Because the corrections imposed at r can be altered at the subsequent resolution, this above procedure is repeated iteratively until convergence or a maximum number of iterations is reached. According to our experience, a highly acceptable behavior of the algorithm can be obtained even with a single iteration.

4.4. *Grouping of Shapes*

As can be deduced from Section 4.3, the new multi-resolution strategy provides an important degree of freedom to the algorithm that could appreciably affect the final result of the segmentation: the grouping of structures at each level of resolution. Beyond the general ideas suggested in the previous section, the method of how objects are grouped together at intermediate resolutions remains an open question.

In the context of hierarchical modeling of multi-object structures, the definition of an adequate framework to establish the optimal configuration represents an interesting and active area of research. In the m-reps-based multi-object statistical approach of Pizer et al.[21] and Lu et al.[22] the modeling of inter-object relationships is established in terms of proximity under the assumption that nearby elements are highly correlated. They also assume that the objects have been previously ordered by decreasing level of stability. Similarly, the hierarchical method proposed by Camara et al.[23] also requires a specific order for the segmentation of the thoracic and abdominal structures. Although Camara suggests some ordering criteria, such as structure recognition simplicity or relationship robustness, no information about the ordering process is provided. Rao et al.[24] tries to deduce potential relationships between sub-cortical brain structures based on the information provided by canonical correlation analysis. However, the application of this algorithm is restricted to establishing correlation between pairs of objects in a single-resolution environment.

One possible strategy to define an adequate grouping of objects is to perform pilot experiments that test different configurations. However, the number of possible configurations can be considerably high when working with a large number

Table 1. Hierarchical Statistical Modeling Configurations

Resolution r	Subsets S_s^r		
	Grouping I	Grouping II	Grouping III
5	$S_1^5 = (1,2,3,4,5,6,7,8)$	$S_1^5 = (1,2,3,4,5,6,7,8)$	$S_1^5 = (1,2,3,4,5,6,7,8)$
4	$S_1^4 = (1,2,3,4,5,6); S_2^4 = (7,8)$	$S_1^4 = (1,2,3,4,5,6,7,8)$	$S_1^4 = (1,3,5,7); S_2^4 = (2,4,6,8)$
3	$S_1^3 = (1,3,5); S_2^3 = (2,4,6); S_3^3 = (7,8)$	$S_1^3 = (1,2,5,6); S_2^3 = (3,4); S_3^3 = (7,8)$	$S_1^3 = (1,3,5,7); S_2^3 = (2,4,6,8)$
2	$S_1^2 = (1,5); S_2^2 = (2,6); S_3^2 = (3);$ $S_4^2 = (4); S_5^2 = (7,8)$	$S_1^2 = (1,5); S_2^2 = (2,6); S_3^2 = (3);$ $S_4^2 = (4); S_5^2 = (7,8)$	$S_1^2 = (1,5); S_2^2 = (2,6); S_3^2 = (3);$ $S_4^2 = (4); S_5^2 = (7); S_6^2 = (8)$
1	$S_1^r = (1); S_2^r = (2); S_3^r = (3); S_4^r = (4)$	$S_1^r = (1); S_2^r = (2); S_3^r = (3); S_4^r = (4)$	$S_1^r = (1); S_2^r = (2); S_3^r = (3); S_4^r = (4)$
0	$S_5^r = (5); S_6^r = (6); S_7^r = (7); S_8^r = (8);$	$S_5^r = (5); S_6^r = (6); S_7^r = (7); S_8^r = (8);$	$S_5^r = (5); S_6^r = (6); S_7^r = (7); S_8^r = (8);$

of objects. To reduce the number of possible groupings, listed below are a set of conditions that are of great utility for creating valid configurations that exploit the potential advantages of the new multi-resolution approach:

- The set of objects must be modeled as a whole set at coarser resolutions (e.g., $r = 5$ and $r = 4$) to ensure the overall coherence of the multi-object structure.
- The number of objects in each subset must be reduced as the resolution and, therefore, the level of detail, of the contours rises.
- Two objects that have been modeled separately, i.e., in different subsets, at a specific level of resolution should not be jointly modeled at finer levels.
- Those subsets based on relationships of proximity or symmetry, such as $(\mathbf{x}_1^3, \mathbf{x}_5^3)$ or $(\mathbf{x}_1^3, \mathbf{x}_3^3)$ appear a priori to be more logical choices than others that involve more distant objects, such as $(\mathbf{x}_1^3, \mathbf{x}_4^3)$.
- Additional constraints based on the underlying topology of the multi-object structure can also be used to define feasible groupings. Thus, once one is aware of the common boundary between the upper ventricle and the caudate nucleus, a possible overlap between them could be prevented if they are modeled jointly up to a specific level of resolution, e.g., $r = 2$ (Fig. 4(d)).

Table 1 shows three possible hierarchical configurations designed according to the general ideas described above. The configurations behaviour is discussed in Section 5.

5. Results and Discussion

To complete the study, the behavior of the new approach, which we refer to as Active Hierarchical Shape Model (AHSM), the algorithm is also compared with classical ASM and with two of the most popular variants of this method. The first method is the multi-object version of the hierarchical approach proposed by Davatzikos et al.[9,10] (MO-HASM). The second method is the nonlinear version of ASM (NL-ASM) presented by Twining and Taylor[25].

5.1. *Experimental Set-up*

The tests were performed on a database of 87 brain MRI studies, with each corresponding to a different patient, obtained with an acquisition equipment of 1.5 T and a gradient field strength of 45 mT. The images have been obtained using the following acquisition protocol in the axial plane: field of view 300 mm; section thickness 0.9 mm; repetition time 1160 ms; and echo time 4.05 ms. The database has approximately the same number of male and female cases. All of the cases correspond to healthy patients with no evidence of stroke or severe Alzheimer's disease. Prior to working with these images, it is convenient to define a common coordinate system by means of Talairach transform.

The multi-object shape of interest is composed of the 8 structures of the lateral ventricle, the putamen and the caudate nucleus (Fig. 1(c)). Each object has been manually delineated by experts on images of 382×472 pixels, using 64 landmarks to define each contour, i.e., 512 landmarks per shape (see $\mathbf{x}^0$ at Fig. 3). This human-guided segmentation will be used as ground truth for the accuracy assessment of the tested algorithms. In particular, two different error measures are used, the overlapping ratio (Ω) and the symmetric point-to-curve error[26]. The above overlap measure can be defined as

$$\Omega = \frac{TP}{TP + FP + FN} \tag{16}$$

where TP (true positive) indicates the area correctly classified as an object, i.e., the area of the segmented object that matches the actual area, FP (false positive) corresponds to the area incorrectly classified as belonging to the object and FN (false negative) represents the area of the target object that remains unclassified. On the other hand, the point-to-curve error is defined as follows. Let $\mathbf{x}_1$ and $\mathbf{x}_2$ represent the target shape and the segmentation provided the algorithm, respectively. The mean point-to-contour distance from $\mathbf{x}_1$ to $\mathbf{x}_2$ is computed and averaged with the mean point-to-contour distance from $\mathbf{x}_2$ to $\mathbf{x}_1$, making this measure symmetric.

When dealing with statistical shape models built from a number of sample shapes, it is very interesting to relate these indicators of accuracy with the size of the training set. This study allows us to analyze the HDLSS problem for each one of the algorithms. To this end, the images of the aforementioned 87 studies were divided into two sets, the training and the test set, so that both contain the same proportion of male and female cases and the same patients' age distribution. In turn, the sets of training shapes were arranged in sets of different sizes. To minimize the potential bias effect caused by a particular selection of training shapes, different subsets were considered when building the statistical models for a given size of the training set. The average behavior of these subsets give more reliable information about the real effect that the number of training shapes has on the accuracy of the algorithm. In particular, 7 different sizes for the training set were considered, namely, 43, 35, 30, 25, 20, 15 and 10, building for each one 1, 2, 2, 3, 3, 4 and 4 subsets, respectively.

The variability explained by each statistical shape model is 98% of that observed in the training set, setting the flexibility parameter to $\beta = 2$. The wavelet based multi-resolution decomposition framework was configured with 6 levels of resolution

($R = 5$), using the Linear B-Spline wavelet basis because of its close linkage to the typical join-the-dots approach used to describe shapes in the context of PDM. Of course, there are many other possible wavelet bases; however, pilot experiments demonstrated the good behavior of the linear B-spline one without the need for use of other bases with higher numbers of vanishing moments such as Daubechies-7. The three hierarchical configurations tested are detailed in Table 1.

With regard to the statistical appearance models, they were built according to the original model described in Section 2.2, defined by the mean and the covariance matrix of gray-level profiles of fixed length, normal to the boundary and centered at each landmark. The length of these profiles was set to 11 pixels, 5 to each side of the landmark, defining a search space of 23 pixels (6 to each side) during the landmark updating process.

5.2. *Results*

Table 2 shows the accuracy of the four tested algorithms in terms of the point-to-curve error for the different sizes of training sets considered. The new hierarchical segmentation algorithm, AHSM, provides a systematic improvement in accuracy for the three different configurations described in Table 1. The accuracy improvement even hold true when a large number of training cases were used; i.e., when the HDLSS problem was minimal.

As the size of the training set decreases, the HDLSS problem becomes critical. The traditional statistical modeling of ASM is unable to adequately capture the underlying population of shapes, which leads to an increase in the segmentation error, as Fig. 7 graphically illustrates. The new hierarchical statistical shape modeling of AHSM, however, provides an efficient description of the patterns of variation providing an accurate and robust segmentation algorithm even with a training set of 10 samples. Because of the great similarity between the results obtained for the three configurations of AHSM only data from the first configuration is graphically represented for clarity. Although the MO-HASM algorithm does not show an improvement as significant as AHSM, its average segmentation error is notably better than that obtained with the classical ASM for up to 20 training cases. Beyond this training size, both ASM and MO-HASM, show a similar behavior. The results for NL-ASM also show a slight reduction in error over the original implementation of ASM. Unlike classical ASM, NL-ASM adopts a nonlinear version of PCA,

Table 2.   Point-to-Curve Segmentation Error: $\mu \pm \sigma$ (pixels)

# Trn. Cases	ASM	MO-HASM	NL-ASM	AHSM-Gr.I	AHSM-Gr.II	AHSM-Gr.III
43	3.69 ± 8.44	2.62 ± 4.34	3.02 ± 5.85	1.38 ± 0.54	1.32 ± 0.56	1.39 ± 0.61
35	4.00 ± 8.61	3.02 ± 5.96	3.42 ± 6.50	1.36 ± 0.64	1.28 ± 0.48	1.34 ± 0.57
30	3.35 ± 7.23	3.20 ± 5.47	3.18 ± 4.88	1.46 ± 0.54	1.33 ± 0.49	1.39 ± 0.57
25	3.73 ± 7.82	3.11 ± 5.55	3.73 ± 6.55	1.47 ± 0.54	1.39 ± 0.52	1.46 ± 0.66
20	5.46 ± 10.17	3.91 ± 6.78	4.19 ± 7.35	1.51 ± 0.93	1.51 ± 0.59	1.55 ± 0.73
15	4.15 ± 7.71	4.29 ± 7.01	4.24 ± 6.56	1.68 ± 1.13	1.69 ± 0.68	1.69 ± 0.69
10	8.01 ± 12.26	7.54 ± 10.89	8.00 ± 14.37	2.03 ± 1.05	2.10 ± 1.01	2.09 ± 1.75

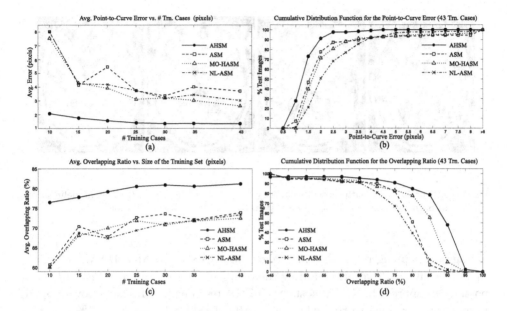

Fig. 7. (a) Evolution of the point-to-curve segmentation error with the size of the training set. (b) Cumulative distribution function of the point-to-curve error when using the largest training set (43 cases). (c) Evolution of the overlapping ratio with the size of the training set. (d) Cumulative distribution function of the overlapping ratio when using the largest training set (43 cases).

Table 3. Avg. Overlapping Ratio: $\mu \pm \sigma$ (%)

# Trn. Cases	ASM	MO-HASM	NL-ASM	AHSM-Gr.I	AHSM-Gr.II	AHSM-Gr.III
43	73.90 ± 17.05	72.49 ± 11.18	73.37 ± 12.61	81.12 ± 6.80	80.87 ± 6.49	80.60 ± 6.45
35	72.11 ± 18.65	71.83 ± 13.23	71.92 ± 15.20	80.56 ± 7.21	79.30 ± 6.58	80.71 ± 6.05
30	73.60 ± 15.01	70.80 ± 13.99	71.16 ± 13.42	80.88 ± 7.27	79.80 ± 6.72	80.78 ± 5.90
25	72.64 ± 16.62	71.87 ± 13.46	69.38 ± 14.63	80.52 ± 6.45	79.59 ± 6.57	80.09 ± 5.88
20	67.79 ± 22.27	69.99 ± 15.35	67.38 ± 16.71	79.20 ± 9.29	79.35 ± 7.27	78.35 ± 6.97
15	70.39 ± 16.75	68.08 ± 16.83	68.78 ± 15.82	77.83 ± 10.73	76.38 ± 7.39	77.83 ± 6.82
10	60.68 ± 26.57	60.12 ± 26.61	60.02 ± 27.16	76.51 ± 9.54	74.55 ± 10.34	74.53 ± 10.03

which is known as Kernel PCA (KPCA). The presence of nonlinearities in the patterns of variations of shape and the ability of KPCA to process these nonlinear transformations could explain the slight improvement obtained with NL-ASM. The above analysis is completed with Fig. 7(b), which shows the cumulative distribution function of the point-to-curve error of the three algorithms when using the largest training set.

Fig. 7(c), and (d) show the behavior of the algorithms from the alternative perspective of the overlapping ratio (see (16)), whose numerical values are detailed in Table 3. Unlike the point-to-curve error, the higher the value of the overlapping ratio is, the more accurate the segmentation. While the same conclusions concerning the robustness and accuracy of AHSM can be extracted in this new error measure, it is worth noting how the previous improvement provided by MO-HASM and NL-ASM in terms of the point-to-curve distance vanishes. That is, in terms of the

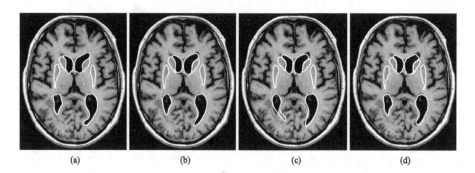

Fig. 8. MR brain image with severe asymmetry in the lateral ventricles. (a) Manual delineation. (b) AHSM Segmentation. (c) ASM segmentation. (d) MO-HASM segmentation.

average overlapping ratio, the three algorithms, ASM and MO-HASM, provide a similar behavior. However, regarding the cumulative distribution in Fig. 7(d), it is possible to appreciate how almost 78% of the test images present an overlapping ratio greater or equal to 80% when using MO-HASM, whereas only 51% and 40% of the cases obtain this accuracy for the ASM and NL-ASM respectively. This value rises to almost 85% for AHSM, which systematically provides better results.

Although some of these conclusions, such as the noticeable improvements obtained with AHSM, are fairly obvious, they have been statistically verified by means of a paired t-test with the typical alpha value of 5%, including the Bonferroni correction into the statistical test to take into account the different sizes of the training set.

Let us illustrate the benefits of the new hierarchical segmentation approach with the particular MR brain image of Fig. 8(a). This image corresponds to a case with severe asymmetry of the lateral ventricles, i.e., significant neuroanatomical differences between the left and right sides. An accurate segmentation and identification of this relatively common radiological finding $(5-12\%[27])$ is of vital importance for an adequate neurological diagnosis because its formation is an expected pathological result in the setting of space-occupying lesions, intracranial bleeding, recent infarction and trauma[28]. In the particular set of 87 brain MRI studies that composes our database, a total of 7 cases with severe asymmetry were observed ($\sim 8\%$) and we attempted to maintain this ratio when building the aforementioned training sets of different sizes.

In Fig. 8(c), it is possible to observe the segmentation result obtained by means of the original ASM when using the largest training set available. Because all the objects are modeled jointly at their highest level of resolution in ASM, the statistical shape model is unable to efficiently characterize the particularity of the asymmetry. As a consequence, the inferior horn of the left lateral ventricle is incorrectly segmented, forcing the generation of a more symmetrical shape. Fig. 8(b) shows the shape provided by AHSM, whose hierarchical decomposition of the statistical shape model efficiently segment minority cases such as this on. The alternative hierarchical formulation of MO-HASM is also able to deal with cases showing severe asymmetry of the lateral ventricles (Fig. 8(d)). However, the independent modeling of the bands in which the shapes are decomposed generates certain inaccuracies in the contours, which are particularly appreciable in those objects with a less defined appearance, such as the putamen.

Finally, it is worth pointing out the computational cost increase associated with both hierarchical approaches, AHSM and MO-HASM, and the nonlinear version NL-ASM. Unlike classical ASM, AHSM and MO-HASM require additional mathematical operations to calculate the wavelet decomposition and reconstruction of shapes. As deduced form the general multi-resolution framework presented in Section 3, the calculus of the wavelet transform basically consists of a series of matrix products, which increase the time for segmenting a new image. For the particular experimental set-up detailed in Section 5.1, AHSM implies an increase in the computational cost of around 12%. Because the multi-object version of HASM involves a larger number of transformations[10], this increase increases up to 50% for MO-HASM. For NL-ASM, the segmentation time increases by approximately 160%. The peculiarities of KPCA prevent the use of simple and fast techniques to constrain shape variability (Section 2.1) and, instead, force the use of more expensive alternatives, such as gradient ascent[25]. Only those operations involved in the segmentation process are computed here because the construction of the statistical shape models are performed only once during the training stage.

6. Summary and Conclusions

Over the years, statistical models of shapes such as ASM have demonstrated their usefulness and versatility to deal with the segmentation of multi-object anatomical structures, a frequent and challenging task in the field of medical imaging. In this paper we present a new algorithm for the hierarchical modeling of multi-object structures, which is able to efficiently characterize both the inter-object relationships and the particular localities of each object.

Based on the wavelet transform, a new multi-resolution framework is presented. Due to the simple and efficient matrix notation used, the framework can decompose any kind of multi-object structure, both 2D and 3D, at several levels of resolution. Unlike classical approaches such as ASM, this multi-scale decomposition of shapes allows us to create specific statistical shape models that characterize those inter-object associations defined at each level of resolution. The goal of this strategy is twofold: to reduce the HDLSS problem and to model the localities of the objects efficiently.

To demonstrate the benefits of this new approach, the segmentation of subcortical structures in axial cross sectional MR brain images was addressed. The experimental results obtained reveal how the new hierarchical algorithm provides not only a systematic improvement of the segmentation accuracy but also a remarkable robustness with the size of the training set, i.e., reducing the HDLSS problem. The ability of the new hierarchical modeling to successfully characterize minority neuroanatomical singularities such as the asymmetry of the lateral ventricle was also tested. The algorithm was compared to three different approaches and provided systematically better results than the classical ASM, the multi-object extension of a previous hierarchical approach proposed by Davatzikos et al.[9], and the nonlinear version of ASM, NL-ASM[25].

In some particular anatomical structures such as the brain, prior human knowledge about the inter-objects relationships may be particularly useful to define valid hierarchical configurations. The experimental tests performed in this study reveal that different valid configurations can be defined to obtain excellent results based on a set of simple conditions. However, despite the generality and versatility of AHSM, the absence of automatic grouping techniques could hinder its use when working with structures with a large number of objects, or when the interaction between objects is more uncertain. The development of such techniques is one of our main concerns for the future.

Appendix A. Extension to 3*D*

Although the notation and the framework presented in this study is completely general, the tests presented in this text are restricted to the 2D case because of the availability of images to work with. This case proves the potential benefits of AHSM. However, the HDLSS problem becomes more pressing as the complexity of the relationships between objects and the number of landmarks increases. Thus a further study in 3D would be of great interest in the future. In this regard, the seminal work of Lounsbery et al.[17] results of great interest providing a convenient multi-resolution framework to obtain the analysis and synthesis filters for meshes with subdivision connectivity. In particular, the structures depicted in Fig. 9 were obtained using the octahedron as a reference mesh, with a 4-to-1 splitting step, and a lifter butterfly scheme for triangular meshes[29]. The method proposed by Praun and Hoppe[30] was employed to parametrize each structure onto the octahedron. The original data to create Fig. 9 were obtained from the Internet Brain Segmentation Repository[31].

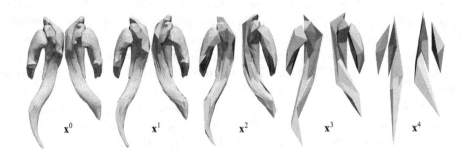

Fig. 9. Fine-to-coarse representation of the set of subcortical brain structures in 3D.

References

1. H. Hahn, "Computer-assistance in neuroimaging: From quantitative image analysis to computer-aided diagnosis," in *Proc. (IEEE) International Symposium on Biomedical Imaging: From Nano to Macro (ISBI'10)*, april 2010, p. 275.
2. M. Atkins and B. Mackiewich, "Fully automatic segmentation of the brain in MRI," *IEEE Trans. Med. Imag.*, vol. 17, no. 1, pp. 98–107, feb. 1998.
3. P. Brambilla, A. Hardan, S. U. di Nemi, J. Perez, J. C. Soares, and F. Barale, "Brain anatomy and development in autism: review of structural MRI studies," *Brain Research Bulletin*, vol. 61, no. 6, pp. 557–569, 2003.
4. M. Kass, A. Witkin, and D. Terzopoulos, "Snakes: Active contour models," *Int. J. Comput. Vis.*, vol. 1, no. 4, pp. 321–331, 1988.
5. T. F. Cootes, C. J. Taylor, D. H. Cooper, and J. Graham, "Active shape models—their training and application," *Comput. Vis. Image Underst.*, vol. 61, no. 1, pp. 38–59, 1995.
6. B. van Ginneken, M. B. Stegmann, and M. Loog, "Segmentation of anatomical structures in chest radiographs using supervised methods: a comparative study on a public database," *Med. Image Anal.*, vol. 10, no. 1, pp. 19–40, feb. 2006.
7. P. D. Allen, J. Graham, D. J. J. Farnell, E. J. Harrison, R. Jacobs, K. Nicopolou-Karayianni, C. Lindh, P. F. van der Stelt, K. Horner, and H. Devlin, "Detecting reduced bone mineral density from dental radiographs using statistical shape models," *IEEE Trans. Inf. Technol. Biomed.*, vol. 11, no. 6, pp. 601–610, nov. 2007.
8. A. F. Frangi, D. Rueckert, J. A. Schnabel, and W. J. Niessen, "Automatic construction of multiple-object three-dimensional statistical shape models: application to cardiac modeling," *IEEE Trans. Med. Imag.*, vol. 21, no. 9, pp. 1151–1166, sept. 2002.
9. C. Davatzikos, X. Tao, and D. Shen, "Hierarchical active shape models, using the wavelet transform," *IEEE Trans. Med. Imag.*, vol. 22, no. 3, pp. 414–423, march 2003.
10. J. Cerrolaza, A. Villanueva, and R. Cabeza, "Multi-shape - hierarchical active shape models," in *Proc. International Conference on Image Processing, Computer Vision, and Pattern Recognition (IPCV'11)*, July 2011.
11. A. Tsai, W. Wells, C. Tempany, E. Grimson, and A. Willsky, "Mutual information in coupled multi-shape model for medical image segmentation," *Med. Image Anal.*, vol. 8, no. 4, pp. 429–445, dec. 2004.
12. M. B. Stegmann, R. Fisker, and B. K. Ersbøll, "On properties of active shape models," Informatics and Mathematical Modelling, Technical University of Denmark, DTU, Richard Petersens Plads, Building 321, DK-2800 Kgs. Lyngby, Tech. Rep., 2000, (Available from http://www2.imm.dtu.dk/pubdb/views/edoc download.php/125/pdf/imm125.pdf).
13. B. van Ginneken, A. F. Frangi, J. J. Staal, B. M. ter Haar Romeny, and M. A. Viergever, "Active shape model segmentation with optimal features," *IEEE Trans. Med. Imag.*, vol. 21, no. 8, pp. 924–933, aug. 2002.
14. A. Haar, "Zur theorie der orthogonalen funktionensysteme," *Mathematische Annalen*, vol. 26, no. 3, pp. 331–371, 1910.
15. I. Daubechies, *Ten lectures on wavelets*. Philadelphia, PA, USA: Society for Industrial and Applied Mathematics, 1992.
16. M. Akay, "Wavelet applications in medicine," *IEEE Spectr.*, vol. 34, no. 5, pp. 50–56, may 1997.
17. M. Lounsbery, T. DeRose, and J. Warren, "Multiresolution surfaces of arbitrary topological type," Department of Computer Science and Engineering, University of Washington, Tech. Rep., 1994.

18. A. Finkelstein and D. H. Salesin, "Multiresolution curves," in *Proc. SIGGRAPH'94*. New York, NY, USA: ACM, 1994, pp. 261–268.

19. E. J. Stollnitz, T. D. Derose, and D. H. Salesin, *Wavelets for computer graphics: theory and applications*. San Francisco, CA, USA: Morgan Kaufmann Publishers Inc., 1996.

20. Z. Azimifar, P. Fieguth, and E. Jernigan, "Wavelet shrinkage with correlated wavelet coefficients," in *Proc. (IEEE) International Conference on Image Processing (ICIP'01)*, vol. 3, no. aug., 2001, pp. 162–165.

21. S. M. Pizer, J. yeon Jeong, C. Lu, K. Muller, and S. Joshi, "Estimating the statistics of multi-object anatomic geometry using inter-object relationships," in *Proc. Workshop on Deep Structure, Singularities and Computer Vision, Springer LNCS*, 2005.

22. C. Lu, S. Pizer, S. Joshi, and J.-Y. Jeong, "Statistical multi-object shape models," *Int. J. Comput. Vis.*, vol. 75, pp. 387–404, 2007.

23. O. Camara, O. Colliot, and I. Bloch, "Computational modeling of thoracic and abdominal anatomy using spatial relationships for image segmentation," *Real-Time Imaging*, vol. 10, pp. 263–273, August 2004.

24. A. Rao, P. Aljabar, and D. Rueckert, "Hierarchical Statistical Shape Analysis and Prediction of Sub-Cortical Brain Structures," *Medical Image Analysis*, vol. 12, no. 1, pp. 55–68, Feb. 2008. [Online]. Available: http://dx.doi.org/10.1016/j.media.2007.06.006

25. C. J. Twining and C. J. Taylor, "Kernel principal component analysis and the construction of non-linear active shape models," in *BMVC*, 2001.

26. R. Davies, C. Twining, and C. Taylor, *Statistical Models of Shape*. Springer-Verlag, 2008.

27. H. Grosman, M. Stein, R. C. Perrin, R. Gray, and E. L. St Louis, "Computed tomography and lateral ventricular asymmetry: clinical and brain structural correlates." *Can. Assoc. Radiol. J.*, vol. 41, no. 6, pp. 342–6, 1990.

28. Y. Kiroglu, N. Karabulut, C. Oncel, B. Yagci, N. Sabir, and B. Ozdemir, "Cerebral lateral ventricular asymmetry on CT: how much asymmetry is representing pathology?" *Surgical and Radiologic Anatomy*, vol. 30, pp. 249–255, 2008.

29. N. Dyn, D. Levine, and J. A. Gregory, "A butterfly subdivision scheme for surface interpolation with tension control," *ACM Trans. Graph.*, vol. 9, no. 2, pp. 160–169, Apr. 1990.

30. E. Praun and H. Hoppe, "Spherical parametrization and remeshing," *ACM Trans. Graph.*, vol. 22, no. 3, pp. 340–349, Jul. 2003.

31. The Internet Brain Segmentation Repository (IBSR). Available from http://www.cma.mgh.harvard.edu/ibsr/.

CHAPTER 19

ADVANCED PDE-BASED METHODS FOR AUTOMATIC QUANTIFICATION OF CARDIAC FUNCTION AND SCAR FROM MAGNETIC RESONANCE IMAGING

Durco Turco and Cristiana Corsi[*]

Department of Electric, Electronic and Information Engineering
"Guglielmo Marconi" (DEI), University of Bologna, Italy
[*]E-mail: cristiana.corsi3@unibo.it

This chapter will focus on the application of geometric deformable models based on partial differential equations (PDEs) for cardiac magnetic resonance imaging data processing. In particular we present two possible segmentation approaches: the basic level set model and a "region-based" level set model. We applied them for left and right ventricular chamber segmentation and extraction of volumes and derived functional parameters. The application of these shape independent models directly in the three dimensional domain to data acquired with a 3D imaging system could potentially achieve the clinical need for correct and complete interpretation of ventricular morphology and pathology and for fast quantification of cardiac chamber volumes, ventricular function and myocardial scar in various situations. The two models have been detailed described in the chapter and the results obtained applying them to cardiac magnetic resonance data are also presented.

1. PDEs in Medical Image Segmentation

In the past years the use of partial differential equations (PDEs) in medical image analysis has become a rising research topic and it has been applied in a multitude of different applications such as filtering, registration, matching, segmentation and tracking. In particular, medical images segmentation is a difficult task due to variability of anatomical shapes and variation in image quality and classical segmentation techniques fail when applied to medical data analysis. In literature many approaches based on PDEs addressed these difficulties with promising results: deformable models have been extensively studied and widely used for medical image segmentation.

They were proposed for use in computer vision by Terzopoulos [1] who introduced the theory of continuous multidimensional deformable models in a Lagrangian dynamics setting based on deformation energies in the form of generalized splines. The basic idea of these models relies on the deformation of a template to extract image features. For a complete review on deformable models in medical image analysis refer to McInerney [2].

Basically there are two types of deformable models: parametric deformable models and geometric deformable models. Parametric deformable models have several formulations (energy-minimizing, dynamic forces, external forces) and have been applied successfully in a wide range of applications; however, they have two main limitations. First, dynamic re-parameterization could be necessary in situations where the initial model and the desired object boundary differ greatly in size and shape and, while 2D re-parameterization requires moderate computational overhead, 3D re-parameterization requires complicated and computationally expensive methods. Moreover, this approach difficultly deals with topological adaptation because new parameterization should be constructed whenever the topology change occurs, which requires sophisticated schemes.

Geometric deformable models [3;4] provide a solution to address the limitations of parametric deformable models. These models are based on curve evolution theory [5-8] and the level set methods [9;10]. In particular, curves and surfaces are evolved using only geometric measures, independently from a parameterization, therefore, the evolving curves and surfaces can be represented implicitly as a level set of a higher-dimensional function. As a result, topology changes can be handled automatically.

The original idea behind the level set methodology is very simple. Given an interface φ in R^n bounding an open region Ω, we wish to analyze and compute its motion under a velocity field $\mathbf{F}$. To achieve this result the idea [9] was to define in R^{n+1} a Lipschitz and continuous function $\Phi(\mathbf{x},t)$ that represents the interface φ as the set where $\Phi(\mathbf{x},t)=0$. Consequently the interface can be detected for all later time by locating the set $\varphi(t)$ for which Φ vanishes. The function Φ has the following properties:

- $\Phi(\mathbf{x},t)<0$ for $\mathbf{x} \in \Omega$
- $\Phi(\mathbf{x},t)>0$ for $\mathbf{x} \notin \Omega$
- $\Phi(\mathbf{x},t)=0$ for $\mathbf{x} \in \partial\Omega=\varphi(t)$

Therefore we embed the propagating front φ as the zero level set of a higher dimensional function Φ called *level set function* and the motion is analyzed by convecting the Φ values with the vector field $\mathbf{F}$. The elementary front evolution equation is:

$$\frac{\partial \Phi}{\partial t} + \mathbf{F} \cdot \nabla \Phi = 0 \qquad (1)$$

Actually only the normal component of the speed vector **F** is needed:

$$F_N = F \cdot \frac{\nabla \Phi}{|\nabla \Phi|}$$

and eq. (1) becomes:

$$\frac{\partial \Phi}{\partial t} = F_N \cdot |\nabla \Phi|$$

with initial condition $\Phi(\mathbf{x},0)=\Phi_0$. The expression of the speed function **F** changes with the application field and it can depend on position, shape, geometry, curvature of the interface, time and external forces. We stress that this model is easy to implement in the presence of boundary singularities, topological changes such as breaking and merging, and in 2 or 3 dimensions because their formulation can be directly extended to 3D. A thorough treatment on evolving curves and surfaces using the level set representation can be found in [10].

In this chapter we will focus on the application of different type of geometric deformable segmentation models to extract clinically useful information about anatomic structures imaged through cardiac magnetic resonance imaging.

2. Cardiac Magnetic Resonance Imaging

Magnetic resonance imaging is becoming a standard technique for the assessment of cardiac function, morphology and structure [11-13]. Echocardiography remains the generally accepted modality for cardiac evaluation but in many cases it does not provide images with enough information for an accurate cardiac assessment. In these cases, literature suggests magnetic resonance imaging as the technique that could warrant a correct diagnosis of the disease.

Magnetic resonance imaging has been shown to have several technical advantages in comparison to other standard diagnostic testing procedures. It is a non-invasive technique that uses no ionizing radiation and there are no known clinically significant side effects. Magnetic resonance imaging is effective for the evaluation of the cardiac structure because it can produce high resolution images of the cardiac chambers and it is considered a three dimensional imaging technique. Moreover the use of fast gradient echo sequences allows to assess global and regional ventricular contractile function. However, it has been shown to have several disadvantages: it requires more patient cooperation than other tests and imaging time is longer than other diagnostic imaging systems, it is incompatible with various medical and life support devices and installation and operation of the equipment is expensive.

Cardiac magnetic resonance data were obtained using a 1.5 Tesla scanner (General Electric) with a phased-array cardiac coil. Electrocardiogram-gated localizing spin-echo sequences were used to identify the long-axis of the heart. Steady-state free precession (FIESTA) dynamic gradient-echo mode was then used to acquire images during 12-second breath-holds. Cine-loops were obtained in 6 to 10 short-axis slices, 9 mm slice thickness with no gaps between slices and a temporal resolution of 20 frames per cardiac cycle.

3. Methods for Ventricular Volume Estimation

In computer vision we are interested in the extraction of a shape which is then analyzed and understood. In particular, in medical imaging, we want to isolate and identify anatomical structures or eventually external masses from the background image and, once a particular shape is segmented, we can compute volumes, surface area or geometric characteristics leading to the recognition and classification of the detected shape. This problem can be accomplished in the level set framework, with the advantage of being capable of detecting complex morphology and topological variations and independent of geometrical assumptions or modeling.

3.1. *The basic level set model*

In medical imaging, the basic level set model relies on the work of Malladi and colleagues [4]: starting from a seed, the front grows and stops at the boundary of the object we desire to detect. Let's consider a volumetric data $I(x,y,z):V \subset R^3 \rightarrow R^2$. The proposed algorithm is build in two steps. In the first step an edge indicator function $g(x,y,z)$ as proposed by Perona [14] is defined as:

$$g(x,y,z) = \frac{1}{1 + |\nabla(G_\sigma * I(x,y,z))|}$$

where $G_\sigma * I$ denotes the image convolved with a Gaussian smoothing filter whose characteristic width is σ:

$$G_\sigma(x,y,z) = \frac{1}{\sigma\sqrt{\pi}} e^{-\left(\frac{|(x,y,z)|}{\sigma}\right)^2}$$

The term $\nabla(G_\sigma * I(x,y,z))$ is zero essentially everywhere in the image with the exclusions of the regions where the image gradient changes rapidly. Therefore the function $g(x,y,z)$ is used to detect local edges, being close to unity far from the boundaries and to zero near changes in the image gradient (see fig. 1, middle panel). Let's outline that the proposed edge indicator could be replaced by a more sophisticated and robust edge detector (for example according to the phase signature (edge shape) rather than intensity gradient information [15;16]).

In the second step a curve evolution inside the object is implemented, where the curve speed is tuned by the edge indicator (see fig. 1, right panel) to stop the evolving curve on the boundaries of the desired object. The speed function used for the evolution of the interface is:

$$F = g(|\nabla I|) \text{div} \frac{\nabla \Phi}{|\nabla \Phi|} - \varepsilon \nabla g(|\nabla I|) \cdot \nabla \Phi$$

Therefore, the evolution equation can be written as:

$$\begin{cases} \dfrac{\partial \Phi}{\partial t} = |\nabla \Phi| g(|\nabla I|) \text{div} \dfrac{\nabla \Phi}{|\nabla \Phi|} - \varepsilon \nabla g(|\nabla I|) \cdot \nabla \Phi & \text{in } V \times]0, \infty[\\[2mm] \Phi(t, x, y, z) = \min(\Phi_0) & \text{in } \partial V \times]0, \infty[\\[2mm] \Phi(0, x, y, z) = \Phi_0 & \text{in } x \in V \end{cases} \quad (2)$$

The first parabolic term on the right side moves the curve in the normal direction with a speed equal to the curvature of level curves H=div($\nabla \Phi / |\nabla \Phi|$) weighted by the edge indicator g($|\nabla I|$); it represents a geometric diffusion slowed by the function g where the image has a high gradient and it makes the graph of Φ smooth far from the edges with a minimal smoothing of the edge itself. The second term corresponds to a pure passive advection of the curve along the underlying velocity field -∇g that is a vector field pointing always towards the existing local boundaries. The behavior of the terms g and -∇g in the 2D space are graphically explained in fig. 1.

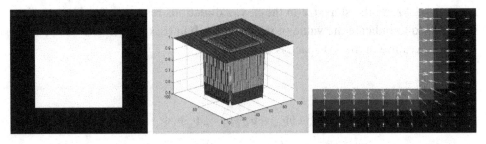

Figure 1. For the image in the left panel the function g is plotted in the middle panel and a zoom of the vector field -∇g is shown in the right panel.

The constant ε in eq. (2) is added to increase the evolution speed in order to attract the curve towards the boundary. After the definition of the initial condition Φ_0 inside the desired region, following eq. (2), the interface grows and stops at the shape boundaries when the geometry dependent term balances the advection term.

Once the equation has reached the stability, simply counting the number of voxels inside the detected boundaries we compute the volume of the anatomical structure. Moreover the detected interface can be easily represented using rendering techniques.

3.1.1. *Initial condition setting*

The two terms in eq. (2) act only close to the local edges, therefore the evolution of the level set function has to start close to the interface. The idea is to use as initial condition for the PDE evolution, an hypersurface (a surface for a contour detection and a 4D function for a surface detection) starting from some feature points close to the boundaries.

In the 2D space, the initial condition for the evolution of the PDE, is obtained computing the signed distance function from a polygon whose vertices are user defined close to the border of the structure we want to detect. This signed distance function is computed in such a way that the function assumes negative values inside the polygon and positive ones outside.

In the 3D case, the same procedure is repeated for few slices of the volumetric data. To build up the three dimensional function a linear interpolation among the initialized slices was performed to fill up the entire volume.

3.1.2 *Numerical implementation*

In order to derive a numerical algorithm one has to consider discretizations of space and time. Consider a rectangular uniform grid in space-time; the grid is the set of points $(t_n, x_i, y_j, z_k) = (n\Delta t,\ i\Delta x,\ j\Delta y,\ k\Delta z)$ where Δt is the time step size and Δx, Δy and Δz are the step size in the x, y, z directions respectively. The notation Φ^n_{ijk} is used to indicate the value of the function Φ in (t_n, x_i, y_j, z_k).

The curvature in the 3D space is defined as:

$$H = \operatorname{div}\frac{\nabla\Phi}{|\nabla\Phi|} =$$

$$= \frac{(\Phi_{yy} + \Phi_{zz})\Phi_x^2 + (\Phi_{xx} + \Phi_{zz})\Phi_y^2 + (\Phi_{yy} + \Phi_{xx})\Phi_z^2 - 2\Phi_x\Phi_y\Phi_{xy} - 2\Phi_x\Phi_z\Phi_{xz} - 2\Phi_z\Phi_y\Phi_{zy}}{(\Phi_x^2 + \Phi_y^2 + \Phi_z^2)^{\frac{3}{2}}}$$

and the parabolic term of eq. (2) is approximated using centered schemes [4]. The second term on the right side of eq. (2) is approximated through upwind schemes for hyperbolic terms in which, depending on the sign of each component of g, the upwind scheme is computed in the corresponding direction:

$$\nabla g \cdot \nabla \Phi = \max \left(g_{ijk}^{0x},0\right)D_{ijk}^{-x} + \min \left(g_{ijk}^{0x},0\right)D_{ijk}^{+x} + \max \left(g_{ijk}^{0y},0\right)D_{ijk}^{-y} + \min \left(g_{ijk}^{0y},0\right)D_{ijk}^{+y} + \max \left(g_{ijk}^{0z},0\right)D_{ijk}^{-z} + \min \left(g_{ijk}^{0z},0\right)D_{ijk}^{+z}$$

where the operator D represents the finite difference operator applied to Φ_{ijk}^{n} following centered, forward or backward schemes depending on the symbols in the superscript (0, +, - respectively).

The temporal discretization used to approximate equation (2) utilizes the Euler forward finite difference scheme. Therefore the complete first order scheme used to approximate the whole equation is:

$$\Phi_{ijk}^{n+1} = \Phi_{ijk}^{n} + \Delta t \left(\begin{array}{c} g_{ijk} H_{ijk}^{n} \left(D_{ijk}^{0x^2} + D_{ijk}^{0y^2} + D_{ijk}^{0z^2}\right)^{1/2} + \\ - \varepsilon[\max \left(g_{ijk}^{0x},0\right)D_{ijk}^{-x} + \min \left(g_{ijk}^{0x},0\right)D_{ijk}^{+x} + \\ + \max \left(g_{ijk}^{0y},0\right)D_{ijk}^{-y} + \min \left(g_{ijk}^{0y},0\right)D_{ijk}^{+y} + \\ + \max \left(g_{ijk}^{0z},0\right)D_{ijk}^{-z} + \min \left(g_{ijk}^{0z},0\right)D_{ijk}^{+z}] \end{array} \right)$$

The narrow band implementation of level set methods was adopted to make the algorithm more efficient [17].

3.1.3. *Data analysis*

The analysis of the cardiac magnetic resonance data is performed in few steps. First, a fully automated 3D reconstruction of the volumetric data was performed from the short-axis slices. For each frame, a 3D dataset was generated using tri-linear interpolation, while taking into account slice thickness, the number of slices and the spacing between them. An example of the 3D reconstruction from the acquired short axis cardiac magnetic resonance slices is shown in fig. 2.

This resulted in a dynamic representation of the entire heart. This dynamic display was used to select end-diastolic and end-systolic frames, which were visually determined as the largest and smallest left ventricular cavities in the 3D space.

Then, the basic level set model previously described was applied to these frames to extract endocardial end-diastolic and end-systolic volumes, epicardial end-diastolic volume and derived parameters such as ejection fraction and mass. Moreover, the performance of the model were tested to estimate right ventricular volume at end-diastole.

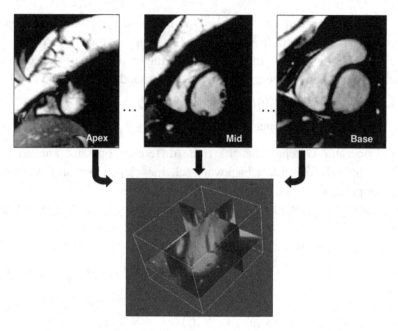

Figure 2. 3D reconstruction of a 3D magnetic resonance imaging dataset from a stack of short axis slices (top panels) in a compact orthogonal view (bottom panel).

3.1.4. *Results*

The time required to analyze a single dataset, including data retrieval, 3D interpolation, frame selection, surface initialization, correction and computation of volumes was approximately 5 minutes on a personal computer (Pentium II, 755MHz, 512Mb RAM) of which only 30 seconds were required for the computations once user interaction was complete. These analyses were performed using Matlab 6 Release 12.1 software (MathWorks).

In figs. 3 and 4 we show two examples of the initialization procedure to detect respectively right and left ventricular endocardial surfaces.

By superimposing the extracted surface on the original data, the user can evaluate the reliability of the detection in any plane, as shown in fig. 5.

Segmented surfaces at end-diastole (left panels) and end-systole (right panels) for the left ventricle (top panels) and right ventricle (bottom panels) are reported in fig. 6.

The procedure for the epicardial surface detection is shown in fig. 7, together with the final result of the segmentation.

Visual verification of the position of the detected surfaces necessary for mass estimation is shown in fig. 8.

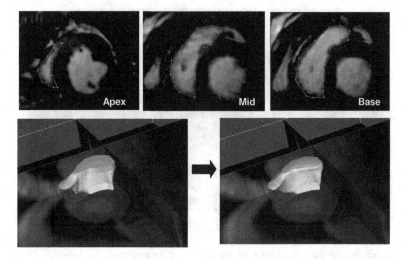

Figure 3. Example of manually initialized right ventricular endocardial boundaries in three short-axis planes at end-diastole (top panels). The initial surface for the evolution (left) and the final detected surfaces (right) are shown in the bottom panels.

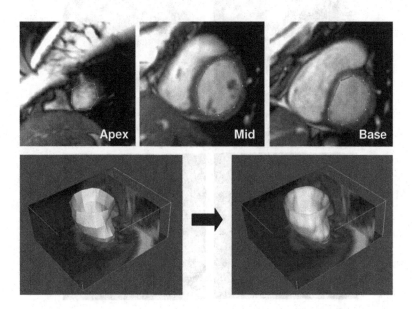

Figure 4. Example of manually initialized left ventricular endocardial boundaries in three short-axis planes at end-diastole (top panels). The initial surface for the evolution (left) and the final detected surfaces (right) are shown in the bottom panels.

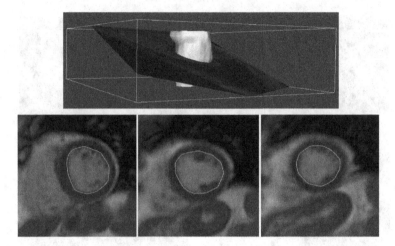

Figure 5. Examples of the contouring of the extracted surfaces on the original data to allow verification of the correctness of the detection in any arbitrary cross-sectional plane (top panel) and in multiple short-axis slices (bottom panels).

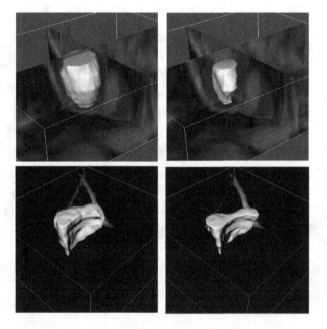

Figure 6. Examples of detected surfaces for end-diastolic (left panels) and end-systolic (right panels) frames of the same magnetic resonance data, are shown, for both left ventricle (top panels) and right ventricle (bottom panels).

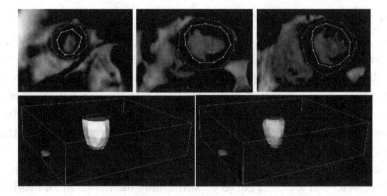

Figure 7. Initial left ventricle epicardial surface (bottom left panel) obtained by joining the selected points (top panels), and the final calculated epicardial surface (bottom right panel) shown in semi-transparent display with the endocardial surface inside.

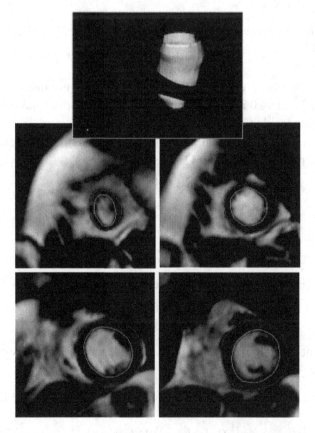

Figure 8. Example of the detected left ventricular endocardial and epicardial surfaces (top), and corresponding short-axis cross-sections from apex to base (bottom panels, from left to right). This display allowed visual verification of the position of the calculated endocardial and epicardial surfaces in multiple planes.

3.2. *The "region-based" level set model*

In this paragraph we propose a different approach for cardiac magnetic resonance data segmentation. The previous method is "edge-based" that is it evolves a curve with a speed function depending on a pre-computed edge indicator. Chan and Vese proposed a different model [18] based on a "region-based" approach in which the speed of curve evolution involves integral quantities (like mean values of the gray level image pixels inside and outside the curve) instead of differential quantities (like image gradient).

Following the Chan and Vese formulation, let's consider an image $I(x,y):\Omega \subset R^2 \to R^2$ and a closed curve C partitioning the image in an inside Ω_i and outside Ω_o. These two regions have piecewise-constant intensities and the object to be detected is represented by the region inside C. They consider the energy functional $F(c_1,c_2,C)$ and they aim to minimize the functional:

$$F(c_1, c_2, C) =$$
$$= \mu \cdot length\ (C) + v \cdot area\ (inside\ (C)) +$$
$$+ \lambda_1 \int_{inside\ (C)} |I(x,y) - c_1|^2 dxdy + \lambda_2 \int_{outside\ (C)} |I(x,y) - c_2|^2 dxdy$$

where c_1 and c_2 are the averages of the image I respectively inside and outside C, and λ_1, λ_2, $\mu \geq 0$ and $v \geq 0$ are fixed parameters. The length of the curve C and the area of the region inside C are two regularizing terms.

In the Chan and Vese formulation, the curve C is represented by the zero level set of a Lipschitz function $\Phi:\Omega \to R$ such that:

$$\begin{cases} C = \{(x,y) \in \Omega : \Phi(x,y) = 0\} \\ inside\ (C) = \{(x,y) \in \Omega : \Phi(x,y) < 0\} \\ outside\ (C) = \{(x,y) \in \Omega : \Phi(x,y) > 0\} \end{cases}$$

Using the Heaviside function H(z) and the Dirac function d(t):

$$H(z) = \begin{cases} 1 & \text{if } z \geq 0 \\ 0 & \text{if } z < 0 \end{cases} \qquad \delta(z) = \frac{d}{dz}H(z),$$

and their slight regularized versions δ_ε and H_ε respectively, they express the energy [18] as:

$$F(c_1, c_2, \Phi) = \mu \int_\Omega \delta_\varepsilon(\Phi(x,y))|\nabla\Phi(x,y)|dxdy + v \int_\Omega H_\varepsilon(\Phi(x,y))dxdy +$$

$$+ \lambda_1 \int_{inside\ (C)} |I(x,y) - c_1|^2 H_\varepsilon(\Phi(x,y))dxdy + \tag{3}$$

$$+ \lambda_2 \int_{outside\ (C)} |I(x,y) - c_2|^2 (1 - H_\varepsilon(\Phi(x,y)))dxdy$$

By keeping the function Φ fixed and minimizing eq. (3) with respect c_1 and c_2 they write the values of the two constants:

$$c_1(\Phi) = \frac{\int_\Omega I(x,y) H(\Phi(x,y)) dxdy}{\int_\Omega H(\Phi(x,y)) dxdy} \qquad c_2(\Phi) = \frac{\int_\Omega I(x,y)(1 - H(\Phi(x,y))) dxdy}{\int_\Omega H(\Phi(x,y)) dxdy}$$

If the curve has empty interior and exterior respectively, $c_1(\Phi)$=average(I) in $\{\Phi \geq 0\}$ and c_2=average(I) in $\{\Phi < 0\}$.

Now, keeping c_1 and c_2 fixed, and minimizing the energy with respect to Φ, they deduced the associated Euler–Lagrange equation for Φ:

$$\begin{cases} \dfrac{\partial \Phi}{\partial t} = \delta_\varepsilon(\Phi)\left[\mu \operatorname{div} \dfrac{\nabla \Phi}{|\nabla \Phi|} - v - \lambda_1(I - c_1)^2 + \lambda_2(I - c_2)^2 \right] & \text{in } \Omega \times]0, \infty[\\[4mm] \Phi(0, x, y) = \Phi_0(x, y) & \text{in } \Omega \\[4mm] \dfrac{\delta_\varepsilon(\Phi)}{|\nabla \Phi|} \dfrac{\partial \Phi}{\partial n} = 0 & \text{on } \partial\Omega \end{cases} \qquad (4)$$

where n denotes the exterior normal to the boundary.

In our method we keep this region-based approach presented by Chan and Vese and we embed in the segmentation model the a priori knowledge of statistical distribution of grey levels of magnetic resonance data [19]. The gray levels are assumed to be uncorrelated and independently distributed, therefore they are characterized by their respective probability density function (pdf) p(I). For cardiac magnetic resonance data the pdf can be described considering the Poisson noise:

$$p(I) = \frac{e^{-\lambda} \lambda^{I(x,y)}}{I(x,y)!}$$

where $\lambda \geq 0$.

The probability of the random field inside and outside the curve C is respectively $P_i = \Pi_{\Omega i(C)} p(I)$ and $P_o = \Pi_{\Omega o(C)} p(I)$. The likelihood function given by the product of the inner and the outer probability $P[I|C] = P_i P_o$ [20] will have the maximum in correspondence of the object we want to detect in the image.

Using the log function that is strictly increasing, the maximum value of the likelihood function, if it exists, will occur at the same points as the maximum value of $l(I,C) = \log(P[I|C])$ (log likelihood function). Therefore we obtain:

$$l(I, C) = \log \ P_i + \log \ P_o =$$

$$= - \int_{\Omega_i(C)} I(x, y) dxdy \ \log \left(\frac{1}{A_i} \int_{\Omega_i(C)} I(x, y) dxdy \right) +$$

$$- \int_{\Omega_o(C)} I(x, y) dxdy \ \log \left(\frac{1}{A_o} \int_{\Omega_o(C)} I(x, y) dxdy \right)$$

where A_i and A_o are the average values of I inside and outside Ω, respectively.

To perform the image segmentation, we maximize the log likelihood function with respect to the variation of the curve C; in particular for the Poisson pdf, following [21] we derive the parameter λ and the log likelihood function results:

$$F = \mu \cdot length \ (C) + \left[\begin{array}{c} \left(\int_{\Omega_i(C)} I(x, y) dxdy \right) \log \left(\frac{1}{A_i} \int_{\Omega_i(C)} I(x, y) dxdy \right) \\ + \left(\int_{\Omega_o(C)} I(x, y) dxdy \right) \log \left(\frac{1}{A_o} \int_{\Omega_o(C)} I(x, y) dxdy \right) \end{array} \right] \tag{5}$$

To compute the first variation of eq. (5) it is useful to introduce the auxiliary function $\Phi:\Omega \to R$ with the same properties described in the Chan and Vese formulation and the log likelihood function can be rewritten as:

$$F = \mu \cdot \int_{\Omega} \delta(\Phi(x, y)) |\nabla \Phi| dxdy +$$

$$+ \left[\begin{array}{c} \left(\int_{\Omega} I(x, y) H(\Phi)(dxdy \right) \log \left(\frac{1}{A_i} \int_{\Omega_i} I(x, y) H(\Phi) dxdy \right) \\ + \left(\int_{\Omega} I(x, y) (1 - H(\Phi)) dxdy \right) \log \left(\frac{1}{A_o} \int_{\Omega} I(x, y) (1 - H(\Phi)) dxdy \right) \end{array} \right]$$

considering [18]:

$$A_i = \int_{\Omega} H(\Phi(x, y)) dxdy \qquad A_o = \int_{\Omega} (1 - H(\Phi(x, y))) dxdy$$

and

$$length \ \{\Phi = 0\} = \int_{\Omega} |\nabla H(\Phi)| dxdy = \int_{\Omega} \delta(\Phi) |\nabla \Phi| dxdy$$

In order to compute the associated Euler-Lagrange equation for the unknown function Φ slightly regularized versions of the function H and δ_0, denoted as H_ε and δ_ε as $\varepsilon \to 0$ are considered:

$$0 = \delta(\Phi) \left[\begin{array}{c} \mu div \dfrac{\nabla \Phi}{|\nabla \Phi|} - \left(I \log(\dfrac{1}{A_i} \int_{\Omega_i} I dx dy) \right) + \\[2ex] + \dfrac{A_i I - \int_{\Omega_i} I dx dy}{A_i} - I \log(\dfrac{1}{A_o} \int_{\Omega_o} I dx dy) + \dfrac{A_o I - \int_{\Omega_o} I dx dy}{A_o} \end{array} \right]$$

The first term on the right hand is a parabolic term and evolves the curve in the normal direction with a speed equals to the Euclidean curve.

In the level set model, the Euler-Lagrange equation for Φ acts only locally, on few level curves around $\Phi=0$. To extend the evolution to all level sets, $\delta(\Phi)$ is replaced with $|\nabla \Phi|$ [22]. The associated level set flow is:

$$\left\{ \begin{array}{ll} \dfrac{\partial \Phi}{\partial t} = |\nabla \Phi| \left[\begin{array}{c} \mu div \dfrac{\nabla \Phi}{|\nabla \Phi|} - \left(I \log(\dfrac{1}{A_i} \int_{\Omega_i} I dx dy) + \dfrac{A_i I - \int_{\Omega_i} I dx dy}{A_i} \right) + \\[2ex] - \left(I \log(\dfrac{1}{A_o} \int_{\Omega_o} I dx dy) + \dfrac{A_o I - \int_{\Omega_o} I dx dy}{A_o} \right) \end{array} \right] & in\ \Omega \times]0, \infty[\\[8ex] \Phi(0, x, y) = \Phi_0(x, y) & in\ \Omega \\[4ex] \dfrac{\delta_\varepsilon(\Phi)}{|\nabla \Phi|} \dfrac{\partial \Phi}{\partial n} = 0 & on\ \partial \Omega \end{array} \right.$$

(6)

where $\Phi(0,x,y)$ is the initial function with the property that its zero level set corresponds to the position of the initial front. Typically is defined as:

$$\Phi(0, x, y) = \pm d$$

where d is the signed distance function from each point to the initial front [10].

The evolution process will stop when the region probability terms of the inside regions equal the terms of outside regions, up to regularization of boundaries.

When working with level set and Dirac function, in order to prevent that the level set function becomes too flat or too steep, a standard procedure is to reinitialize Φ to the signed distance function to its zero level curve as in [21;23]. This can be seen as a rescaling and regularization. The re-initialization is computed solving the following evolution equation:

$$\begin{cases} \dfrac{\partial \Psi}{\partial t} = \text{sign}(\Phi(t))\left(1 - |\nabla \Psi|\right) \\ \Psi(0, x, y) = \Phi(t, x, y) \end{cases} \tag{7}$$

where $\Phi(t,x,y)$ is the solution of eq. (6) at time t. Then the new $\Phi(t,x,y)$ will be Ψ, such that Ψ is obtained at the steady state of eq. (7). The solution $\Psi(t,x,y)$ will have the same zero level set of the $\Phi(t,x,y)$, and everywhere $|\nabla\Phi|$ will converge to 1. In this way, any topological changes due to pop up of new regions, are prevented and new regions can be generated only by the splitting of an existing contour and not by the arising of new maxima in the level set function.

To simplify the comprehension of the reader, the region-based model has been presented in the 2D domain. In the 3D domain we study the evolution of a surface and the associated level set flow in the 3D domain is computed in a similar manner.

3.2.1. *Numerical implementation*

Since we applied this method in the 3D domain, in this section we show how to approximate equation (7) with finite differences in the 3D space.

Consider a rectangular uniform grid in space-time; the grid is the set of points $(t_n, x_i, y_j, z_k) = (n\Delta t, i\Delta x, j\Delta y, k\Delta z)$ where Δt is the time step size and Δx, Δy and Δz are the step size in the x, y, z directions respectively. The notation Φ^n_{ijk} is used to indicate the value of the function Φ in (t_n, x_i, y_j, z_k).

The mean curvature can be written as previously described in the paragraph 3.1.2 and the parabolic term of equation (7) is approximated using centered schemes:

$$Hg = |\nabla\Phi|\, div\, \frac{\nabla\Phi}{|\nabla\Phi|} =$$

$$= \left[\frac{\left(D^{0yy}_{ijk} + D^{0xx}_{ijk}\right)D^{0z^2}_{ijk} + \left(D^{0yy}_{ijk} + D^{0zz}_{ijk}\right)D^{0x^2}_{ijk} + \left(D^{0zz}_{ijk} + D^{0xx}_{ijk}\right)D^{0y^2}_{ijk}}{D^{0x^2}_{ijk} + D^{0y^2}_{ijk} + D^{0z^2}_{ijk}} + \right.$$

$$\left. + \frac{-2D^{0x}_{ijk}2D^{0y}_{ijk}2D^{0xy}_{ijk} - 2D^{0x}_{ijk}2D^{0z}_{ijk}2D^{0xz}_{ijk} - 2D^{0z}_{ijk}2D^{0y}_{ijk}2D^{0zy}_{ijk}}{D^{0x^2}_{ijk} + D^{0y^2}_{ijk} + D^{0z^2}_{ijk}} \right]$$

where the operator D represents the finite difference operator applied to Φ^n_{ijk} following centered, schemes (superscript 0).

In the second term on the right side of eq. (7), $|\nabla\Phi|$ is approximated through upwind schemes:

$$G = |\nabla\Phi| = \left[\begin{array}{l} \left(\max\left(D^{-x}_{ijk},0\right)\right)^2 + \left(\min\left(D^{+x}_{ijk},0\right)\right)^2 + \left(\max\left(D^{-y}_{ijk},0\right)\right)^2 + \\ + \left(\min\left(D^{+y}_{ijk},0\right)\right)^2 + \left(\max\left(D^{-z}_{ijk},0\right)\right)^2 + \left(\min\left(D^{+0z}_{ijk},0\right)\right)^2 \end{array} \right]^{\frac{1}{2}}$$

where the operator D represents the finite difference operator applied to Φ^n_{ijk} following forward or backward schemes depending on the symbols in the superscript (+ and - respectively).

The temporal discretization used to approximate the equation utilizes the Euler forward finite difference scheme. Therefore the complete first order scheme used to approximate the whole equation is:

$$\Phi^{n+1}_{ijk} = \Phi^n_{ijk} + \Delta t \left\{ \mu H g\left(\Phi^n_{ijk}\right) - G\left(\Phi^n_{ijk}\right) \left[\begin{array}{l} I_{ijk}\,\log\left(\dfrac{1}{A_i\left(\Phi^n_{ijk}\right)} \displaystyle\sum_{ijk\in V} I_{ijk} \right) + \\[2mm] + \dfrac{A_i\left(\Phi^n_{ijk}\right)I_{ijk} - \displaystyle\sum_{V_i} I_{ijk}}{A_i\left(\Phi^n_{ijk}\right)} + \\[2mm] - I_{ijk}\,\log\left(\dfrac{1}{A_o\left(\Phi^n_{ijk}\right)} \displaystyle\sum_{ijk\in V} I_{ijk} \right) + \\[2mm] - \dfrac{A_o\left(\Phi^n_{ijk}\right)I_{ijk} - \displaystyle\sum_{V_o} I_{ijk}}{A_o\left(\Phi^n_{ijk}\right)} \end{array} \right] \right\}$$

3.2.2. *Data analysis*

As for the previous method, a fully automated 3D reconstruction of the volumetric data was performed from the cardiac magnetic resonance short-axis slices. For each frame, a 3D dataset was generated using tri-linear interpolation, while taking into account slice thickness, the number of slices and the spacing between them. This resulted in a dynamic representation of the entire heart from which end-diastolic and end-systolic frames were visually determined as the largest and smallest left ventricular cavities in the 3D space. To these frames the region-based level set model was applied to extract endocardial end-diastolic and end-systolic volumes.

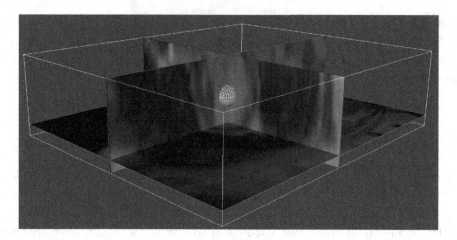

Figure 9. Zero level set of the initial condition for the evolution of the PDE.

In our application, the initial condition for the PDE evolution is obtained by simply selecting a point in the 3D data and building an hypersphere that assumes negative values inside and positive values outside this function and whose zero level is the sphere that after the evolution will correspond to the final detected surface. The zero level set of the initial condition for the evolution of the PDE is graphically presented in fig. 9: the user selects one point in the 3D space and the program compute an hypersphere whose zero level is the sphere shown in the figure. Moreover, the method was automatically applied to all the data in the cardiac cycle to obtain the volume-time curve.

3.2.3. *Results*

The time required to analyze a single dataset, including data retrieval, 3D interpolation, frame selection, surface initialization and computation of each volume was less than 1 minutes on a AMD Athlon (TM) XP 2800+ AT/AT compatible 512 MB RAM. The automatic analysis of the entire cardiac cycle required less than 5 minutes. These analyses were performed using Matlab 6 Release 12.1 software (MathWorks). An examples of the evolution of the zero level surface on a short axis slice is shown in fig. 10.

Examples of the contours extracted from the 3D detected surface, superimposed to the original short-axis cardiac magnetic resonance slices are shown in figs. 11 and 12.

Segmented surfaces at end-diastole and end-systole for the left ventricle are reported in fig. 13.

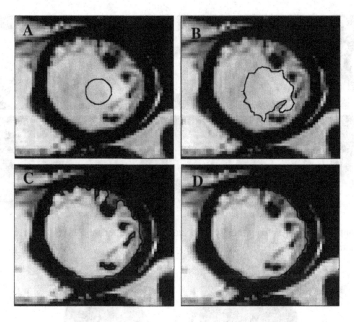

Figure 10. 2D display of the evolution on a cardiac magnetic resonance short axis slice: initial zero level (A) and the evolution after 5 (B) and 10 seconds (C) and the final detected zero level (D) superimposed to the corresponding cardiac magnetic resonance plane.

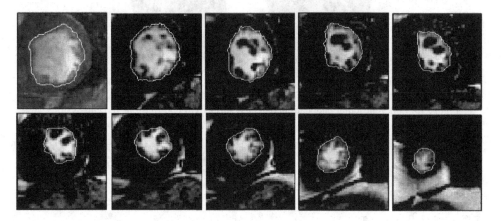

Figure 11. Contours extracted from the 3D detected surface, superimposed to the original short-axis cardiac magnetic resonance slices.

Two examples of the volume time curve computed for two subjects automatically applying the region-based method to all frames throughout the cardiac cycle is presented in fig. 14.

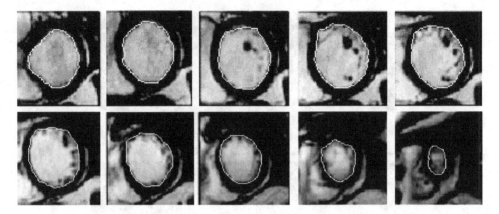

Figure 12. Contours extracted from the 3D detected surface, superimposed to the original short-axis cardiac magnetic resonance slices.

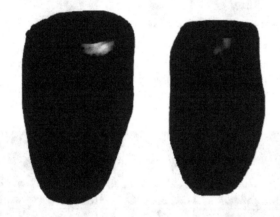

Figure 13. Left ventricular endocardial detected surfaces at end-diastole and end-systole.

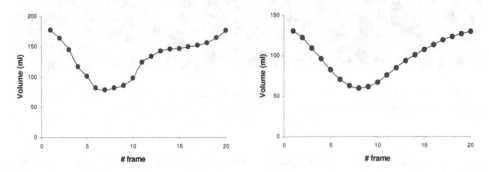

Figure 14. Volume- time curve computed automatically applying the region-based method to the cardiac magnetic resonance data for two subjects.

4. Scar Quantification

The previously described methods can be applied for myocardial scar quantification from late gadolinium enhancement cardiac magnetic resonance imaging (LGE-CMRI) imaging. This is the technique of choice to detect myocardial scars and assess myocardial viability.

In clinical practice, this analysis is performed qualitatively or by manually tracing the enhanced area in each acquired slice. Applying these methods based on PDEs, the myocardium can be automatically identified from steady-state free precession (SSFP) images and registered on LGE-CMRI data. Scar tissue inside the myocardium can be defined as myocardium with a defined signal intensity and quantified on each slice.

A fast region-based global segmentation has been applied for endocardium detection on the SSFP sequence in the same instant of time in which LGE-CMRI data was acquired. To identify the epicardial boundary we applied a basic edge-based level-set model to search the image from the endocardium outwards. The detected surfaces were registered on the LGE-CMRI data, considering the different acquisition parameters, to study the myocardium signal intensity to automatically extract scar location and extent.

In fig. 15 we show an example of an automatically detected scar in one patient in the lateral segment:

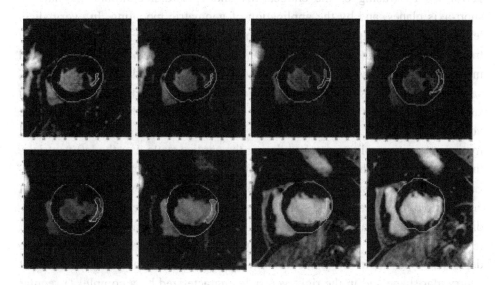

Figure 15. Example of an automatically detected scar in the lateral segment at different LV levels in one patient.

5. Discussion

Segmentation of medical images is a difficult and challenging task. Classical segmentation techniques applied to medical data usually fail for several reasons: for example, distribution of intensity values corresponding to one anatomical structure may vary throughout the structure, defeating intensity-based segmentation techniques or the strength of an edge at the boundary of a structure may vary or be weak relative to the texture inside the object creating difficulties for gradient-based boundary detection methods.

The widely recognized efficacy of level set models arises from their ability to segment images of anatomic structures by exploiting constraints derived from the image data together with other a priori knowledge about the shape or the location of the structure. Many recent studies [24-30] show that they are capable of adapting to the variability of biological structures over time and across different individuals and they support highly intuitive interaction mechanisms that allow medical doctors to bring their expertise to support the model-based image interpretation task. In both the models proposed in this chapter we don't exploit the a priori knowledge about the shape of the anatomical structure because ventricular shapes can be affected by diseases and can change in an unpredictable manner and we want the model to be independent from this knowledge.

In clinical practice, cardiac magnetic resonance datasets segmentation, is performed by tracing of the endocardial and epicardial contours on multiple short-axis planes, and by the application of geometric modeling. In every slice, left ventricular and right ventricular endocardial contours are semi-automatically traced frame-by-frame, with the papillary muscles included in the cavities, and manually corrected when necessary to optimize the boundary position. Then, ventricular volume is computed throughout the cardiac cycle using a disk-area summation method (modified Simpson's rule). End-diastolic and end-systolic volumes (EDV and ESV, respectively) are determined as the maximum and minimum cavities volume reached during the cardiac cycle. For the left ventricle, these volumes are then used to compute the ejection fraction as 100*(EDV-ESV)/EDV. For mass, left ventricular epicardial boundaries are then traced at end-diastole in each slice and mass is computed as the difference between end-diastolic epicardial and endocardial volumes times the mass density constant (1.05 g/cc). These procedures are subjective, tedious, operator-experience dependent and could be inaccurate in presence of asymmetries in the left ventricular shape and in the right ventricle characterized by a complex, irregular and widely variable morphology [11;12;31].

The use of techniques that do not rely on geometrical assumptions or modeling and work directly in the three dimensional domain could be the solution to overcome these limitations.

The two proposed techniques applied for the computation of volumes, ejection fraction and mass from cardiac magnetic resonance data fulfill these requirements and seem to provide a possible solution by directly calculating volumes and mass from endocardial and epicardial surfaces detected in the 3D space without any a priori knowledge of the shape of the object and without the use of geometric modeling. Moreover the level set formulation guarantees numerical stability and topological flexibility. Importantly, the results of these analyses could involve not only ventricular function, being available endocardial and epicardial surfaces from which volumes at ED and ES, stroke volume, ejection fraction, and mass can be derived, but also systolic and diastolic parameters could be easily derived and quantified as well as scar location and extent from the automatic dynamic analysis throughout the cardiac cycle.

The basic level set model requires an initialization step. Manual initialization of endocardial and epicardial boundaries is relatively quick and simple but could introduce some subjectivity in the volume, EF and mass measurements [32]. For the region-based level set method the initialization consists of only one point inside the cardiac chamber and the segmentation is completely automatic for the entire cardiac cycle therefore it is considerably less exacting than manual segmentation. Moreover, the results obtained comparing volumes and mass estimates [32;33] with the ones obtained by manually tracings show that these models provide accurate results.

6. Conclusion

In this chapter two mathematical models and computational algorithms based on level set methods to segment cardiac magnetic resonance imaging data have been presented. These approaches allow segmentation and reconstruction not only of the left ventricle but also of topologically complex anatomical structures such as the right ventricle, as well as automated endocardial and epicardial surface detection for scar location and extent quantification.

We showed that true volumetric analysis of cardiac magnetic resonance data for global quantitative assessment of ventricular function without the limitations of 2D imaging or 2D-based analysis of 3D data is feasible and these volumetric approaches hold promise for clinical applicability. The use of PDE-based techniques is an interesting and consolidate research topic and we believe that because of the advantages of these methods, their use will become routine in the clinical practice in the near future.

References

[1] M. Kass, A. Witkin, and D. Terzopoulos, "Snakes: Active contour models," *Int. J. Computat. Vis.*, vol. 1, pp. 321-331, 1988.

[2] T. McInerney and D. Terzopoulos, "Deformable models in medical image analysis: a survey," *Med. Image Anal.*, vol. 1, no. 2, pp. 91-108, June1996.

[3] V. Caselles, F. Catte, T. Coll, and F. Dibos, "A geometric model for active contours," *Numerische Mathematik*, vol. 66, pp. 1-31, 1993.

[4] R. Malladi, J. A. Sethian, and B. C. Vemuri, "Shape modeling with front propagation - A level set approach," *IEEE PAMI*, vol. 17, no. 2, pp. 158-175, Feb.1995.

[5] L. Alvarez, F. Guichard, P. L. Lions, and M. Morel, "Axioms and fundamental equations of image processing," *Archive for Rational Mechanics and Analysis*, vol. 123, no. 3, pp. 199-257, 1993.

[6] B. B. Kimia, A. Tannenbaum, and S. W. Zucker, "Shapes, shocks, and deformations I: the components of two-dimensional shape and the reaction-diffusion space," *Int. J. Comp. Vis.*, vol. 15, pp. 189-224, 1995.

[7] R. Kimmel, A. Amir, and A. M. Bruckstein, "Finding shortest paths on surfaces using level set propagation," *IEEE PAMI*, vol. 17, no. 6, pp. 635-640, 1995.

[8] G. Sapiro and A. Tannenbaum, "Affine invariant scale-space," *Int. J. Comp. Vis.*, vol. 11, no. 1, pp. 25-44, 1993.

[9] S. Osher and J. A. Sethian, "Fronts propagating with curvature-dependent speed - Algorithms based on Hamilton-Jacobi formulations," *Journal of Computational Physics*, vol. 79, no. 1, pp. 12-49, Nov.1988.

[10] J. A. Sethian, *Level set methods and fast marching methods*. Cambridge: Cambridge University Press, 1999.

[11] M. C. Dulce, K. Friese, A. Albrecht, B. Hamm, P. Buttner, and K. J. Wolf, "Variability and reproducibility in the determination of left-ventricular heart volume by cine-MR. A comparison of measurement methods," *Rofo*, vol. 155, no. 2, pp. 99-108, Aug.1991.

[12] P. M. Pattynama, H. J. Lamb, E. A. Van der Velde, E. E. van der Wall, and De Roos A., "Left ventricular measurements with cine and spin-echo MR imaging: a study of reproducibility with variance component analysis," *Radiology*, vol. 187, no. 1, pp. 261-268, Apr.1993.

[13] H. Thiele, I. Paetsch, B. Schnackenburg, A. Bornstedt, O. Grebe, E. Wellnhofer, G. Schuler, E. Fleck, and E. Nagel, "Improved accuracy of quantitative assessment of left ventricular volume and ejection fraction by geometric models with steady-state free precession," *J. Cardiovasc. Magn Reson.*, vol. 4, no. 3, pp. 327-339, 2002.

[14] P. Perona and J. Malik, "Scale-space and edge detection using anisotropic diffusion," *IEEE PAMI*, vol. 12, pp. 629-639, 2005.

[15] M. Mulet-Parada and J. A. Noble, "2D+T acoustic boundary detection in echocardiography," *Med. Image Anal.*, vol. 4, no. 1, pp. 21-30, Mar.2000.

[16] G. I. Sanchez-Ortiz, G. J. T. Wright, N. Clarke, J. Declerk, A. Banning, and J. A. Noble, "Automated 3D echocardiography analysis compared with manual delineation and MUGA," *IEEE TMI*, vol. 21, no. 9, pp. 1069-1076, 2002.

[17] D. Adalsteinsson and J. A. Sethian, "A fast level set method for propagating interfaces," *Journal of Computational Physics*, vol. 118, no. 2, pp. 269-277, 1995.

[18] T. F. Chan and L. Vese, "Active contours without edges," *IEEE Transactions on Image Processing*, vol. 10, no. 2, pp. 266-277, 2001.

[19] A. Sarti, C. Corsi, E. Mazzini, and Lamberti C., "Maximum likelihood segmentation of ultrasound images with Rayleigh distribution," in press ed 2005.

[20] A. Azzalini, *Statistical inference based on the likelihood*. New York: Chapman and Hall, 1996.

[21] C. Chesnaud, P. Refrigier, and V. Boulet, "Statistical region snake-based segmentation adapted to different physical noise model," *IEEE PAMI*, vol. 21, no. 11, pp. 1145-1157, 1999.

[22] H. Zhao, T. F. Chan, B. Merriman, and S. Osher, "A variational level set approach to multiphase motion," *Journal of Computational Physics*, vol. 127, pp. 179-195, 1996.

[23] M. Sussman, P. Smereka, and S. Osher, "A level set approach for computing solutions to incompressible two-phase flow," *Journal of Computational Physics*, vol. 119, pp. 146-159, 1994.

[24] S. Joshi, S. Pize, P. T. Fletcher, P. Yushkevich, A. Thall, and J. S. Marron, "Multiscale deformable model segmentation and statistical shape analysis using medial descriptors," *IEEE TMI*, vol. 21, no. 5, pp. 538-550, 2002.

[25] N. Paragios, "A level set approach for shape-driven segmentation and tracking of the left ventricle," *IEEE TMI*, vol. 22, no. 6, pp. 773-776, 2003.

[26] A. Tsai, A. J. Yezzi, W. Wells, C. Tempany, D. Tucker, A. Fan, W. E. Grimson, and A. Willsky, "A shape-based approach to the segmentation of medical imagery using level sets," *IEEE TMI*, vol. 22, no. 2, pp. 137-154, 2003.

[27] J. Yang and J. S. Duncan, "3D image segmentation of deformable objects with joint shape-intensity prior models using level sets," *Med. Image Anal.*, vol. 8, no. 3, pp. 285-294, 2004.

[28] J. Yang, L. H. Staib, and J. S. Duncan, "Neighbor-constrained segmentation with level set-based 3-D deformable models," *IEEE TMI*, vol. 23, no. 8, pp. 940-948, 2004.

[29] K. Kadir, H. Gao, A. Payne, J. Soraghan, and C. Berry, "LV wall segmentation using the variational level set method (LSM) with additional shape constraint for oedema quantification," *Phys Med Biol* vol. 57, no. 19, pp. 6007-23, 2012.

[30] M. Ammar, S. Mahmoudi, M. A. Chikh, and A. Abbou, "Endocardial border detection in cardiac magnetic resonance images using level set method," *J Digit Imaging*, vol. 25(2), pp. 294-306, 2012.

[31] P. M. Pattynama, H. J. Lamb, E. A. Van der Velde, R. J. van der Geest, E. E. van der Wall, and De Roos A., "Reproducibility of MRI-derived measurements of right ventricular volumes and myocardial mass," *Magn Reson. Imaging*, vol. 13, no. 1, pp. 53-63, 1995.

[32] C. Corsi, C. Lamberti, O. Catalano, P. MacEneaney, D. Bardo, R. M. Lang, E. G. Caiani, and V. Mor-Avi, "Improved quantification of left ventricular volumes and mass based on endocardial and epicardial surface detection from cardiac MR using level set methods," *J Am Soc Echocardiography*, vol. in press 2005.

[33] O. Catalano, C. Corsi, S. Antonaci, G. Moro, M. Mussida, M. Frascaroli, M. Baldi, E. Caiani, C. Lamberti, and F. Cobelli, "Improved reproducibility of right ventricular volumes and function estimation from cardiac magnetic resonance images using level-set models," *Magn Reson Med*, vol. 57(3), pp. 600-5, 2007.

CHAPTER 20

AUTOMATED IVUS SEGMENTATION USING DEFORMABLE TEMPLATE MODEL WITH FEATURE TRACKING[*]

Prakash Manandhar[1,*] and Chi Hau Chen[2,†]

[1]*University of Massachusetts Dartmouth and Integra Co.*
[2]*University of Massachusetts Dartmouth*
E-mail: pmanandhar@umassd.edu
†*E-mail: cchen@umassd.edu*

Intravascular Ultrasound (IVUS) has been established as a useful tool for diagnosis of coronary heart disease (CHD). Recent developments have opened the possibility of using IVUS to create a 3D map from which preventative prediction of CHD can be attempted. Segmentation of IVUS images is an important step in this process. However reliable automated segmentation has been elusive, in part because of the variety of image features that are invariably present in the image that distract from the main segmentation objectives. Active contour models (ACM)s have been used successfully for automated segmentation of IVUS images. However, the accuracy of the segmentation is still not adequate for clinical use. Here we describe a new approach of a constrained deformable template model (DTM) that improves on the standard ACM algorithm by (1) detecting distracting image features (2) using tracking algorithms to get a better estimate of the positions of these features (3) including the knowledge of these positions to eliminate distortions in the ACM due to these features. In addition, semantic constraints are inbuilt into the DTM so that computational time is not wasted in improbable segmentation results.

A 3-D IVUS image segmentation display is presented. Our results show that this is a promising approach to achieving fully automated segmentation with accuracy comparable to manual segmentation.

1. Introduction

Starting with its introduction in the late 1980s [1], Intravascular Ultrasound (IVUS) has been used successfully as a diagnostic tool for various coronary heart diseases. More recently, the IVUS technique has been used for "vascular profiling" where a 3D representation of the coronary artery is formed by

---

[*]Adapted from Chapter 4.3 in Handbook of PRCV, vol. 4, WSPC, 2010.

combining a series of IVUS images with location data from x-ray angiography. This process is an accurate and reproducible [2], but labor-intensive since a single profile can consist of thousands of IVUS frames. Automated segmentation algorithms have been improving. However, a fully automated algorithm that achieves accuracy at the level of manual segmentation has been elusive. Numerous automated IVUS segmentation algorithms have been reported ranging from knowledge-based graph search [3], texture-based [4], active-contour models [5] or a combination of these techniques [6]. These techniques do not directly address the presence of artefacts in the typical IVUS image, of which two of the major ones are due to the guidewire and the catheter (Fig. 2) [7].

Observation of the manual segmentation by human experts hinted that the experts are well aware of the presence of these artefacts and actively allowed for their effects to create a good segmentation. Additionally, the positions of the artefacts are strongly correlated between adjacent frames which provide further hints for the segmentation process. Here we present evidence that detecting artefacts and tracking them to later compensate is a good strategy for increased accuracy in automated segmentation.

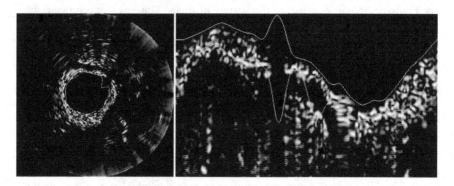

Fig. 1. Distortion in contour initialization due to guidewire and its shadow (The left side shows a cross-sectional slice in normal view while the right side is 'polar' view). The contour initialization was done using the algorithm described in [5].

Blood vessels are composed of several layers of tissues. The lumen through which blood flows is surrounded by the intima, which is surrounded by the media and then the adventitia. The media and adventitia are separated by the external elastic membrane (EEM). In addition there can be deposits of plaque of different types within the intimal layer. Multilayered tissue creates an ultrasound image that is non-trivial to interpret. Adding to this complexity is the scatter from flowing blood in the lumen.

2. Guidewire detection and tracking

A guidewire (usually 0.038 inch) is inserted and manipulated inside the blood-vessel to the point of interest. The IVUS catheter is threaded over the guidewire, either co-axially or in a monorail fashion. The guidewire in the monorail system creates an acoustic shadow (along with a bright reverberation from the metal wire itself). When an interventionalist is in an interactive diagnosis session, the IVUS catheter can be rotated to reveal the hidden area, however in a pullback sequence, this cannot be done [8].

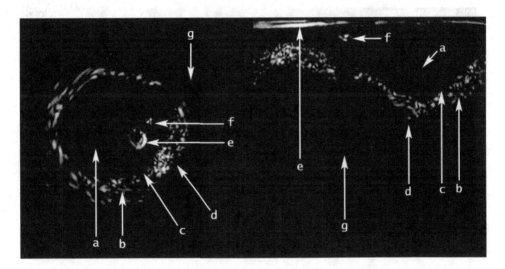

Fig. 2. Typical IVUS image (left: rectangular view, right: polar view) showing (a) lumen (b) media (c) intima (d) EEM (e) catheter artefact (f) guidewire artefact (g) guidewire shadow.

The guidewire feature was investigated from all frames of 2 different pull-back sequences consisting of about 10,000 frames in total. A typical frame of data is presented in Fig. 2. It can be seen that close to the catheter (low r-index, refer to Fig. 10) the guide wire produces a distinct echo-dense region with reverberations followed by a long narrow shadow region. As it is possible to have shadow regions due to other features such as calcified deposits and branches in the vessels, the salient features of the guidewire artefact were identified. Based on this a template matching algorithm was implemented where a series of templates consisting of Gaussian blobs at various r-index positions were matched with slices of the image. However, this only resulted in 80% accuracy for guidewire position. A simpler method of ordering "energy" levels in a certain radial range, combined with tracking produced better results.

Since the guidewire is a continuous wire, it can be expected from the nature of the physical process that the change in guidewire position in subsequent frames is minimal. Often, to reduce the effects of the moving heart an ECG set is gathered simultaneously with the IVUS data. The IVUS frames are then 'gated' so that only the frames from the same part of the cardiac cycle are considered. This means that a majority of the data is discarded. We found that using the full data set is helpful in tracking the guidewire position since changes in position are minimal between adjacent frames.

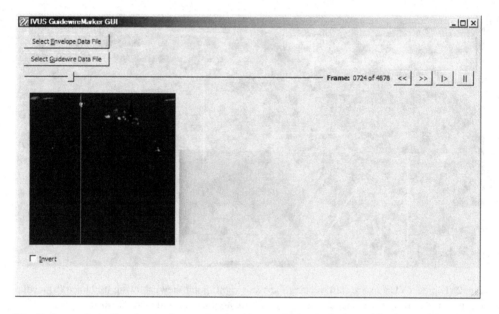

Fig. 3. Screenshot of custom software developed to quickly mark the guidewire position in an IVUS pullback sequence. After the user loads the data file and the guidewire marker file which contains, for each frame a flag indicating whether the guidewire has been marked or not and if yes, the position of the guidewire. The when the mouse pointer is inside the image area, a line follows the pointer and when the user clicks the position is marked the frame moves forward; existing marks are shown in a different color. This allows the user to quickly mark a large number of frames – at the rate of about 5000 frames in several hours.

To study the character of the data a reference set of data where the guidewire position was manually marked was needed. Since this data is not typically recorded during routine manual segmentation, custom software was designed to quickly mark the guidewire position in a pullback sequence manually (Fig. 3). Four typical pullback sets consisting of about 5000 frames were marked using this software. Various statistics of the vectors along the guidewire area were compiled from these data to determine an appropriate algorithm for accurate guidewire detection and tracking algorithm. Fig. 5 shows the manually marked guidewire position for a particular pullback sequence. Analysis of the data showed that the guidewire position can be considered to be an autoregressive process where the next position is the previous position plus white Gaussian noise. This suggests the use of tracking the guidewire using Kalman filtering, however the presence of clutter meant that there were significant places in regions where there were shadows other than caused by the guidewire. Using the ConDensation algorithm gave much better results (Table 1). Comparison between the vectors with guidewire and without guidewire in the manually marked data showed that a simple process to compare the intensity values after radius index from $r_{min} = 50$ and $r_{max} = 200$ might be just as effective as using a template matching algorithm. Indeed the simpler algorithm was able to track the guidewire with improved accuracy (Table 1). N hypotheses (where $N = 5$) were generated using the following ordering method:

$$x_{n,t} = \min_{\theta,n} \sum_{r=r_{min}}^{r_{max}} f(r,\theta); \; n = 1,2,...N$$

where

$f(r,\theta)$ is   the image pixel value at radius r and angle θ

t is   the frame index

$x_{n,t}$ is   the nth hypothesis that the guidewire is located at $\theta = x_{n,t}$

Multiple observation hypotheses generated by this process are fed into a particle filtering tracking algorithm [9] based on a variation of the conditional density propagation (ConDensation) tracking algorithm [10]. This algorithm performs better than the Kalman filtering algorithm and can handle multiple hypotheses simultaneously due to extensive clutter (Fig. 4). The accuracy of the results was evaluated by considering the difference in θ between the tracked guidewire position and the manually marked position.

We tried several different methods for guidewire tracking and a variation of the ConDensation algorithm that we have named particle filtering with weighted tunneling has given us the best results. In this algorithm the Bayesian reasoning box in Fig. 4 gives higher weight to the more probable observations and lower weights to the less likely ones. Additionally a "tunneling probability" is also included which keep the possibility that all the observations are false taking into account the probability of non-detection. This probability allows the guidewire estimates from the previous frames to carry on even when none of the new observations match. Table 1 compares results between choosing the best hypothesis without tracking and using various tracking algorithms and shows that particle filtering with weighted tunneling is clearly a more robust method.

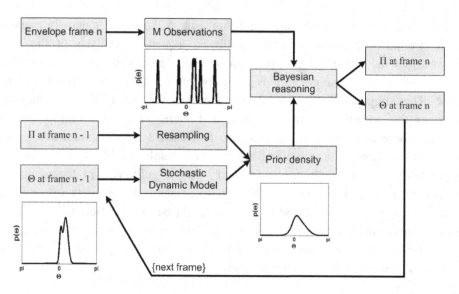

Fig. 4. Conditional density tracking (a.k.a. sequential Monte Carlo particle filtering [11]) used for accurate tracking of guidewire in cluttered observation. Θ and Π are the sets of samples (particles) and their probability weights. The dynamic model that we have used is an AR-1 model where the estimate for the next iteration is assumed to be the estimate for the present iteration with some noise added. Re-sampling and applying the stochastic model diffuses the PDF of the prior and also prevents degeneracy. Note the presence of many peaks in the observation density due to 'clutter'. The observation and prior are combined to get the new densities from which the new estimate of guidewire position can be derived in a maximum-apriori (MAP) sense or by taking the expectation of the distribution.

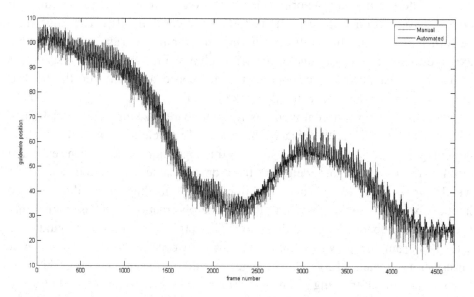

Fig. 5. Match between ConDensation tracking estimate and manual marked guidewire position.

Table 1. Comparison of error rates among various algorithms that we developed for guidewire tracking. BL – baseline algorithm just chooses the best estimate from the observation of the current frame. KP – Kalman filtering with position model is a Kalman filter implementation where the next guidewire position is estimated to be the previous position with Gaussian noise. KV – similar to KP, but includes a velocity model. PF – simple particle filtering without tunneling. PT – particle filtering with tunneling. PW – particle filtering with tunneling and weighting of observations. Details of the algorithm implementation have been left out as they are out of the scope of this chapter.

Dataset	Frames	Error >±10						Error >±5					
		BL	KP	KV	PF	PT	PW	BL	KP	KV	PF	PT	PW
1	5211	18	3	11	14	28	16	406	367	490	704	805	494
		0.35%	0.06%	0.21%	0.27%	0.54%	0.31%	7.79%	7.04%	9.4%	13.51%	15.44%	9.48%
2	4691	88	99	100	136	10	2	311	286	389	596	535	275
		1.88%	2.11%	2.13%	2.90%	0.21%	0.04%	6.63%	6.10%	8.29%	12.71%	11.40%	5.86%

3. Catheter position and vessel diameter estimate using the Circular Hough Transform (CHT)

"Ring-down" artefacts observed as bright halos of variable thickness surround the catheter. These are produced by acoustic oscillations in the transducer and obscure the area immediately adjacent to the transducer [7].

The image is easier to segment when the catheter lies near the centre of the lumen so that it is not touching the vessel intima. A human observer can quite easily determine the catheter position and identify regions within the image where the ring-down artefacts can reduce the certainty of conclusions about the position of the intima and the other vessel wall layers.

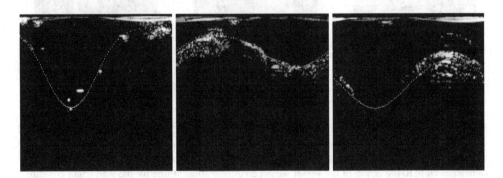

Fig. 6. Circular Hough Transform results for three different catheter positions. These results also show how the ring-down artefacts can be a hindrance in subsequent active contour model processing. For example in the second the third figure the catheter is sufficiently close to the lumen wall that the active contour model is highly likely to get confused distorting the final result.

Although it is clear that the lumen is most often not a perfect circle, it was found that in most frames the circle approximation does provide an approximate location of the catheter with respect to the vessel wall. Rosales [12] also use a circular model for tracking the catheter position within the vessel, while Gil [13] use an eclipse template. A circle only has three parameters (centre coordinates and radius), an eclipse has 5 parameters which dramatically expands the search space increasing the time and memory resources needed for the algorithm. Since we are not considering the result of this step to be the final segmentation and still need to apply the deformable model, a circular model does suffice in our case. Huang [14] have also found tracking of CHT parameters directly in the Hough domain across video frames using a ConDensation like probabilistic data association filter, to be feasible for real time tracking of circular objects in clutter for robotic vision. Elsewhere, French [15] have found tracking in the Hough space to be suitable for vehicle tracking using parallel lines.

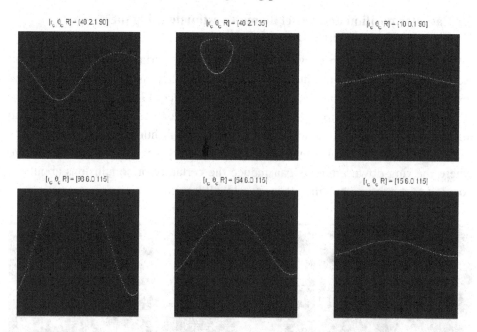

Fig. 7. Simulated catheter position and vessel radius variations. Note that for the catheter to be within the vessel, the radius of the vessel has to be greater than the radial position of the center of the catheter; the top center image shows an example of a violation of this principle. When the catheter is close to the center of the vessel we get an almost straight line for the wall (right column), while an a highly curved structure means that the catheter is positioned close to the vessel wall.

Fig. 7 shows the trace of the shape of the curve for circles in polar co-ordinates. These traces are very similar to the vessel wall outlines we see in the polar IVUS images hinting that CHT in the polar domain might be a good process to identify them.

Since the guidewire position has already been estimated, the image regions distorted by the guidewire can be ignored while performing the Hough transform. This reduces the resources required by the algorithm and increases the accuracy of the method. Fig. 8 depicts a case where the CHT fails to find the correct wall when there is too much distraction from the guidewire artifact. Inclusion of the guidewire position knowledge corrected the mistake in the CHT output.

Fig. 6 shows some results of the application of CHT to IVUS images. Observation of the catheter position shows that it is also highly correlated between adjacent frames. The ConDensation algorithm is general enough to track more than one parameter at once. Incorporation of tracking along with avoidance of artefacts by using results from guidewire tracking shows a marked improvement in registration of vessel wall without error (Fig. 8).

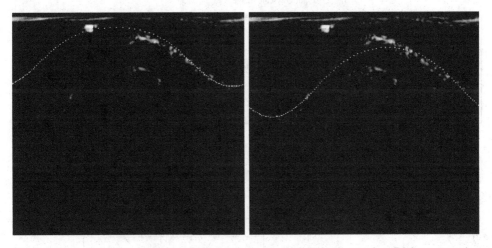

Fig. 8. Left – error in registration by CHT due to presence of guidewire artefact. Right – correction of this error by incorporation of unreliable data avoidance with guidewire tracking.

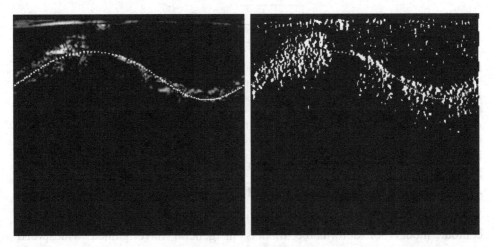

Fig. 9. Left: CHT result superimposed over original frame image. Right: the Sobel edge detected image with adaptive threshold based on which the CHT is performed.

Curve fitting algorithms are usually applied on binary images and their statistical performance has also been evaluated based on the assumption of a binary image [16]. It is possible to directly work on the grayscale image, however to reduce the effect of noise and focus on the changes in intensity rather than on constant graylevel areas. We have used an adaptive Sobel method to create the binary image from the envelope data (Algorithm 1).

Algorithm 1 Sobel edge filter with adaptive thresholding

$$
\begin{aligned}
f_i & : \quad \text{input grayscale image} \\
f_b & : \quad \text{output binary image} \\
H & = \begin{bmatrix} 1 & 2 & 1 \\ 0 & 0 & 0 \\ -1 & 2 & -1 \end{bmatrix} \text{(vertical Sobel edge filter)} \\
t & = 1.05 \text{ (threshold ratio)} \\
f & = H * f_i \\
m & = \text{median}(f) \\
f_b & = f > (t \times m)
\end{aligned}
$$

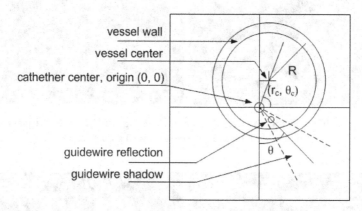

Fig. 10. Geometry of tracked parameters. The angle at which guidewire artefact appears (θ) is tracked using particle filtering (or ConDensation) algorithm with observations generated by ordering of energy values along data vectors as described in the text (section 2). The parameters (R, r_c, θ_c) corresponding to the position and radius of the vessel wall modeled as a circle are tracked separately using a similar particle filtering method with observations generated by ordering bins in a Circular Hough Transform space. All parameters are indexed into bins, for example θ is indexed into 256 bins of $360/256 = 1.4$ degrees.

4. Deformable template model for IVUS

Since its introduction in the late 1980s in the computer vision literature, active contour models or deformable models in general have gained widespread popularity in the medical image processing community [17].

Here we devise a deformable template model with a goal to refine the contour estimated by the CHT in the previous step so that a more accurate contour for the lumen and adventitia are produced. There are some additional constraints that need to be satisfied at all times, so that the artefacts do not disturb the contour and some natural domain constraints are satisfied:

1. extra edges and gradients in the gap due to the guidewire and other gaps due to branches should be avoided
2. extra edges due to the catheter should be avoided
3. the catheter should always be located inside the lumen
4. the lumen should always be located inside the EEM

Data Structure 1 IVUS template

Constants:
- N [Integer, power of 2]: number of pixels in IVUS image in the r and theta directions, so that we have a NxN image [N == 256].
- M [Integer, power of 2]: number of node points per contour. [M == 8].
- delM [Integer, power of 2]: = N/M
- rMin, rMax [Integer, rMin < rMax < N]: rMin [== 30] defines the region close to the catheter where catheter artefacts are prominent. rMax [== 225] defines the region far away from catheter where there is no usable data.
- minWall [Integer]: minimum radial distance between lumen and adventitial giving a minimum thickness of vessel wall.
- gradSigma [Real]: parameter for Gaussian smoothing to be applied before calculating the gradient.
- gwPos [Integer between 1 and N]: location of guidewire. This parameter is initialized once for each frame.
- circleParams [Real x Real x Real]: triplet giving r_c (center of catheter radial co-ordinate), theta_c (center of catheter theta co-ordinate) and R (radius of vessel). This parameter is initialized once for each frame, and then is used to initialize luNodes and avNodes.

Variables:
- luNodes, avNodes [array of M integers]: r indices of lumen and adventitia respectively. Together these form the 2M parameters to be optimized in a constrained space.

The problem of adding hard constraints has been dealt with variously in the literature. For example, Fua [18] have devised an optimization method where the gradient is projected onto the constraint to speed up convergence in the direction of the constraint. They have argued that the simpler method of just including a penalty in the cost function results in an ill behaved optimization problem with poor convergence and also requires careful consideration for commensurate choice of weights. Jain [19] show that a global model based approach is suitable for ensuring consistency due to constraints and bridging between gaps in the model. The deformable template model that we have devised has served as a good example of these properties. In addition, compared to a simple active contour model, we have achieved good convergence while minimizing the number of parameters to be optimized.

We have used a template model based on closed 3rd degree B-splines [20]. The method has been extended by encoding into the model parameters for two separate contours: lumen and EEM in the same template and then optimizing simultaneously. The constraints defined above are naturally incorporated in this approach. The deformable template model data structure is listed in box: Data Structure 1. It is convenient to choose M and N to be powers of 2 for computational convenience and simplicity in algorithms. The node points are uniformly divided along the theta direction, with the distance between them as delM (this is simplified if N and M are both powers of 2). A larger M allows the contours to follow the features more closely, but this also means the smoothness of the resulting curve is compromised. A small M results in a contour that is too smooth. By choosing an appropriate M, we are in effect implementing an internal energy function in the traditional snake model [20]. A multi-resolution approach can also be implemented by varying M, minWall and gradSigma.

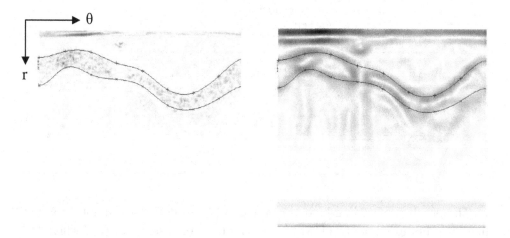

Fig. 11. Result of fitting deformable template model with two contours – lumen (top) and EEM (bottom). The cost function is actually calculated on the Derivative of Gradient image (right). The left image is the actual frame data.

```
Algorithm 2 Deformable template optimization

T: optimized template = optimize (f: image frame, To: old template)
fg = DoG (f, gradSigma) : take the derivative of Gaussian
initializeNodes : see Algorithm 4
del = 1 : search stepsize
Iterate until no change in current cost
        1.  For each node (n[i]) in luNodes and avNodes check
            (sequencially) minimum cost of n[i] + del, n[i] - del, and
            n[i], avoiding the rMin, rMax and minWall constraints and
            assign the lowest cost to luNodes or avNodes respectively
        2.  For each node pair (l[i], a[i]) in (luNodes, avNodes) check
            (sequencially) minimum combined cost of (l[i] + del, a[i] +
            del), (l[i] - del, a[i] - del) and (l[i], a[i]), subject to
            the constraints. Assign lowest cost as new contours
```

```
Algorithm 3 Generate exclusion mask

Ze = exclusionMask (T: template)
Ze = zero matrix of size T.N x T.N
Ze = 1 where r <= T.rMin and r >= T.rMax
Ze = 1 where theta is between plus or minus thWidth (= 10) of T.gwPos
```

```
Algorithm 4 Initialize Nodes

delR = 10 is the spacing between the circle and initial luNodes and
avNodes initialization

c  = r_c*r_c - R*R
th = array of M theta values equally spaced from -pi to pi
b  = -2*r_c*cos(th - theta_c)
r  = round((b + sqrt(b*b - 4*c))/2)
luNodes = r - delR; avNodes = r + delR
if luNodes[i] < rMin, luNodes[i] = rMin
if avNodes[i] > rMax, avNodes[i] = rMax
```

```
Algorithm 5 Cost function for template model optimization

c : Real = cost (nodes: luNodes or avNodes, fg: NxN gradient image)
r_array = interpolate between nodes and round to get from list of nodes
to radius index of the contour for all theta.
c = negative of sum over theta of fg[r_array[theta], theta]] except at
exclusion mask positions generated by Algorithm 3.
```

Although B-splines are more naturally implemented as control points, we use nodes (nodes pass through the B-spline curve, while control points do not) to simplify the process of initializing and updating the contours. An efficient algorithm described in [21] is used to convert between the representations and also to interpolate between the nodes. These give rise to the cost function (Algorithm 5) to be optimized along with the frame data. The frame data is processed through a Derivative of Gaussian filter [22] to eliminate speckle noise effects to get a gradient map; costs are calculated as line integrals on this map (Fig. 11). Note that we use the negative of the integral so that we have a minimization problem.

Once we have the cost function, we perform a gradient descent search on the parameters until the cost can no longer be reduced. This simple greedy approach [23] produces good results since the approximation of the vessel wall from which we start is already a good approximation. (Refer to box: for more details.) Note that in each iteration we are tweaking each of the 2M parameters in turn towards decreasing cost. In effect we are following a space alternating gradient descent method similar to the space alternating expectation maximization algorithm described in [24]. In our case, we are also simultaneously enforcing geometric constraints to further constrain the search space. It is also possible to do a true gradient descent or conjugate gradient search and it is also possible to do a true gradient descent or conjugate gradient search. Brigger [20] outline a method to achieve this when we have B-spline nodes as parameters, by first converting them to control points and taking the necessary partial derivatives with respect to these parameters. However, due to the large parameter space and the presence of noise in the gradient, we find that this method is less effective than a space alternating search.

Improvements in the search strategy can be made by incorporating non-greedy steps in the search process, or by incorporating more flexible greedy steps onto the process. An example of the former could be the incorporation of large jumps in non-optimal directions every few iterations which can be backtracked if no optimal solution is found in that direction. An example of the later could be to incorporate search at `2*del` and `10*del` positions away from the current positions into each iteration. We have left these improvements for further work.

5. Concluding Remarks

Comparing the traditional snake based method with our deformable template method, it can be seen that the contours are not distracted (Fig. 9, Fig. 11) due to the presence of the guidewire or catheter artifact (compare with Fig. 1). Additionally, these contours converged from the CHT based initialization in only 10 iterations, compared to several hundred iterations required for the inferior results in Fig. 1. As the template model is severely constrained according to domain knowledge, it is not surprising that better results can be obtained in fewer iterations.

Fig. 12 summarizes the entire dataflow pipeline combining the various methods outlined in this chapter. It is conceivable that further improvements in the results can be achieved if errors due to convergence to local minima in the final step of fitting the deformable contour model can be removed. One possible way to achieve this is to use a deformable surface model and fit across frames. Godbout [25] describe one such approach that can be adopted to fit the method described in this chapter.

In summary, deformable template models where the model embodies the constraints due to the domain can be a feasible way to modify the simple active contour model. Tracking by particle filtering of multiple features can be a feasible preprocessing step for improving accuracy of segmentation by deformable models by simply changing the cost function to reflect data about the position of the tracked features. This can be especially helpful when the features to be tracked are persistent across frames and their positions correlated between frames. Fig. 10 depicts the parameters that are tracked in the current implementation in relation to the geometry of the problem. Further improvements could be made by tracking more parameters. For example the radial location of the guidewire location can be tracked along with the angle at which the guidewire artefact occurs. The tracking algorithm can also be further refined since we know that the motion of the catheter within the vessel and the guidewire with respect to the catheter is cyclic in nature resulting from the beating heart.

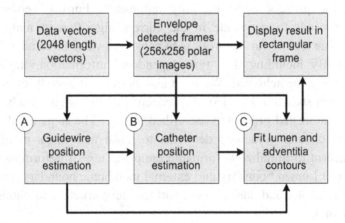

Fig. 12. Dataflow in our automated IVUS segmentation algorithm showing its three major components: (A) Guidewire position estimation (B) Catheter position estimation and (C) lumen and adventitia contour fitting using a deformable template model. All three processes get their data from the envelope detected frame. Steps (B) and (C) use the data from (A) to create a data unreliability region where data in the envelope frame is not used (to avoid distortion due to artefacts). The contours (deformable template parameters) in (C) are initialized with data from (B), the deformable template then optimizes its precise position with data from the envelope frame.

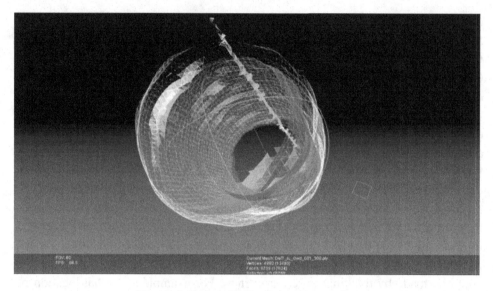

Fig. 13. A display of 3-D segmentation results.

We have outlined a framework for fully automated IVUS image segmentation from a pullback sequence which can potentially overcome the limitations of current methods. However, a very high accuracy level in all the frames is required if the process is to be fully automated. Further verification and improvement needs to me made in the current algorithm to make it fit for clinical use. One area of further work is to consider two or three adjacent images at one time. By including the "time-dependent" information, more accurate segmentation may be achieved. We have also performed a study of 3-D display (with a snapshot shown in Fig. 13) of a sequence of 300 images each segmented by using the automated procedure described above. The steps involved for the 3-D construction are: guidewire detection to make next steps more accurate, Hough transform to initialize deformable template, use of deformable template model to detect Lumen boundary and external membrane boundary, representing boundaries as point cloud, and Poisson surface reconstruction to obtain surfaces from point cloud.

With 2-D display some results for various cases are shown in Figs. 14 and 15. While the fully automated segmentation results in these figures are near to what we would expect from manual segmentation, there is room for improvement. Verification using manually segmented data is required for full evaluation.

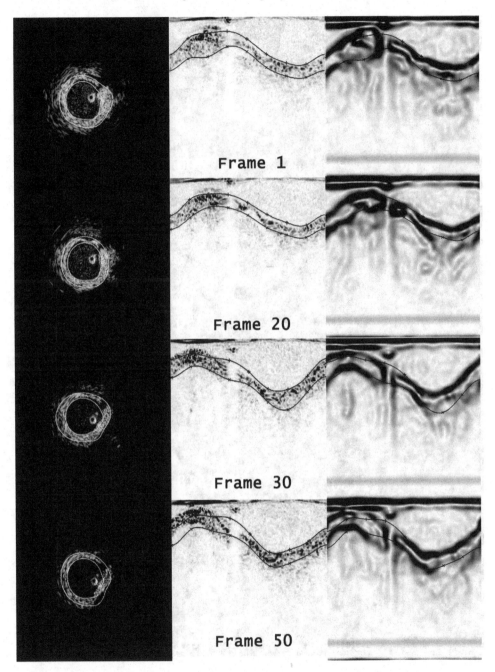

Fig. 14. Several representative frames of fully automated segmentation. In frame 50, there is a non-uniform rotational distortion and the algorithm was successful in smoothing over this distortion. Left column: segmentation result plotted on rectangular image, middle column: segmentation result plotted on polar image (image inverted for clarity), right column: segmentation results plotted on gradient image.

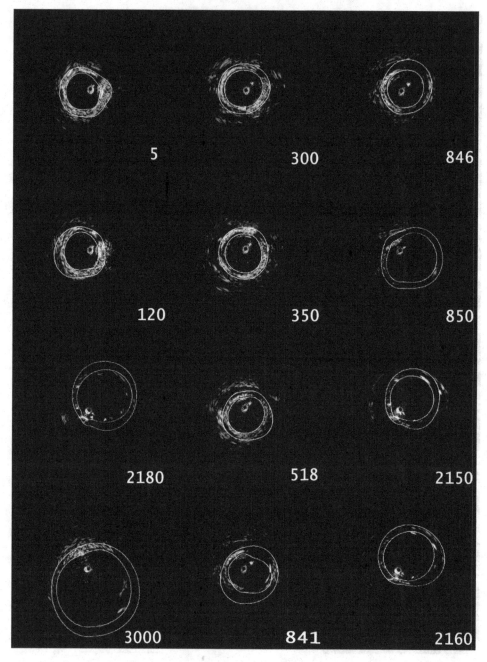

Fig. 15. A selection of segmentation results from a pull-back sequence. The segmentation is mostly correct but can miss parts of the intima or EEM pointing to room for improvement.

Acknowledgements

We thank the help of Gail MacCallum, Michelle Lucier and Nicholas Cefalo of the Vascular Profiling Laboratory at the Brigham & Women's Hospital, Boston, MA for their help with the IVUS image data.

References

[1] P. Yock, D. Linker, O. Saether, H. Thapliyal, J. Arenson, N. White and others, "Intravascular Two-Dimensional Catheter Ultrasound: Initial Clinical Studies," *Circulation*, vol. 78, pp. 11-21, 1988.

[2] A. U. Coskun, Y. Yeghiazarians, S. Kinlay, M. E. Clark, O. J. Ilegbusi, A. Wahle, M. Sonka, J. J. Popma, R. E. Kuntz, C. L. Feldman and P. H. Stone, "Reproducibility of coronary lumen, plaque, and vessel wall reconstruction and of endothelial shear stress measurements in vivo in humans," *Catheterization and Cardiovascular Interventions*, vol. 60, pp. 67-78, 2003.

[3] M. Sonka, X. Zhang, M. Siebes, M. Bissing, S. Dejong, S. Collins and C. McKay, "Segmentation of intravascular ultrasound images: a knowledge-basedapproach," *Medical Imaging, IEEE Transactions on*, vol. 14, pp. 719-732, 1995.

[4] M. Papadogiorgaki, V. Mezaris, Y. Chatzizisis, I. Kompatsiaris and G. Giannoglou, "A fully automated texture-based approach for the segmentation of sequential IVUS images," in *13th International Conference on Systems, Signals & Image Processing (IWSSIP 2006), Budapest, Hungary*, 2006, pp. 461-464.

[5] G. D. Giannoglou, Y. S. Chatzizisis, V. Koutkias, I. Kompatsiaris, M. Papadogiorgaki, V. Mezaris, E. Parissi, P. Diamantopoulos, M. G. Strintzis and N. Maglaveras, "A novel active contour model for fully automated segmentation of intravascular ultrasound images: In vivo validation in human coronary arteries," *Comput. Biol. Med.*, vol. 37, pp. 1292-1302, 2007.

[6] D. Gil, A. Hernandez, O. Rodriguez, J. Mauri and P. Radeva, "Statistical Strategy for Anisotropic Adventitia Modelling in IVUS," *IEEE Trans. Med. Imaging*, vol. 25, pp. 768, 2006.

[7] G. Mintz, S. Nissen, W. Anderson, S. Bailey, R. Erbel, P. Fitzgerald, F. Pinto, K. Rosenfield, R. Siegel, E. Tuzcu and others, "ACC Clinical Expert Consensus Document on Standards for Acquisition, Measurement and Reporting of Intravascular Ultrasound Studies (IVUS). A report of the American College of Cardiology Task Force on Clinical Expert Consensus Documents," *J. Am. Coll. Cardiol.*, vol. 37, pp. 1478-1492, 2001.

[8] P. Neglén, "Venous stenting using intravascular ultrasound," in *Noninvasive Vascular Diagnosis*, 2nd ed. A. F. AbuRahma and J. J. Bergan, Eds. London: Springer, 2007, pp. 406-413.

[9] S. Das, D. Lawless, B. Ng and A. Pfeffer, "Factored particle filtering for data fusion and situation assessment in urban environments," in *Information Fusion, 2005 7th International Conference on*, 2005,

[10] M. Isard and A. Blake, "CONDENSATION—Conditional Density Propagation for Visual Tracking," *International Journal of Computer Vision*, vol. 29, pp. 5-28, 1998.

[11] M. Arulampalam, S. Maskell, N. Gordon, T. Clapp, D. Sci, T. Organ and S. Adelaide, "A tutorial on particle filters for online nonlinear/non-GaussianBayesian tracking," *Signal Processing, IEEE Transactions on [See also Acoustics, Speech, and Signal Processing, IEEE Transactions on]*, vol. 50, pp. 174-188, 2002.

[12] M. Rosales, P. Radeva, O. Rodriguez-Leor and D. Gil, "Modelling of image-catheter motion for 3-D IVUS," *Med. Image Anal.*, 2008.

[13] D. Gil, P. Radeva, J. Saludes and J. Mauri, "Automatic segmentation of artery wall in coronary IVUS images: aprobabilistic approach," *Computers in Cardiology 2000*, pp. 687-690, 2000.

[14] C. M. Huang, C. W. Lai and L. C. Fu, "Visual tracking with probabilistic data association filter based on the circular hough transform," in *Robotics and Automation, 2006. ICRA 2006. Proceedings 2006 IEEE International Conference on*, 2006, pp. 4094-4099.

[15] A. French, S. Mills and T. Pridmore, "Condensation tracking through a hough space," in *Pattern Recognition, 2004. ICPR 2004. Proceedings of the 17th International Conference on*, 2004.

[16] K. Kanatani, "Statistical Optimization for Geometric Fitting: Theoretical Accuracy Bound and High Order Error Analysis," *International Journal of Computer Vision*, vol. 80, pp. 167-188, 2008.

[17] T. McInerney and D. Terzopoulos, "Deformable models in medical image analysis: a survey," *Med. Image Anal.*, vol. 1, pp. 91-108, 1996.

[18] P. Fua and U. Brechbuehler, "Imposing hard constraints on soft snakes," *LECTURE NOTES IN COMPUTER SCIENCE*, pp. 495-506, 1996.

[19] A. K. Jain, Y. Zhong and M. P. Dubuisson-Jolly, "Deformable template models: A review," *Signal Process*, vol. 71, pp. 109-129, 1998.

[20] P. Brigger, J. Hoeg and M. Unser, "B-spline snakes: a flexible tool for parametric contour detection," *Image Processing, IEEE Transactions on*, vol. 9, pp. 1484-1496, 2000.

[21] M. Unser, A. Aldroubi and M. Eden, "B-spline signal processing. II. Efficient design and applications," *Signal Processing, IEEE Transactions on [See also Acoustics, Speech, and Signal Processing, IEEE Transactions on]*, vol. 41, pp. 834-848, 1993.

[22] M. Sonka, V. Hlavac and R. Boyle, *Image Processing, Analysis, and Machine Vision.*, 2nd ed. PWS Pub., 1999, pp. 770.

[23] T. H. Cormen, C. E. Leiserson, R. L. Rivest, C. Stein and T. H. Cormen, *Introduction to Algorithms.*, 2nd ed. MIT Press, 2001, pp. 1180.

[24] J. Fessler and A. Hero, "Space-alternating generalized expectation-maximization algorithm," *Signal Processing, IEEE Transactions on [See also Acoustics, Speech, and Signal Processing, IEEE Transactions on]*, vol. 42, pp. 2664-2677, 1994.

[25] B. Godbout, J. A. de Guise, G. Soulez and G. Cloutier, "3D elastic registration of vessel structures from IVUS data on biplane angiography1," *Acad. Radiol.*, vol. 12, pp. 10-16, 2005.

INDEX

Call for Book Proposals

Direct your submissions to *cchen@umassd.edu*

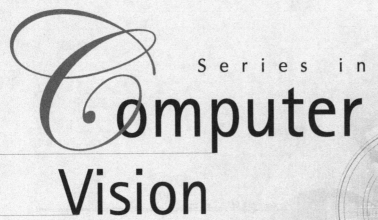

Series in

Computer Vision

Series Editor

C.H. CHEN

Professor Emeritus
Department of Electrical and Computer Engineering
University of Massachusetts Dartmouth, USA

In recent years, there has been significant progress in computer vision in theory and methodology and enormous advancement on the application front, accompanied by rapid progress in vision systems and technology.

It is hoped that this book series in computer vision can capture most of the important and recent progress and results in computer vision. The target audiences cover researchers, engineers, scientists and professionals in many disciplines including computer science and engineering, mathematics, physics, biology, and medical areas, etc.

Topics include (but not limited to)

- Computer vision theory and methodology (algorithms)

- Computer vision applications in biometrics, biomedicine, etc biometrics, biomedicine, etc

- Robotic vision

- New vision sensors, software and hardware systems and technology

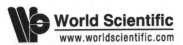
World Scientific
www.worldscientific.com

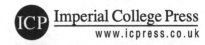
ICP Imperial College Press
www.icpress.co.uk

Preferred Publisher of Leading Thinkers